Phytotherapy
DESK REFERENCE
Michael Thomsen Msc, ND, DBM

Disclaimer

The information in this book is intended as a practical guide to the use of herbal extracts in clinical practice. It is not intended as a substitute for competent advice and guidance by a qualified health practitioner. The author and publisher accept no liability for any claims arising from the use of any medicine or strategy discussed in this book.

Acknowledgements

Thank you to my life partner and fellow herbalist, Erin Collins, for content editing, and to Alex Thomsen and Madeleine Delany, for proofreading and editing. No herbal medicine supplier had any editorial influence over the content of this book. Botanical illustrations are from Köhler's Medizinal-Pflanzen, a German herbal written principally by Hermann Adolph Köhler (1834–1879, physician and chemist), and edited after his death by Gustav Pabst. The work was first published in the late 19th century by Franz Eugen Köhler. Ginkgo images by the author.

Copyright

Published by

Michael Thomsen
www.phytotherapydeskreference.com
ISBN 9781801520010

This edition printed under licence by Aeon Books Ltd 2022

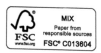

Contents

Introduction

About this book

This book has been designed as a reliable desk reference for the busy herbalist. It contains short, precise descriptions of 233 of the most commonly used herbs in Western Herbal Medicine. It is not designed as an exhaustive materia medica with detailed descriptions of the herbs. Practitioners not familiar with the herbs should seek additional information elsewhere.

The intention of this text is to provide practitioners with a limited number of reliable therapeutic actions with some reliable indications for each herb, with the information organised in such a way as to be a valuable clinical tool.

The short monographs also provide the main active constituents, the qualities of the herbs, known drug interactions and any caution or contraindications in addition to the recommended dosage for liquid extracts.

As a quick reference index, the herbs have been grouped together under their therapeutic actions and indications. These lists are of course not exhaustive and may be expanded with time. They do, however, include the actions and indications on which most authors agree on. Information on the herbs has come from accepted textbooks (see bibliography) and published articles.

Some references are included and more can be found in the online version at phytotherapydeskreference.com.au

Energetics

For many herbalists, the introduction of Chinese and Indian herbs into the modern practice of phytotherapy has renewed their interest in the energetics of herbs.

To further support the exploration of the energetics of herbal medicine, the qualities and occasionally tastes of the herbs have been included in the monographs.

The information on the energetics of the herbs has come primarily from Culpeper, Bensky and Holmes (see bibliography). Culpeper and others grade the degree of intensity: *Zingiber officinale* (ginger) is thus hot in the third degree, whereas *Achillea millifolium* (yarrow) is only warm in the first degree. It has not always

been possible to access such information, and any further suggestions are welcome. It is not straightforward to reconcile interpretations of the energetics of a particular herb from a variety of authors, thus for some herbs the qualities are not included. We welcome any suggestions from the reader that may help to clarify the concept of qualities or energetics of herbs.

Updated botanical names

Agropyron repens (couch grass) has been renamed *Elymus repens*.

Cimicifuga racemosa (black cohosh) has been renamed *Actea racemosa*.

Eupatorium purpureum (gravel root, sweet Joe-Pye weed) has been renamed *Eutrochium purpureum*.

Coleus forskolii (makandi) has been renamed *Plectranthus barbatus*.

Commiphora molmol (myrrh) has been renamed *Commiphora myrrha*.

Common names

When Chineses and Indian herbs were introduced into Western herbal medicine over the last few decades, their common names were often referred to by just their genus names; these include astragalus, schisandra, boswelia and withania, to name a few.

I encourage all herbalists to memorise the binomial botanical names but also pay respect to the cultures from which these medicinal plants come from and learn their common names. Of course, there are often a multitude of common names across a region. I have tried to include the major common names, especially the Chinese and Indian names. Apologies to our international readers, the common names I have chosen may not always be the ones you are familar with.

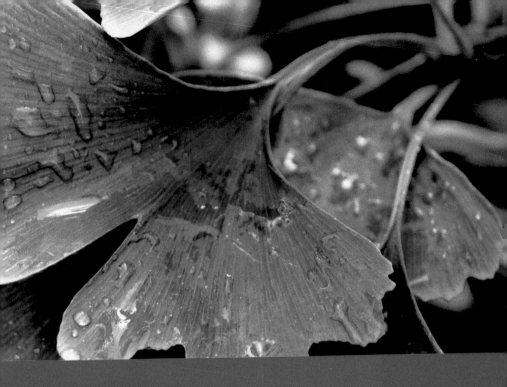

Therapeutic Dosages

Phytotherapy Desk Reference

Dosages

The dosages listed are adult dosages.

It is recommended that the lower end of the dosage range be used initially, especially if the particular herb is unfamiliar to you.

As a rule of thumb, use 20% of the adult dose for infants, 30% for children two to six years of age and 50% for children under 12.

If you are unsure about using a particular herb in children: don't. Not all herbs are suitable for children.

To improve the flavour, add 10% liquorice or flavouring mixture to the formulation.

Essential oils or extracts of peppermint and fennel can also be used to improve the flavour greatly, as can the use of glycerol extracts.

The dosages provided are the average or typical dosages used in Australia and are very broad, as the dosage of a medicine is, of course, product related.

It is therefore essential that you check the dosage range as recommended by the manufacturer of the actual product you are using.

A

African geranium, umckaloabo	Pelargonium sidoides	20–40 ml per week
Agrimony	Agrimonia eupatoria	20–30 ml per week
Albizia, sirisha	Albizia lebbeck	25–60 ml per week
Alder buckthorn	Rhamnus frangula	20–40 ml per week
Aloe vera (gel), bitter aloes (resin)	Aloe ferox	See manufacturer
American ginseng	Panax quinquefolium	7–40 ml per week
Anantamul, Indian sarsparilla	Hemidesmus indicus	30–60 ml per week
Andrographis, kalmegh	Andrographis paniculata	20–40 ml per week
Angelica	Angelica archangelica	10–20 ml per week
Aniseed	Pimpinella anisum	20–40 ml per week
Arjuna	Terminalia arjuna	15–40 ml per week
Arnica	Arnica montana	External use only
Ashwaghanda, winter cherry	Withania somnifera	40–90 ml per week
Astragalus, milk vetch	Astragalus membranaceus	30–60 ml per week
Atractylodes, bai zhu	Atractylodes macrocephala	25–50 ml per week

B

Bacopa, brahmi	Bacopa monnieri	40–90 ml per week
Bai zhu	Atractylodes macrocephala	25–50 ml per week
Baikal skullcap	Scutellaria baicalensis	30–60 ml per week
Barberry	Berberis vulgaris	20–40 ml per week
Basak, vasaka, Malabar nut	Justicia adhatoda	10–25 ml per week
Bayberry, candleberry, wax myrtle	Myrica cerifera	15–40 ml per week
Bearberry	Arctostaphylos uva-ursi	30–60 ml per week
Bei-Wuweizi	Schisandra chinensis	30–60 ml per week
Beth root, birth root	Trillium erectum	10–30 ml per week
Bilberry, blueberry	Vaccinium myrtillus	20–40 ml per week
Bistort	Bistorta officinalis	20–30 ml per week
Bitter melon, bitter gourd	Momordica charantia	20–30 ml per week
Black cohosh, squawroot, snakeroot	Actaea racemosa	10–20 ml per week
Black cumin	Nigella sativa	30–80 ml per week
Black haw, sweet viburnum	Viburnum prunifolium	10–30 ml per week
Black horehound	Ballota nigra	10–20 ml per week
Black walnut	Juglans nigra	10–40 ml per week
Bladderwrack	Fucus vesiculosus	30–60 ml per week
Blessed or holy thistle	Cnicus benedictus	20–40 ml per week
Blue cohosh	Caulophyllum thalictroides	10–20 ml per week
Blue flag	Iris versicolor	20–40 ml per week
Boldo	Peumus boldus	5–15 ml per week
Boneset, feverwort	Eupatorium perfoliatum	20–40 ml per week
Boswellia, olibanum, frankincense	Boswellia serrata	See monograph
Brahmi	Bacopa monnieri	40–90 ml per week
Bryony	Bryonia dioica	8–25 ml per week
Buchu	Agathosma betulina	20–30 ml per week
Bugleweed, gypsy wort	Lycopus spp.	20–40 ml per week
Bupleurum, sickle-leaved hare's ear	Bupleurum falcatum	25–60 ml per week
Burdock	Arctium lappa	20–25 ml per week
Burr marigold	Bidens tripartita	40–80 ml per week
Butcher's broom, box holly	Ruscus aculeatus	30–50 ml per week
Butternut bark, white walnut	Juglans cinerea	25–50 ml per week

C

Calendula, marigold	Calendula officinalis	10–30 ml per week
Californian poppy	Eschscholzia californica	20–40 ml per week
Californian buckthorn	Rhamnus purshiana	20–40 ml per week
Cat's claw	Uncaria tomentosa	30–80 ml per week
Catnip, catmint, jing jie	Nepeta cataria	25–50 ml per week
Celery seed, karafs	Apium graveolens	20–40 ml per week
Centaury	Centaurium erythraea	20–40 ml per week
Chamomile, German chamomile	Matricaria chamomilla	20–40 ml per week
Chaste tree, chasteberry	Vitex agnus-castus	5–20 ml per week
Chen pi, mandarin, tangerine	Citrus reticulata	25–50 ml per week
Chickweed succus	Stellaria media	20–40 ml per week
Chilli, cayenne	Capsicum spp.	1–3 ml per week
Chinese rhubarb	Rheum palmatum	10–30 ml per week
Cinnamon, cassia bark, rou gui	Cinnamomum verum	20–40 ml per week
Clivers, cleavers	Galium aparine	30–50 ml per week
Cloves	Syzygium aromaticum	10–15 ml per week
Coleus, makandi	Plectranthus barbatus	40–90 ml per week
Coltsfoot	Tussilago farrara	See monograph
Comfrey	Symphytum officinale	See monograph
Orange caterpillar fungus	Cordyceps militaris	20–40 ml per week
Corn silk, maize	Zea mays	20–40 ml per week
Corydalis	Corydalis ambigua	30–60 ml per week
Couch grass	Elymus repens	20–40 ml per week
Cramp bark	Viburnum opulus	10–30 ml per week
Cranesbill	Geranium maculatum	15–35 ml per week

D

Da Huang, Chinese rhubarb	Rheum palmatum	10–30 ml per week
Damiana	Turnera diffusa	20–40 ml per week
Dan shen (Mandarin), red root sage	Salvia miltiorrhiza	25–50 ml per week
Dandelion leaf, pu gong ying	Taraxacum officinale folia	40–80 ml per week
Dandelion root	Taraxacum officinale radix	20–40 ml per week
Dang shen, codonopsis	Codonopsis pilosula	30–60 ml per week
Daruharidra, Indian barberry	Berberis aristata	20–40 ml per week
Devil's claw	Harpagophytum procumbens	20–40 ml per week
Dill	Anethum graveolens	20–40 ml per week
Dong ling cao	Isodon rubescens	30–70 ml per week
Dong quai, dang gui	Angelica polymorpha	30–60 ml per week

E

Echinacea	Echinacea spp.	20–40 ml per week
Elder, elderflower	Sambucus nigra	20–40 ml per week
Elecampane	Inula helenium	20–40 ml per week
Eleuthero	Eleutherococcus senticosus	20–55 ml per week
Euphorbia	Euphorbia hirta	5–15 ml per week
European angelica, angelica	Angelica archangelica	10–20 ml per week
Eyebright	Euphrasia officinalis	20–40 ml per week

F

False unicorn root, helonias	Chamaelirium luteum	15–40 ml per week
Fennel	Foeniculum vulgare	20–40 ml per week
Fenugreek	Trigonella foenum-graecum	15–30 ml per week
Fern-leaf biscuit root	Lomatium dissectum	15–40 ml per week
Feverfew	Tanacetum parthenium	5–10 ml per week
Figwort	Scrophularia nodosa	20–40 ml per week
Fringe tree, old man's beard	Chionanthus virginicus	20–40 ml per week
Fumitory	Fumaria officinalis	10–30 ml per week

G

Garlic	Allium sativum	40–80 ml per week
Gentian	Gentiana lutea	5–15 ml per week
Ginger	Zingiber officinale	5–20 ml per week
Ginseng, ren shen	Panax ginseng	7–14 ml per week
Globe artichoke	Cynara scolymus	15–30 ml per week
Glossy privet, nu zhen zi, joteishi	Ligustrum lucidum	30–80 ml per week
Goat's rue	Galega officinalis	30–60 ml per week
Golden root, rose root, arctic root	Rhodiola rosea	20–40 ml per week
Goldenrod	Solidago virgaurea	20–40 ml per week
Goldenseal	Hydrastis canadensis	15–30 ml per week
Gotu kola, brahmi, Indian pennywort	Centella asiatica	20–40 ml per week
Grape vine, grapeseed extract	Vitis vinifera	20–40 ml per week
Gravel root, Joe Pye weed	Eutrochium purpureum	15–30 ml per week
Graviola, soursop, guanábana	Annona muricata	40–80 ml per week
Greater celandine	Chelidonium majus	5–15 ml per week
Greater galangal, Thai ginger	Alpinia galanga	5–15 ml per week
Green tea	Camellia sinensis	20–40 ml per week
Ground ivy	Glechoma hederacea	20–40 ml per week
Guaiacum	Guaiacum officinale	5–15 ml per week
Gum weed	Grindelia camporum	10–20 ml per week
Gumar, meshashringi	Gymnema sylvestre	30–75 ml per week

H

Hawthorn	Crataegus monogyna	20–40 ml per week
He shou wu, fo-ti	Reynoutria multiflora	50–90 ml per week
Heartsease, wild pansy, viola	Viola tricolor	20–40 ml per week
Hoelen, China root	Poria cocos	40–80 ml per week
Hops	Humulus lupulus	10–30 ml per week
Horny goat weed	Epimedium sagittatum	20–45 ml per week
Horopito	Pseudowintera colorata	10–30 ml per week
Horse chestnut	Aesculus hippocastanum	15–40 ml per week
Horseradish	Armoracia rusticana	25–50 ml per week
Horsetail	Equisetum arvense	20–40 ml per week
Huanglian, makino	Coptis chinensis	20–50 ml per week
Hydrangea	Hydrangea arborescens	20–80 ml per week
Hyssop	Hyssopus officinalis	15–30 ml per week

I

Indian tobacco	Lobelia inflata	4–12 ml per week
Inula	Inula racemosa	30–60 ml per week

Isatis, ban lan gen, woad	Isatis tinctoria	25–70 ml per week
Ivy leaf, English ivy	Hedera helix	5–10 ml per week

J

Jamaican dogwood	Piscidia piscipula	20–40 ml per week
Jiaogulan, xiancao	Gynostemma pentaphyllum	20-40 ml per week
Juniper	Juniperus communis	10–20 ml per week
Jujube	Zizyphus spinosa	30–90 ml per week

K

Kava	Piper methysticum	20–60 ml per week
Kawakawa, New Zealand peppertree	Macropiper excelsum	20–60 ml per week
Kola nut, cola nut	Cola spp.	12–25 ml per week
Kudzu	Pueraria lobata	25–90 ml per week
Kutki	Picrorhiza kurroa	10–20 ml per week

L

Lady's mantle	Alchemilla vulgaris	30–50 ml per week
Lavender	Lavandula angustifolia	15–30 ml per week
Lemon balm, Melissa	Melissa officinalis	20–40 ml per week
Licorice, liquorice, gan cao	Glycyrrhiza spp.	20–40 ml per week
Lily of the valley	Convallaria majalis	10–20 ml per week
Lime tree, linden	Tilia cordata	15–30 ml per week

M

Ma-huang	Ephedra sinensis	20-60 ml per week
Magnolia, hou po	Magnolia officinalis	20–70 ml per week
Maidenhair	Ginkgo biloba	20–40 ml per week
Makandi	Plectranthus barbatus	40–90 ml per week
Manuka, tea tree	Leptospermum scoparium	20–60 ml per week
Maritime bark	Pinus pinaster	See monograph
Marshmallow, white mallow	Althaea officinalis	20–40 ml per week
Meadowsweet	Filipendula ulmaria	15–30 ml per week
Milk vetch	Astragalus membranaceus	30–60 ml per week
Mistletoe	Viscum album	20–40 ml per week
Motherwort	Leonurus cardiaca	20–40 ml per week
Mugwort	Artemisia vulgaris	15–30 ml per week
Muira puama	Dulacia inopiflora	10–40 ml per week
Mullein, candlewick plant	Verbascum thapsus	30–60 ml per week
Myrrh	Commiphora myrrha	10–30 ml per week

N

Nettle leaf, stinging nettle	Urtica dioica folia	15–40 ml per week
Nettle root	Urtica dioica radix	30–60 ml per week

O

Oak bark	Quercus robur	20–40 ml per week
Oats, green oats, oat straw	Avena sativa (green)	20–40 ml per week
Oats, groats, oatmeal	Avena sativa (seed)	20–40 ml per week
Old man's beard, songluo	Usnea spp.	50–100 ml per week
Olive tree	Olea europaea	20–50 ml per week
Oregon grape, mountain grape	Berberis aquifolium	20–50 ml per week

P

Parsley root	Petroselinum crispum	40–80 ml per week
Partridgeberry	Mitchella repens	20–40 ml per week
Passion flower	Passiflora incarnata	20–40 ml per week
Pau d'arco, lapacho	Handroanthus impetiginosus	20–50 ml per week
Paw paw, papaya	Carica papaya	15–30 ml per week
Pennyroyal	Mentha pulegium	20–40 ml per week
Peony, white peony, bai shao	Paeonia lactiflora	30–60 ml per week
Peppermint, bo he	Mentha x piperita	10–30 ml per week
Perilla, su zi, shisu	Perilla frutescens	30–70 ml per week
Periwinkle, lesser	Vinca minor	30–50 ml per week
Phyllanthus	Phyllanthus spp.	15–40 ml per week
Plantain, broad-leaved plantain	Plantago major	15–30 ml per week
Pleurisy root, butterfly weed	Asclepias tuberosa	10–20 ml per week
Poke root, pokeweed	Phytolacca americana	1–5 ml per week
Pomegranate	Punica granatum	40–125 ml per week
Prickly ash	Zanthoxylum clava-herculis	10–30 ml per week
Propolis	Propolis	15–30 ml per week
Pulsatilla	Anemone pulsatilla	5–10 ml per week

R

Raspberry leaf	Rubus idaeus	30–80 ml per week
Red clover, trifoil	Trifolium pratense	20–40 ml per week
Rehmannia, sheng di huang	Rehmannia glutinosa	30–60 ml per week
Reishi, lingzhi	Ganoderma lucidum	1.5–3 g daily
Ribwort, narrow-leaved plantain	Plantago lanceolata	20–40 ml per week
Rosehip, dog rose	Rosa canina	20–40 ml per week
Rosemary	Salvia rosmarinus	15–30 ml per week
Rue	Ruta graveolens	10–20 ml per week

S

Saffron	Crocus sativus	10–25 ml per week
Sage	Salvia officinalis	15–30 ml per week
Sarsaparilla	Smilax ornata	20–40 ml per week
Saw palmetto, cabbage palm	Serenoa repens	15–30 ml per week
Schisandra	Schisandra chinensis	30–60 ml per week
Senna pod	Cassia senna	10–40 ml per week
Shatavari	Asparagus racemosus	30–60 ml per week
Shepherd's purse	Capsella bursa-pastoris	20–40 ml per week
Skulcap	Scutellaria lateriflora	15–30 ml per week
Siberian ginseng	Eleutherococcus senticosus	20–55 ml per week
Silver birch	Betula pendula	10–25 ml per week
Slippery elm, red elm	Ulmus fulva	5 g dried herb daily
Sour Chinese date, jujube	Ziziphus jujuba var. spinosa	30–90 ml per week
Soy, soy germ, soy isoflavones	Glycine max	See monograph
St John's wort	Hypericum perforatum	10–40 ml per week
St Mary's thistle, milk thistle	Silybum marianum	30–60 ml per week
Stevia	Stevia rebaudiana	5–10 ml per week
Stone root	Collinsonia canadensis	20–80 ml per week
Sundew	Drosera spp.	10–20 ml per week
Sweet Annie, qing hao	Artemisia annua	20–50 ml per week

T

Teasel root	Dipsacus asper	15–50 ml per week
Thuja, white cedar	Thuja occidentalis	10–20 ml per week
Thyme	Thymus vulgaris	15–40 ml per week
Tienchi ginseng, Yunnan bayou	Panax notoginseng	30–60 ml per week
Tribulus, calthrops	Tribulus terrestris	See monograph
True unicorn root, white colic root	Aletris farinosa	15–40 ml per week
Tulsi, Holy basil	Ocimum tenuiflorum	20–50 ml per week
Turkey tail PSK, PSP	Trametes versicolor	3–6 g daily
Turmeric	Curcuma longa	40–80 ml per week

V

Valerian, heliotrope	Valeriana officinalis	15–40 ml per week
Varuna	Crateva magna	40–90 ml per week
Vervain	Verbena officinalis	20–40 ml per week

W

White dead nettle	Lamium album	20–40 ml per week
White horehound	Marrubium vulgare	15–40 ml per week
Wild cherry, black cherry	Prunus serotina	15–30 ml per week
Wild indigo	Baptisia tinctoria	15–40 ml per week
Wild yam	Dioscorea spp.	20–40 ml per week
Willow bark, white willow	Salix spp.	25–50 ml per week
Willow herb	Epilobium parviflorum	20–40 ml per week
Winter cherry	Withania somnifera	40–90 ml per week
Witch hazel	Hamamelis virginiana	20–40 ml per week
Wood betony	Stachys officinalis	15–30 ml per week
Wormwood, absinthe	Artemisia absinthium	5–20 ml per week

Y

Yarrow	Achillea millefolium	20–40 ml per week
Yellow dock, curled dock	Rumex crispus	15–30 ml per week
Yellow dye root, delboi	Cryptolepis sanguinolenta	30–100 ml per week
Yu xing cao	Houttuynia cordata	10–25 ml per week

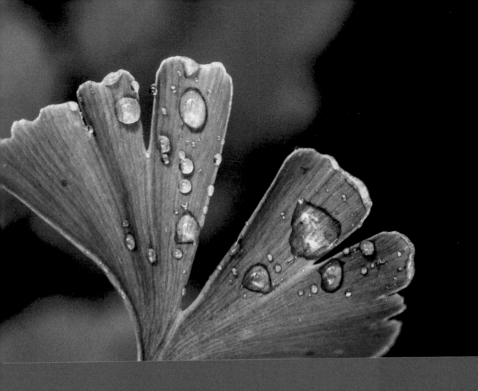

Pregnancy
and Herbs

Phytotherapy Desk Reference

Pregnancy

The majority of herbs are generally considered safe to use during pregnancy, although very few have been thoroughly examined. Treatment during the first trimester, however, should only proceed if absolutely necessary. Treatment at this time is generally only for morning sickness or threatened miscarriage (after medical diagnosis as to the reasons for the threatened miscarriage).

- Avoid known toxic herbs
- Avoid emmenagogues in high doses
- Avoid laxatives in high doses

The following herbs are not recommended in pregnancy or lactation

- Achillea millefolium
- Actaea racemosa
- Aesculus hippocastanum
- Agathosma betulina
- Aloe ferox
- Andrographis paniculata
- Anemone pulsatilla
- Angelica archangelica
- Angelica polymorpha
- Annona muricata
- Arctostaphylos uva-ursi
- Armoracia rusticana
- Artemisia absinthium
- Artemisia annua
- Artemisia vulgaris
- Astragalus membranaceus
- Berberis aquifolium
- Berberis vulgaris
- Bryonia dioica
- Bupleurum falcatum
- Caulophyllum thalictroides
- Chelidonium majus
- Cinnamomum verum
- Collinsonia canadensis
- Commiphora myrrha
- Convallaria majalis
- Coptis chinensis
- Corydalis ambigua
- Crataegus monogyna
- Crateva magna
- Cryptolepis sanguinolenta
- Dulacia inopiflora
- Ephedra sinensis
- Fucus vesiculosus
- Handroanthus impetiginosus
- Harpagophytum procumbens
- Humulus lupulus
- Hydrastis canadensis
- Juniperus communis
- Justicia adhatoda
- Leonurus cardiaca
- Lobelia inflata
- Lycopus spp.
- Mentha pulegium
- Momordica charantia
- Panax notoginseng
- Passiflora incarnata
- Peumus boldus
- Phytolacca americana
- Piscidia piscipula
- Rhamnus frangula
- Rhamnus purshiana
- Ruta graveolens
- Salvia miltiorrhiza
- Schisandra chinensis
- Symphytum officinale
- Tanacetum parthenium
- Terminalia arjuna
- Thuja occidentalis
- Tribulus terrestris
- Tussilago farfara
- Uncaria tomentosa
- Vinca minor
- Viscum album

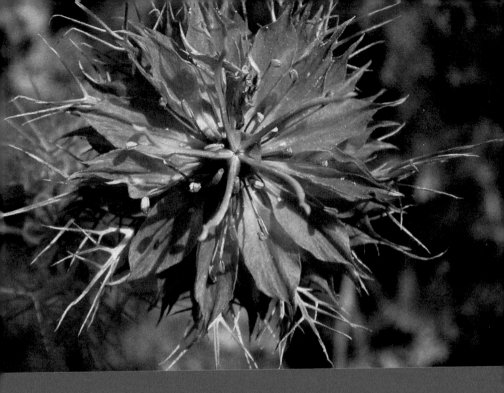

Clinical Monographs

Phytotherapy Desk Reference

Achillea millefolium

Common names: Yarrow

Family: Asteraceae

Part used: Aerial parts

Description: Traditionally used for healing wounds, digestive problems, respiratory infections, and skin conditions. However, its popularity has recently waned. Further research is warranted as a recent study demonstrated a surprising new indication for *A. millefolium* showing that one year administration decreased the annual relapse rate in patients with multiple sclerosis (MS).

Constituents: Azulene, camphor, cineole, essential oil, flavonoids, tannins.

Primary actions: Diaphoretic, Digestive tonic, Emmenagogue.

All actions: Antihaemorrhagic (uterine), Antihypertensive, Antipyretic, Antiseptic (GIT), Aromatic, Bitter tonic, Diaphoretic, Digestive stimulant, Digestive tonic, Styptic/Haemostatic.

Indications:

- Amenorrhoea, Anorexia, Blood stasis, Common cold, Digestive complaints, Dyspepsia, Fever, Hypertension, Inflammation; skin (topically), Menorrhagia, Menstrual irregularity, Muscular tension, Nose bleeds.
- **BHP:** Fever, colds, digestive complaints. Topically for slow healing wounds and inflammatory skin disorders.
- **Commission E:** Loss of appetite, dyspeptic ailments, female pelvic cramping.
- **Other uses:** Also used topically for skin disorders and as a wound closing agent.

Cautions: Avoid in known sensitivity to plants of the Asteraceae (Compositae) family. Arbutin is a mandatory component of *Achillea millefolium*.

Contraindications: Varieties with a high level of thujone are contraindicated in pregnancy.

Qualities: Dry 1st degree, warm 1st degree

Typical dosage: 20–40 ml per week

Actaea racemosa

Synonym or related species: Cimicifuga racemosa

Common names: Black cohosh, squawroot, snakeroot

Family: Ranunculaceae

Part used: Rhizome

Description: Key herb for menopausal symptoms, premenstrual syndrome and dysmenorrhoea. Standardised, clinically tested powdered extracts are available as single preparations.

Constituents: Triterpene glycosides (acetein, cimicifugoside, racemoside), isoflavones, aromatic acids (isoferulic acid, salicylic acid), tannin, resins (cimicifugin), ranunculin, fatty acids, tannins, starch, sugars.

Primary actions: Anti-inflammatory, Selective oestrogen receptor modulator (SERM), Uterine tonic.

All actions: Anti-inflammatory, Antiandrogenic, Anticancer, Antirheumatic, Antispasmodic/ Spasmolytic, Antitussive, CNS depressor, Emmenagogue, Hypothalamic-pituitary-ovarian (HPO) regulator, Sedative, Selective oestrogen receptor modulator (SERM), Uterine tonic, Vasodilator.

Indications:

- Arthritis, Bronchitis, Depression, Dysmenorrhoea, Endometriosis, Fibroids, Hypertension, Menopause, Menopause; symptoms, Neuralgia, Osteoarthritis, Pertussis, Polycystic ovarian syndrome, Rheumatism, Rheumatoid arthritis, Tinnitus.
- **BHP:** Rheumatism, rheumatoid arthritis, intercostal myalgia, sciatica, whooping cough, chorea, tinnitus aurium, dysmenorrhoea, uterine colic. Specific indications: muscular rheumatism, rheumatoid arthritis.
- **Commission E:** Menopausal symptoms, premenstrual syndrome and dysmenorrhoea.
- **ESCOP:** Climacteric symptoms such as hot flushes, profuse sweating, sleep disorders and nervous irritability.
- **WHO:** Treatment of climacteric symptoms such as hot flushes, profuse sweating, sleeping disorders and nervous irritability. Treatment of premenstrual syndrome and dysmenorrhoea.

Cautions: Black cohosh has recently become suspected of being hepatotoxic. The Therapeutic Goods Administration (TGA) reviewed the safety of black cohosh in 2005. The TGA has concluded that the incidence of liver reaction appears to be very low, considering the widespread use of black cohosh. Following the safety review, the TGA decided that medicines containing black cohosh must carry the following label statement: 'Warning: black cohosh may harm the liver in some individuals. Use under the supervision of a healthcare professional.' – TGA, 2007

Evidence

Black cohosh has recently become suspected of being hepatotoxic. The suspicion is based on 69 cases of black cohosh-induced liver disease. A review of the publications of these cases, however, has found them to be of poor quality with major inconsistencies in the data being presented, based on the same patients. Other issues include uncertainty of the black cohosh product used, insufficient adverse event definition, and lack of temporal association and dechallenge, missing or inadequate evaluation of alcohol use, comedication, comorbidity, re-exposure test, and alternative diagnosis. The review concluded that the presented data do not support the reported black cohosh hepatotoxicity, although further research needs to be done to rule out the existence of black cohosh hepatotoxicity as a special disease entity (Teschke 2010).

Contraindications: During pregnancy and lactation, except for assisting birth. Not to be administered to children under the age of 12 years.

Drug interactions: May improve hot flushes associated with tamoxifen. Current evidence does not support an association between black cohosh and increased risk of breast cancer. Results from clinical studies in the alleviation of hot flushes induced by tamoxifen has been mixed (Fritz, Seely et al. 2014).

Black cohosh may decrease the efficacy of cisplatin and carboplatin. Evidence for caution based on a single in vitro study. There is no information about a specific clinical dose at which level a drug interaction may occur. Recommended doses for black cohosh preparations are unlikely to produce a clinically relevant drug interaction with carboplatin. A study examined the effects of black cohosh on chemotherapy in vitro. Black cohosh extracts increased the cytotoxicity of doxorubicin and docetaxel and decreased the cytotoxicity of cisplatin, but did not alter the effects of radiation or 4-hydroperoxycyclophosphamide (4-HC), an analogue of cyclophosphamide that is active in cell culture (Rockwell, Liu et al. 2005). Human studies are needed to determine the clinical relevance of this in vitro study.

Black cohosh has been shown to inhibit CYP3A4 in vitro using human liver microsomes (Sevior, Hokkanen et al. 2010). Esomeprazole is mainly metabolised by CYP2C19 to hydroxy and desmethyl metabolites of esomeprazole. A smaller amount is metabolised by CYP3A4 to esomeprazole sulphone, the main metabolite in plasma. The major metabolites of esomeprazole have no effect on gastric acid secretion. Repeated dosing of esomeprazole inhibits CYP2C19, and the area under the plasma concentration-time curve (AUC) subsequently increases with repeated administration of esomeprazole, especially in patients who are extensive metabolisers of CYP2C19 (AstraZeneca 2009). A pharmacokinetic interaction with black cohosh is likely to occur only in poor esomeprazole metabolisers, as metabolism by CYP3A4 is more important in such individuals. The clinical significance is unknown.

Actein alters the expression of cholesterol biosynthetic genes, but does not inhibit HMG-CoA reductase activity. Black cohosh and actein inhibited the growth of human breast and colon cancer cells and synergized with the statin simvastatin. Combinations of black cohosh with certain classes of statins could enhance their activity, as well as toxicity (Einbond, Soffritti et al. 2018).

References

AstraZeneca (2009). Nexium Product Information.

Einbond, L. S., M. Soffritti, D. D. Esposti, H. A. Wu, M. Balick, H. Ma, S. Redenti and A. Roter (2018). 'A transcriptomic analysis of black cohosh: Actein alters cholesterol biosynthesis pathways and synergizes with simvastatin.' Food Chem Toxicol 120: 356-366.

Fritz, H., D. Seely, J. McGowan, B. Skidmore, R. Fernandes, D. A. Kennedy, K. Cooley, R. Wong, S. Sagar, L. G. Balneaves and D. Fergusson (2014). 'Black cohosh and breast cancer: a systematic review.' Integr Cancer Ther 13(1): 12-29.

Rockwell, S., Y. Liu and S. A. Higgins (2005). 'Alteration of the effects of cancer therapy agents on breast cancer cells by the herbal medicine black cohosh.' Breast Cancer Res Treat 90(3): 233-239.

Sevior, D. K., J. Hokkanen, A. Tolonen, K. Abass, L. Tursas, O. Pelkonen and J. T. Ahokas (2010). 'Rapid screening of commercially available herbal products for the inhibition of major human hepatic cytochrome P450 enzymes using the N-in-one cocktail.' Xenobiotica 40(4): 245-254.

Teschke R 2010, 'Black cohosh and suspected hepatotoxicity: inconsistencies, confounding variables, and prospective use of a diagnostic causality algorithm. A critical review', Menopause, vol. 17, no. 2, pp. 426-40.

Qualities: Cool, dry

Typical dosage: 10–20 ml per week

Aesculus hippocastanum

Common names: Horse chestnut

Family: Hippocastanaceae

Part used: Seeds

Description: The clinical efficacy and safety of an extract (1:5, 50% aqueous ethanol, standardised to contain 50 mg of aescin in 240–290 mg extract at a dose of 100 mg aescin daily), is well documented. The extract improves venous tone and capillary filtration rate.

Constituents: Escin (complex mixture of saponins), flavonoids, lipids, sterols.

Primary actions: Anti-inflammatory, Antioedematous, Venotonic.

All actions: Anti-inflammatory, Antioedematous, Anodyne, Antispasmodic, Venotonic.

Indications:

- Carpal tunnel syndrome, Fluid retention, Fluid retention; premenstrual, Haemorrhoids, Haemorrhoids (topically), Oedema; localised, Varicose veins, Varicose veins (topically), Venous insufficiency, Venous leg ulcers.

- **Commission E:** Symptoms of chronic venous insufficiency such as pain, night cramps, itching or swelling, sensation of heaviness in the legs.

- **ESCOP:** Chronic venous insufficiency and varicosis.

- **WHO:** Internally for treatment of symptoms of chronic venous insufficiency, including pain, feeling of heaviness in legs, nocturnal calf-muscle spasms, itching and oedema. Externally for symptomatic treatment of chronic venous insufficiency, sprains and bruises.

- **Other uses:** Lower leg oedema, chronic venous insufficiency, varicose veins, haemorrhoids, topically for injuries, disease states associated with local tissue oedema (e.g. DVT prophylaxis, carpal tunnel syndrome, Bells palsy, dysmenorrhoea, intervertebral disc lesions, soft tissue injuries, swelling and minor surgery).

Cautions: Do not administer during pregnancy or lactation without medical supervision. Avoid high doses in kidney disease. Oral use may cause gastric irritation (saponins). Consider using enteric-coated tablet. Other adverse reactions include dizziness, headache, nausea, reflux and pruritis.

Contraindications: In cases of known allergy to plants of the Hippocastanaceae family. Do not apply to broken or ulcerated skin. Only mild adverse events were reported in the 17 clinical trials evaluated in a meta-analysis. Also in open clinical trials with over 10,000 participants only a small number of mild adverse events were reported. During 20 years only 15 mild adverse events were reported from the consumption of 447 million daily doses of the horsechestnut extract contained in the product Venostasin.

Qualities: Cooling, drying

Typical dosage: 15–40 ml per week

Agathosma betulina

Synonym or related species: Barosma betulina
Common names: Buchu
Family: Rutaceae
Part used: Leaves
Description: Buchu is an important part of the Khoi-San culture of Africa. It is still used in the Cape as a general tonic and medicine throughout South Africa for its antispasmodic and antipyretic properties in the treatment of cough, colds and flu; as a diuretic for kidney and urinary tract infections; for haematuria and prostatitis, cholera, stomach ailments; rheumatism, gout and bruises; and relief of renal calculus.

Constituents: Essential oil (diosfenol, limonene, menthone), flavonoids (dismin, rutin), mucilage, resin

Primary actions: Antipyretic, Antispasmodic/ Spasmolytic, Diuretic.

All actions: Antidiarrhoeal, Antipyretic, Antiseptic, Antispasmodic/Spasmolytic, Astringent, Bitter tonic, Cholagogue, Digestive tonic, Diuretic.

Indications:

- Cystitis, Dysuria, Gout, Haematuria, Prostatitis, Rheumatism, Urethritis.

Cautions: May cause digestive upset.
Contraindications: During pregnancy
Qualities: Dry, hot
Typical dosage: 20–30 ml per week

Agrimonia eupatoria

Common names: Agrimony
Family: Rosaceae
Part used: Aerial parts
Description: Traditionally used in the treatment of diarrhoea and cystitis, including in children. Pharmacological investigations have also found anti-inflammatory, antinociceptive, hepatoprotective and antidiabetic properties. Drinking a herbal tea for a month was found to improve lipid profiles of subjects.

Constituents: Several phenolic constituents mainly apigenin, kaempferol, and quercetin derivatives, as well as catechin, oligomeric proantocyanidins, and a volatile oil. The most abundant compounds are quercetin glycosides and proantocyanidin trimers (condensed tannins).

Primary actions: Anti-inflammatory, Antidiarrhoeal, Bitter tonic.

All actions: Anti-inflammatory, Anti-inflammatory (urinary), Antidiabetic, Antidiarrhoeal, Antihyperlipidemic, Antinociceptive, Demulcent, Demulcent (urinary), Diuretic, Hepatoprotective.

Indications:

- Anorexia, Colitis, Cystitis, Diarrhoea, Dyslipidaemia, Hypochlorhydria, Liver toxicity.

- **BHP:** Diarrhoea in children, mucous colitis. Grumbling appendicitis. Urinary incontinence and cystitis. As a gargle for acute sore throat and chronic nasopharyngeal catarrh.

- **Other uses:** One month's consumption of agrimony tea in healthy volunteers resulted in significant elevation of plasma total antioxidant capacity and significantly lowered interleukin 6 levels at the end of the intervention. Agrimony tea improved lipid profiles as estimated by increased high density lipoprotein (HDL) cholesterol and HDL cholesterol correlated with adiponectin levels. The results indicate that the plant has potential in improving markers of lipid metabolism, oxidative status and inflammation in healthy adults.

Contraindications: None known
Qualities: Dry 1st degree, hot 1st degree
Typical dosage: 20–30 ml per week

Albizia lebbeck

Synonym or related species: Albizia julibrissin
Common names: Albizia, sirisha
Family: Fabaceae
Part used: Leaves and stem bark
Description: Mainly used for its antiallergic and anti-inflammatory properties in the treatment of allergies, infections and infestations, albizia may also have a role in cancer support. The saponin rich fraction of albizia showed antiproliferative, antiangiogenic and apoptogenic potential using various in vitro models.

Constituents: Albiziasaponins A, B and C, epicatechins, procyanidins B2, B5 and C1, stigmastadienones.

Primary actions: Anti-inflammatory, Antiallergic, Anticancer.

All actions: Anti-inflammatory, Antiallergic, Antiasthmatic, Anticancer, Antihyperlipidemic, Antimicrobial, Antiseptic (GIT), Astringent, Cardiotonic, Immunemodulating.

Indications:

- Allergies/Sensitivities, Asthma, Eczema, Hayfever, Lymphoma treatment; as an adjunct to, Rhinitis, Sinusitis, Urticaria.

- **Other uses:** As an adjunct to lymphoma treatment.

Cautions: Albizia is immunemodulating, not immune suppressive.

Qualities: Cooling, drying

Typical dosage: 25–60 ml per week

Alchemilla vulgaris

Common names: Lady's mantle

Family: Rosaceae

Part used: Aerial parts

Description: Traditionally used for wound healing and for diarrhoea, dysentery and menorrhagia, pharmacological studies have also described cytoprotective and vasdilatory properties suggesting a use in gastrointestinal ulceration and in hypertension.

Constituents: Glycosides (ranunculin), saponins, tannin.

Primary actions: Anti-inflammatory, Antihaemorrhagic (uterine), Wound healing/Vulnerary.

All actions: Anti-inflammatory, Antidiarrhoeal, Antihaemorrhagic (uterine), Antilithic, Antipyretic, Astringent, Cytoprotective, Demulcent (urinary), Emmenagogue, Menstrual cycle regulator, Nervine tonic, Selective oestrogen receptor modulator (SERM), Styptic/Haemostatic, Uterine tonic, Vasodilator, Wound healing/Vulnerary.

Indications:

- Amenorrhoea, Colic; intestinal, Diarrhoea, Dysentery, Dysmenorrhoea, Haemorrhage; post-partum, Hypertension, Insomnia, Leucorrhoea, Menopause, Menopause; symptoms, Menorrhagia, Menstrual irregularity, Pruritus vulvae (douche), Ulcer; gastrointestinal, Wounds, Wounds (topically).

- **BHP:** Diarrhoea, dysentery, passive haemorrhage, menorrhagia. Topically for leucorrhoea and pruritus vulvae (douche).

- **ESCOP:** As an adjuvant in non-specific diarrhoea, gastrointestinal complaints and dysmenorrhoea.

- **Other uses:** Diarrhoea, intestinal colic, menorrhagia, leucorrhoea, amenorrhoea, to

promote contractions during labour, period pain, irregular menstrual cycles, menopausal menorrhagia, urinary incontinence in postmenopausal women, insomnia.

Contraindications: None known

Qualities: Drying and cooling

Typical dosage: 30–50 ml per week

Aletris farinosa

Common names: True unicorn root, white colic root

Family: Liliaceae

Part used: Rhizome and root

Description: Aletris farinosa is a uterine tonic traditionally used for habitual miscarriages, dysmenorrhoea and amenorrhoea. It is, however, an endangered plant in the wild. Consider alternative if not from cultivations.

Constituents: Bitter compound

Primary actions: Antispasmodic/Spasmolytic, Bitter tonic, Uterine tonic.

All actions: Antispasmodic/Spasmolytic, Bitter tonic, Digestive tonic, Uterine tonic.

Indications:

- Adenomyosis, Amenorrhoea, Anorexia, Childbirth recovery, Cystic hyperplasia, Digestive complaints, Digestive weakness, Dyspepsia, Flatulence, Gynaecological disorders, Hysterectomy recovery, Infertility, Menstrual irregularity, Pelvic floor weakness, Pelvic heaviness; congestion, Uterine bleeding; dysfunctional, Weight loss; to assist.

- **BHP:** Anorexia, Dyspepsia; flatulent colic, reported to be useful in threatened miscarriage. Specifically indicated for anorexia with nervous dyspepsia.

- **Other uses:** Anorexia, dyspepsia, flatulence, digestive weakness, sense of pelvic heaviness or congestion, pelvic floor weakness, recovery from hysterectomy or childbirth, gynaecological disorders

Contraindications: None known

Qualities: Warming

Typical dosage: 15–40 ml per week

Allium sativum

Common names: Garlic

Family: Liliaceae

Part used: Bulb

Description: The majority of the clinical trials on the cardiovascular effects of garlic have used supplements that are standardised to alliin or allicin releasing potential. Enteric coating of the tablets or capsules is essential for this type of medicinal garlic. Almost all clinical trials with garlic powder supplements have used a daily dose standardised

19

at 3.6–7.8 mg allicin potential from 7.8–17 mg alliin, which represents 1–2 g of typical raw garlic (Lawson and Hunsaker 2018). Types of medicinal garlic include essential oil, oil macerate, powder, and aged garlic extracts. Preparations with clinical efficacy include Kwai garlic powder and Kyolic aged garlic. Aged garlics like Kyolic contains S-allylcysteine as their main identified S-allyl compound; neither contains active alliinase; and both contain little or no alliin or alliin-derived thiosulfinates or sulfides. Prophylaxic for atherosclerosis, treatment of elevated blood lipid levels, improvement of blood flow in arterial vascular disease (Ried 2020).

Constituents: Fresh garlic contains alliin (odourless amino acid), crushing releases the enzyme alliinase, which converts alliin to allicin. Allicin and γ-glutamyl-S-allylcysteine, as the source of S-allylcysteine, appear to be responsible for the hypotensive effects of garlic.

Primary actions: Antihyperlipidemic, Antihypertensive, Antimicrobial.

All actions: Anthelmintic, Antiatherosclerotic, Antifungal, Antihyperlipidemic, Antihypertensive, Antimicrobial, Antioxidant, Antiparasitic, Antiplatelet, Antiseptic (GIT), Antiviral (systemically), Chemoprotective, Fibrinolytic, Mucolytic, Vasodilator.

Indications:

- Arteriosclerosis, Atherosclerosis, Circulation; peripheral; impaired, Dyslipidaemia, Hypertension, Infection; gastrointestinal system, Infection; respiratory tract.

- **BHP:** Chronic bronchitis, respiratory catarrh, recurrent colds, whooping cough, bronchial asthma and influenza. Specifically indicated for chronic bronchitis.

- **Commission E:** Support to dietary measures for elevated blood lipid levels, preventive for age-dependent vascular changes.

- **ESCOP:** Prophylaxic for atherosclerosis, treatment of elevated blood lipid levels insufficiently influenced by diet, improvement of blood flow in arterial vascular disease. Note traditional use for relief of cough, colds, catarrh and rhinitis.

- **WHO:** Adjuvant to dietetic management of hyperlipidaemia, and prevention of atherosclerotic vascular changes. May be useful in treatment of mild hypertension.

- **Other uses:** Kyolic aged significantly lowered central blood pressure, pulse pressure, pulse wave velocity and arterial stiffness, and improved the gut microbiota, evidenced by higher microbial richness and diversity, with a marked increase in the numbers of Lactobacillus and Clostridia species found following 3 months of supplementation.(Ried 2020)

Cautions: Garlic may cause gastric irritation, allergy, contact dermatitis, and other skin reactions, and increased body odour.

Contraindications: Contraindicated in those with

20

known sensitivity. Prolonged or high doses of fresh raw garlic and allicin-releasing garlic products should not be taken during pregnancy.

Drug interactions: Clinical trials to date have provided no evidence that *Allium sativum* interacts with warfarin. Theoretical interactions are cited due to its antiplatelet activity in vitro. A clinical trial with 10 subjects investigating risk of perioperative bleeding found no change in platelet activity (Beckert, Concannon et al. 2007).

Forty-eight patients were randomised in a double-blind, placebo-controlled study to examine anticoagulant effects in patients taking warfarin. An oral dose of *A. sativum* (aged garlic) or placebo was administered at a dose of 5 ml twice a day (14.7 mg/day) for 12 weeks. There was no evidence of increased bleeding in either group. The results suggest that this dose of *A. sativum* is safe and poses no serious haemorrhagic risk for closely monitored patients on warfarin oral anticoagulation therapy (Macan, Uykimpang et al. 2006).

In 2008, an open-label, three-treatment, randomised crossover clinical trial was undertaken on 12 healthy subjects of known CYP2C9 and VKORC1 genotype to investigate the effect of *A. sativum* and *Vaccinium oxycoccos* (cranberry), on the pharmacokinetics and pharmacodynamics of warfarin. Each received a single dose of warfarin 25 mg alone or were pre-treated with either garlic or cranberry. Warfarin enantiomer concentrations, INR, platelet aggregation and clotting factor activity were measured. Cranberry significantly increased the area under the INR-time curve by 30% when administered with warfarin compared with treatment with warfarin alone. Cranberry did not alter S- or R-warfarin pharmacokinetics or plasma protein binding. Coadministration of garlic did not significantly alter warfarin pharmacokinetics or pharmacodynamics. Both herbal medicines showed some evidence of VKORC1 (not CYP2C9) genotype-dependent interactions with warfarin. Cranberry alters the pharmacodynamics of warfarin with the potential to increase its effects significantly. Coadministration of warfarin and cranberry requires careful monitoring. Coadministration of *A. sativum* at a dose of 4000 mg/day (7.42 mg/day) of allicin did not appear to have a significant effect on warfarin (Mohammed Abdul, Jiang et al. 2008).

Recommendation

Prescribe if indicated or appropriate. Avoid coadministration of doses greater than 4 g/day.

Directions for use

Supervise and monitor patient in collaboration with other prescribers. Monitor the INR more frequently when herbal medicine/supplement is started (e.g., twice weekly) or when dose is altered or discontinued. Patients should be aware of the clinical symptoms associated with minor and major bleeding.

Qualities: Warming

Typical dosage: 40–80 ml per week

References

Beckert BW, Concannon MJ, Henry SL, et al. 2007, 'The effect of herbal medicines on platelet function: an in vivo experiment and review of the literature', Plast Reconstr Surg, vol. 120, no. 7, pp. 2044-50. PMID 18090773

Lawson, L. D., and S. M. Hunsaker. 2018. 'Allicin Bioavailability and Bioequivalence from Garlic Supplements and Garlic Foods', *Nutrients*, 10.

Macan H, Uykimpang R, Alconcel M, et al. 2006, 'Aged garlic extract may be safe for patients on warfarin therapy', J Nutr, vol. 136, no. 3 Suppl, pp. 793S-795S. PMID 16484565

Mohammed Abdul MI, Jiang X, Williams KM, et al. 2008, 'Pharmacodynamic interaction of warfarin with cranberry but not with garlic in healthy subjects', Br J Pharmacol, vol. 154, no. 8, pp. 1691-700. PMID 18516070

Ried, K. 2020. 'Garlic lowers blood pressure in hypertensive subjects, improves arterial stiffness and gut microbiota: A review and meta-analysis', *Exp Ther Med*, 19: 1472-78.

Aloe ferox

Synonym or related species: Aloe barbadensis

Common names: Aloe vera (gel), bitter aloes (resin)

Family: Liliaceae

Part used: Leaf (resin and gel)

Description: The raw aloe leaf is composed of approximately 98.5% water. The remaining solid material contains a range of compounds including organic acids, lignins, phenolic compounds, anthraquinones, and phytosterols. The chemical composition depends on many factors, including extraction processing. The bitter yellow latex (sap) along the margin of the leaf is laxative. The gel is used for wound healing, in particular for burns. Concentrated polysaccharide extracts have immune-stimulating properties.

Constituents: The latex (resin) contains anthraquinone glycosides including barbaloin (aloin A), anthrones, and free anthraquinones. The gel contains mucopolysaccharides including acemannan, an acetylated glucomannan.

Primary actions: Anti-inflammatory, Laxative, Wound healing/Vulnerary.

All actions: Anti-inflammatory, Antimicrobial, Laxative, Wound healing/Vulnerary.

Indications:

- Burns (topically), Constipation, Inflammation; gastrointestinal tract, Inflammation; skin (topically), Irritable bowel syndrome, Radiation; side effects of, Ulcer; gastrointestinal, Wounds (topically).

- **ESCOP:** For short-term use in cases of occasional constipation.

- **WHO:** Short-term treatment of occasional constipation.

- **Other uses:** Constipation (resin), gastrointestinal inflammation, irritable bowel, skin conditions (external application of gel); wounds, burns, inflammation.

Cautions: Not recommended during lactation. Gel: do not use during pregnancy without professional advice. Resin: should not be used excessively or long-term as potassium losses may occur through laxative effects. Aloes should not be given when any undiagnosed acute or persistent abdominal symptoms are present. Caution with other strong laxatives. Adverse effects include burning sensations, dermatitis and mild itching.

Contraindications: Contraindicated in those with known sensitivity. Strong laxatives such as aloe latex are contraindicated during pregnancy, in women attempting to conceive, or for administration to children under 10 years. Intestinal obstruction and stenosis, atony, inflammatory colon diseases, appendicitis, abdominal pain of unknown origin, chronic constipation, haemorrhoids, kidney disorders, severe dehydration states with water and electrolyte depletion.

Drug interactions: Potassium deficiency (from long-term use of laxatives) can potentiate the action of cardiac glycosides and may affect the action of antiarrhythmic agents. Possible beneficial interactions with topical cortisone preparations.

Qualities: Cooling. Moist, warm 2nd degree

Typical dosage: Resin 1:10 10–30 ml per week

Internal dosage (resin extract): 10–30 ml per week (1:10). Internal dosage (gel): fresh from living plant, freeze dried or as stabilised juice as recommended by manufacturer (dosage depends on concentration). Topical dosage: as required.

Alpinia galanga

Common names: Greater galangal, Thai ginger

Family: Zingiberaceae

Part used: Rhizome

Description: Both the crude extracts and pure constituents isolated from the genus Alpinia exhibit a wide range of bioactivities such as anti-cancer, anti-oxidant, anti-bacterial, anti-viral, cardiovascular, and digestive system protective effects. Alpinia galanga combines well with ginger for osteoarthritis.

Constituents: Diarylheptanoids, galangoflavonoids, volatile oil, resin, galangol, kaempferid, galangin and alpinin.

Primary actions: Anti-inflammatory, Digestive stimulant, Gastroprotective.

All actions: Anti-inflammatory, Anti-inflammatory (GIT), Antiallergic, Antibacterial, Anticancer, Antidiabetic, Antiemetic, Antifungal, Antihypertensive, Antimicrobial, Antinociceptive, Antispasmodic (respiratory tract), Carminative, Digestive tonic, Expectorant (general), Gastroprotective, Neuroprotective.

Indications:

- Arthritis, Asthma, Asthma; bronchial, Bronchitis, Catarrh; naso-pharyngeal congestion, Colic; intestinal, Cough, Diabetes, Diarrhoea, Digestive complaints, Dyspepsia, Fever, Gastritis, Hypertension, Infection; bacterial, Infection; fungal, Infection; gastrointestinal system, Infection; respiratory tract, Inflammation; gastrointestinal tract, Inflammation; respiratory tract, Nausea.

Qualities: Warming

Typical dosage: 5–15 ml per week

Althaea officinalis

Common names: Marshmallow, white mallow

Family: Malvaceae

Part used: Leaf and root

Description: The genus name *althaea* comes from the Greek *altho,* to cure. Traditional herbal medicine used as a demulcent preparation for oral or pharyngeal irritation and associated dry cough and for gastrointestinal discomfort. Suitable for children.

Constituents: Mucilage polysaccharides, flavonoid glycosides, phenolic acids, tannins, sugars, amines, fat, calcium oxalate, coumarins and sterols.

Primary actions: Anti-inflammatory (GIT), Antitussive, Emollient.

All actions: Anti-inflammatory (GIT), Anti-inflammatory (urinary), Antilithic, Antimicrobial, Antitussive, Cytoprotective, Demulcent, Diuretic, Emollient, Gastroprotective, Immunomodulator, Wound healing/Vulnerary.

Indications:

- Asthma, Boils (poultice), Bronchitis, Colitis, Cough, Cystitis, Dermatitis, Dyspepsia, Dyspepsia; nervous, Eczema, Gastritis, Gastroenteritis, Infection; urinary tract, Inflammation; gastrointestinal tract, Inflammation; oral cavity, Inflammation; respiratory tract, Pertussis, Respiratory catarrh, Sore throat (gargle), Ulcer (topically), Ulcer; gastrointestinal, Ulcerative colitis, Urethritis, Wounds (topically).

- **BHP:** Root: gastritis, gastric or peptic ulceration, enteritis, inflammation of the mouth or pharynx, respiratory catarrh with irritating cough, cystitis, locally for varicose and thrombotic ulcers. BHC: internal use of root for gastroenteritis, peptic and duodenal ulceration, common and ulcerative colitis, and enteritis. As a mouthwash or gargle for inflammation of mouth and pharynx, as poultice or ointment/cream in furunculosis, eczema and dermatitis. Specific indication: gastric or duodenal ulcer.

- **Commission E:** Internal use of leaf: irritation of oral and pharyngeal mucosa and associated dry cough. Internal use of root: as above, and for mild inflammation of gastric mucosa.

- **ESCOP:** Dry cough, irritations of the oral, pharyngeal, and/or gastric mucosa.

- **WHO:** As a demulcent for symptomatic treatment of dry irritable coughs and irritations of oral and pharyngeal mucosa and as an emollient for wounds and dry skin.

- **Other uses:** Irritation/inflammation of GIT and respiratory tract, poultice for wounds, boils, abscesses and ulcers, gastrointestinal ulcers and ulcerative colitis. Tissue regeneration: *Althea officinalis* extracts and polysaccharides have been shown to up-regulate genes related to cell adhesion proteins and growth; they are effective stimulators of cell physiology of epithelial cells.

Cautions: Use with caution during pregnancy or lactation.

Contraindications: None known

Qualities: Moist, warm 1st degree

Typical dosage: 20–40 ml per week

Andrographis paniculata

Common names: Andrographis, kalmegh

Family: Acanthaceae

Part used: Aerial parts

Description: Andrographis, known as King of Bitters, or kalmegh in India, and Chuan-Xin-Lian in China, is a major traditional herb throughout Asia. Isolated andorgrapholides have been developed as an antiviral medicine for injections. The Swedish Herbal Institute, with the help of leading expert on adaptogens, Prof Panossian, developed and clinically tested the preparation known as *Kan Jang* consisting of andrographis, echinacea and eleuthero for the common cold and influenza. In the last few years there have been reports of allergic reactions to andrographis. The great majority of these have been from methanol or highly concentrated extracts (14–19:1). The TGA Safety review of *Andrographis paniculata* and anaphylactic/allergic reactions from 2015 provides further information, but no details of the individual adverse events reports and no conclusive evidence is provided. Pharmacological investigations have shown andrographis to have anti-inflammatory, antiallergic and hepatoprotective properties.

Constituents: Bitter diterpenoid lactones, especially andrographolides, consisting of aglycones and glucosides, diterpene dimers, flavonoids

Primary actions: Antiviral (systemically), Bitter tonic, Immunomodulator.

All actions: Adaptogen, Anti-inflammatory, Antidiarrhoeal, Antioxidant, Antiparasitic, Antiplatelet, Antipyretic, Antiviral (systemically), Bitter tonic, Cardioprotective, Cholagogue, Choleretic, Digestive tonic, Hepatoprotective, Hepatotonic, Immunomodulator.

Indications:

- Boils, Bronchitis, Cardiovascular disease prevention, Chronic fatigue syndrome, Common cold, Convalescence, Debility, Diarrhoea,

Digestive complaints, Digestive weakness, Dysentery, Dyspepsia, Flatulence, Gastrointestinal tract infestation, Hepatitis, Hypochlorhydria, Immune deficiency, Infection; respiratory tract, Infection; skin, Infection; systemic, Infection; to improve resistance to, Infection; urinary tract, Infection; viral, Influenza, Liver insufficiency, Liver toxicity, Post-viral syndromes, Sinusitis, Warts.

- **WHO:** Prophylaxis and symptomatic treatment of upper respiratory infections, such as the common cold and uncomplicated sinusitis, bronchitis and pharyngotonsillitis, lower urinary tract infections and acute diarrhoea.

Cautions: Since January 2015, the TGA has received a further 70 Australian reports of allergic reactions related to *Andrographis paniculata* and an additional 37 reports of anaphylaxis. For 11 of these cases, the sole suspected medicine contained Andrographis paniculata as the single active ingredient, with 4 of the 11 cases involving anaphylactic reactions.

Large doses of the liquid extract may cause gastric discomfort as it is very bitter.

Contraindications: Contraindicated during pregnancy, and in cases of known allergy to plants of the Acanthaceae family. Bitters are contraindicated in states of hyperacidity, especially duodenal ulcers.

Drug interactions: May potentiate effects of midazolam.

Qualities: Bitter, cold

Typical dosage: 20–40 ml per week

Anemone pulsatilla

Synonym or related species: Pulsatilla vulgaris
Common names: Pulsatilla
Family: Ranunculaceae
Part used: Aerial parts
Description: Traditionally used as a nervine in the treatment of insomnia, tension and neuralgia. Ethanol extract shown to cause relaxation of intestinal smooth muscles.
Constituents: Lactones including ranunculin, protoanemonin, and anemonin as well as triterpene saponins and flavonoids.
Primary actions: Analgesic, Antispasmodic/ Spasmolytic, Emmenagogue.
All actions: Analgesic, Anodyne, Antispasmodic/ Spasmolytic, Diaphoretic, Emmenagogue, Sedative.
Indications:
- Amenorrhoea, Dysmenorrhoea, Endometriosis, Headache, Hyperactivity, Inflammation; ovaries/ testes, Insomnia, Ovarian and uterine pains, Ovulation; painful.

Cautions: The fresh plant is extremely irritating to the skin, gastrointestinal tract and mucous membranes. Allergic reactions have been attributed to pulsatilla.

Contraindications: During pregnancy and lactation

Qualities: Secondary cooling effect, warm
Typical dosage: 5–10 ml per week

Anethum graveolens

Common names: Dill
Family: Apiaceae
Part used: Seeds
Description: Traditional remedy for dyspepsia, gastritis, flatulence and stomach ache. Suitable for children and infants. Pharmacological studies have also found antidiabetic and antihyperlipidaemic properties, although a clinical trial found no beneficial effects on lipid profiles. Small clinical studies suggest a use in supporting labour during regular uterine contractions and for vulvovaginal candidiasis.
Constituents: Volatile oil in seeds contains carvone. Flavonoids, furanocoumarins, coumarins.
Primary actions: Aromatic, Carminative, Galactagogue.
All actions: Antidiabetic, Antihyperlipidemic, Aromatic, Carminative, Digestive tonic, Galactagogue.
Indications:
- Colic; childhood, Diabetes, Dyslipidaemia, Dyspepsia; flatulent, Flavouring.
- **BHP:** Flatulent dyspepsia, tormina. Specific indication: flatulent pain in infants.
- **Commission E:** Dyspepsia: Seed, 3 g; essential oil, 0.1–0.3 g; equivalent preparations.
- **WHO:** Treatment of dyspepsia, gastritis and flatulence and stomach ache.
- **Other uses:** Childhood colic, flatulent dyspepsia.

Qualities: Cooling
Typical dosage: 20–40 ml per week

Angelica archangelica

Synonym or related species: Angelica officinalis
Common names: European angelica, angelica
Family: Apiaceae
Part used: Rhizome and root
Description: Traditionally used in Western herbal medicine for loss of appetite, peptic discomfort such as mild spasms of the gastrointestinal tract, feeling of fullness, and flatulence. Ingredient with *Iberis amara, Melissa officinalis, Matricaria recutita, Carum carvi, Mentha x piperita, Glycyrrhiza glabra, Silybum marianum* and *Chelidonium majus* comprises the clinically validated preparation, STW 5 (*Iberogast*). Also used for nervous disorders including anxiety, anorexia, migraine and other cerebral diseases in India and China.
Constituents: Root: essential oil containing monoterpene hydrocarbons such as 24.5% alpha-pinene, 13.8% delta-3-carene, 10.1% beta-phellandrene, 8.8% p-cymene, 8.4% limonene, and

6.3% sabinene.s, over 20 different furocoumarins including imperatorin, also fatty acids. Seeds have a similar essential oil content to root. Imperatorin, a furanocoumarin, also found in the roots of *Angelica dahurica* and *A. sinensis*, have been shown to have anticancer, anti-inflammatory, cardiovascular protective, antinociceptive and anxiolytic properties.

Primary actions: Anticatarrhal, Circulatory stimulant, Digestive tonic.

All actions: Antispasmodic (respiratory tract), Anxiolytic, Aromatic, Bitter tonic, Carminative, Diaphoretic, Digestive tonic, Diuretic, Expectorant (stimulating), Vasodilator.

Indications:

- Anorexia, Bronchitis, Circulation; peripheral; impaired, Colitis, Digestive complaints, Digestive weakness, Dyspepsia, Dyspepsia; flatulent, Flatulence, Gastrointestinal catarrh, Hypochlorhydria, Infection; respiratory tract, Inflammation; gastrointestinal tract, Inflammatory bowel disease, Insomnia, Nervous exhaustion, Neuralgia (topically), Peripheral vascular disease, Respiratory catarrh, Rheumatism, Ulcer; gastrointestinal.
- **BHP:** Respiratory catarrh, psychogenic asthma, flatulent dyspepsia, anorexia nervosa, rheumatic disease and peripheral vascular disease. Specific indication: bronchitis associated with vascular deficiency.
- **Commission E:** Loss of appetite, peptic discomfort such as mild spasms of the gastrointestinal tract, feeling of fullness, flatulence.
- **Other uses:** Respiratory tract infection, respiratory catarrh, impaired peripheral circulation, gastrointestinal tract inflammation, gastrointestinal catarrh, colitis, gastrointestinal ulcer, digestive weakness, anorexia, flatulence, dyspepsia, insomnia, nervous exhaustion.

Cautions: Furanocoumarins in large doses may lead to photosensitivity and subsequent exposure to UV radiation can lead to photodermatitis.

Contraindications: During pregnancy.

Qualities: Dry 3rd degree, warm 3rd degree

Typical dosage: 10–20 ml per week

Angelica polymorpha

Synonym or related species: Angelica sinensis
Common names: Dong quai, dang gui, Chinese angelica
Family: Apiaceae
Part used: Root

Description: Dang gui is both a general tonic and a uterine tonic, used for a variety of menstrual disorders. Combines with astragalus in a simple formulation for menopausal symptoms. *Danggui Buxue Tang*, as stipulated in AD 1247, calls for a ratio of astragalus to dang gui of 5:1. Dang gui is also a

major herbal medicine for the cardiovascular system; reducing coronary vascular resistance and the total peripheral resistance, as well as increasing blood flow and significantly decreasing myocardial oxygen consumption.

Constituents: Essential oil containing mainly ligustilide and n-butylidene phthalide, coumarins including angelol and angelicone, phenylpropanoids including ferulic acid, angelica polysaccharides, phospholipids. *Angelica polymorpha* has a lower coumarin content than other angelica species.

Primary actions: Anti-inflammatory, Antiarrhythmic, Uterine tonic.

All actions: Anti-inflammatory, Antiarrhythmic, Anticancer, Antiplatelet, Antispasmodic (uterus), Blood tonic, Cardiotonic, Gastroprotective, Hepatoprotective, Immunomodulator, Uterine tonic.

Indications:

- Adenomyosis, Allergies/Sensitivities, Amenorrhoea, Anaemia, Angina pectoris, Arrhythmia, Buerger's disease, Cerebral ischaemia, Cerebrovascular disease, Constipation, Digestive complaints, Dysmenorrhoea, Dysmenorrhoea; congestive, Endometriosis, Hypertension, Infertility, Liver cirrhosis, Menopausal symptoms, Menstrual irregularity, Metrorrhagia, Ovulation; eratic, Palpitations, Premenstrual syndrome.
- **WHO:** Treatment of menstrual disorders such as irregular menstruation, amenorrhoea and dysmenorrhoea. As an analgesic for symptomatic treatment of rheumatic arthralgia, abdominal pain and in the management of postoperative pain. Treatment of constipation, anaemia, chronic hepatitis and cirrhosis of the liver.
- **Other uses:** Cerebral ischaemia, constipation associated with ageing or debility.

Cautions: Furanocoumarins in large doses may lead to photosensitivity and subsequent exposure to UV radiation can lead to photodermatitis.

Contraindications: Contraindicated during pregnancy, particularly in first trimester and in women with a tendency to spontaneous abortion.

Although dang gui has been shown to stimulate growth in tumour cell lines, animal experiments have shown no significant stimulatory activities on tumor growth after 28-day treatments in human breast xenograft or syngeneic mouse breast tumour-bearing mice. However, it should be used with caution in ER-positive breast cancer patients.

Drug interactions: May theoretically interact with antiplatelet and anticoagulant medication. One case report of potentiation of warfarin.

Qualities: Warming, moistening

Typical dosage: 30–60 ml per week

Annona muricata

Common names: Graviola, soursop, guanábana

Family: Annonaceae

Part used: Leaf

Description: Graviola has a long history of medicinal use for treating inflammatory conditions including diabetes, hypertension, insomnia, parasitic infections, and cancer. An extract has been shown to inhibit multiple signalling pathways that regulate metabolism, cell cycle, survival, and metastatic properties in pancreatic cancer cells.

Constituents: Annonaceous acetogenins have been shown to have antitumour, antiparasitic, antiprotozoal, anthelmintic, and antimicrobial properties. Also contains flavonoids (quercetin, isoquercitrin, quercitrin, rutin, and kaempferol) and phenolics acids (gallic, chlorogenic, ellagic and caffeic acids).

Primary actions: Anthelmintic, Anticancer, Antidiabetic.

All actions: Anthelmintic, Antibacterial, Anticancer, Antidepressant, Antifungal, Antihypertensive, Antimicrobial, Antiparasitic, Antispasmodic (muscles), Antiviral (systemically), Astringent, Febrifuge, Nervine tonic, Sedative.

Indications:

*   Cancer; including prevention/supportive treatment, Depression, Diabetes, Digestive complaints, Fever, Hypertension, Indigestion, Infection; bacterial, Infection; respiratory tract, Intestinal worms, Rheumatism.

Contraindications: Avoid in pregnancy: Uterine stimulant activity shown in an rodent study.

Typical dosage: 40–80 ml per week

Apium graveolens

Common names: Celery seed, karafs

Family: Apiaceae

Part used: Seed

Description: Celery has been used in traditional systems of medicine to treat spasm and stomach problems and as diuretic, laxative, and sedative. Often used for gout and arthritis. Karafs is used as an anthelmintic, antispasmodic, carminative, diuretic, laxative, and sedative stimulant in Arabian traditional medicine. Pharmacological examinations have demonstrated hepatoprotective, antidiabetic, antiulcer and anti-inflammatory properties.

Constituents: Volatile oil including apiol, limonene, and phthalides which give the characteristic celery odour; coumarins; furanocoumarins including begapten; fixed oil; flavonoids; phenolic acids. The aroma of the oil is due to the presence of sedanonic anhydride and sedanolide in the seed oil.

Primary actions: Anti-inflammatory, Antirheumatic, Diuretic.

All actions: Anti-inflammatory (musculoskeletal), Anti-inflammatory (urinary), Antioedematous, Antirheumatic, Antiseptic (urinary), Antispasmodic (muscles), Diuretic, Emmenagogue, Hypoglycaemic.

Indications:

*   Arthritis, Colic; intestinal, Cystitis, Flatulence, Fluid retention, Gout, Indigestion, Rheumatism, Urinary tract infecton.

*   **BHP:** Rheumatism, arthritis, gout and inflammation of the urinary tract. Specific indication: rheumatoid arthritis with mental depression.

*   **Other uses:** Gout, oedema, rheumatism, arthritis, indigestion, flatulence, intestinal colic, urinary tract infection, cystitis, urinary lithiasis.

Cautions: Considered safe in normal dosage. May cause allergic reactions (rarely). Furanocoumarins in large doses may lead to photosensitivity, and subsequent exposure to UV radiation can lead to inflammation. Do not administer during pregnancy or lactation without professional supervision.

Contraindications: Kidney disease (apiol is toxic to kidneys). Avoid high-dose preparations in pregnancy.

Drug interactions: May decrease the efficacy of thyroxine replacement therapy (case report). May reduce gastrointestinal symptoms associated with NSAIDs.

Qualities: Cold

Typical dosage: 20–40 ml per week

Arctium lappa

Common names: Burdock

Family: Asteraceae

Part used: Root

Description: Traditionally, fresh macerated leaves were wrapped around the painful body parts of patients with rheumatism. This can create an urticarial reaction which was considered to be even more beneficial (not recommended). A leaf infusion also used to treat skin diseases, insect bites, itching and scratches, stomach ulcer and gastritis; gargle for mouth infections, and also used for bladder stones, eczema, gallstones, gout, and skin afflictions.

The root is traditionally used as a blood purifier for rheumatism, inflammation, and to to stimulate urinary and hepato-biliary function.

Constituents: Phenolcarbonic acids and tannins: The fresh root contains 1.9% up to 3.65% polyphenols with chlorogenic acid, isochlorogenic acid and caffeic acid. Sulfur-containing polyacetylenes (thiophenes) including arctinal and arctinol. Lignans including neoarctin A and the lignanolide arctiin. Triterpenes, fatty acids, polysaccharides, aliphatic hydrocarbons, pyrazines sesquiterpenes, baicalin and a small amount of essential oil.

Primary actions: Anti-inflammatory, Antirheumatic,

25

Depurative/Alterative, Diuretic.

All actions: Anti-inflammatory, Choleretic, Depurative/Alterative, Diuretic.

Indications:

- Acne, Anorexia, Arthritis, Boils, Cancer; including prevention/supportive treatment, Eczema, Gout, Inflammation; gastrointestinal tract, Psoriasis, Urticaria.

- **BHP:** Cutaneous eruptions, rheumatism, cystitis, gout, anorexia nervosa. Specific indication: Eczema, especially in dry and desquamatory phase. Psoriasis. Combines well with Rumex crispus and Trifolium pratense.

Cautions: Avoid in patients with known sensitivity to plants in the Asteraceae (Compositae) family.

Contraindications: None known.

Qualities: Bitter, cooling

Typical dosage: 20–25 ml per week

Arctostaphylos uva-ursi

Common names: Bearberry

Family: Ericaceae

Part used: Leaf

Description: Primarily used for inflammatory diseases and mild, uncomplicated infections of the urinary tract. The ability of bearberry leaf to act against urinary infections is believed to be the result of action of free hydroquinone cleaved from the arbutin molecule in the urinary tract. It has been experimentally proven that pH value of the urine sample is very important for its antibacterial activity. Antibacterial effect of arbutin was increased and prolonged in alkaline urine pH 8 (when compared to the urine sample at pH 6). Administer with an alkaline preparation. However, this is not required for infections with E. coli as the bacteria will deconjugate arbutin and liberate the toxic hydroquinone. The free hydroquinone damages bacterial cells by destabilisation of its membranes. E. coli is the most frequent cause of urinary infections. *Neisseria gonorrhoeae* and *Chlamydia trachomatis* are clinically important infectious causes of urethritis.

Constituents: Flavonoids, iridoids, hydroquinone glycosides (mainly arbutin), tannins and terpenoid

Primary actions: Antimicrobial, Antiseptic (urinary), Diuretic.

All actions: Anti-inflammatory (urinary), Antilithic, Antimicrobial, Antiseptic, Antiseptic (urinary), Astringent, Diuretic.

Indications:

- Calculi; kidney and bladder, Cystitis, Dysuria, Lithuria, Prostatitis, Pyelitis, Urethritis.

- **BHP:** Cystitis, urethritis, dysuria, pyelitis, and lithuria. Specific indication: acute catarrhal cystitis with dysuria and highly acid urine.

- **ESCOP:** Uncomplicated infections of the lower urinary tract such as cystitis, when antibiotic

treatment is not considered essential.

- **WHO:** Internally, as a mild urinary antiseptic for moderate inflammatory conditions of the urinary tract and bladder, such as cystitis, urethritis and dysuria.

Cautions: Safety profile of crude extract of bearberry leaves in rabbits has been investigated. Dry ethanolic extract (DER 11:1; extraction solvent ethanol, concentration not specified) was administered orally for 90 days in male and female rabbits and haematology, biochemistry parameters and histopathology changes were analysed after 90 days. Gender-based variations were observed in haematological, kidney function, liver function, cardiac enzymes and lipids profile. Urine samples revealed the same results as those of standard and control drug. No significant pathology was observed in heart, stomach, liver and kidney tissues of rabbits, treated with bearberry extract in a dose of 25 mg/kg per day.

References: Saeed F, Mehjabeen S, Sikandar K S, Jahan N, Ahmad M. Diuretic and Anti-urolithic activity of Some Crude Extracts. Int J Pharmacogn Phytochem Res 2015, 7(1):128-131

Arbutin is a mandatory component of Arctostaphylos uva-ursi. Arbutin is not specifically scheduled in the Poisons Standard but has a cross-reference to hydroquinone in the index of the Poisons Standard. The concentration of arbutin in the medicine must be no more than 25 mg/kg or 25mg/L or 0.0025% unless used on the hair.

Contraindications: Kidney disorders, pregnancy, lactation and for children under 12 years.

Qualities: Cold

Typical dosage: 30–60 ml per week

Armoracia rusticana

Synonym or related species: Armoracia lapathifolia

Common names: Horseradish

Family: Brassicaceae

Part used: Fresh or dried root and leaves

Description: Horseradish is traditionally used to treat respiratory tract and sinus infections. Tablets containing 200 mg nasturtium (*Tropaeoli majoris*) powder and 80 mg horseradish root powder at a dose of 6 tablets daily is also used for the prophylactic treatment of chronically recurrent urinary tract infections.

Constituents: Volatile oils: glucosinolates (mustard oil glycosides), coumarins, phenolic acids, ascorbic acid, asparagin, resin, peroxidase enzymes

All actions: Antiseptic (respiratory tract), Circulatory stimulant, Decongestant, Digestive stimulant.

Indications:

- Bronchitis, Catarrh; naso-pharyngeal congestion, Circulation; peripheral, Hayfever, Infection; urinary tract, Sinusitis.

- **Commission E:** Catarrh of the respiratory tract,

supportive therapy for infections of urinary tract, externally for minor muscle aches.

- **Other uses:** Respiratory mucous, hayfever, bronchitis, sinusitis, nasal congestion, impaired peripheral circulation.

Cautions: Excessive intake may cause irritation (stomach, respiratory tract and kidneys); avoid in people with stomach and intestinal ulcers and kidney disorders, and in children under 4 years. Very strong tasting.

Contraindications: Mustard oils released upon crushing are potentially toxic; therefore doses exceeding dietary intakes are contraindicated during pregnancy.

Qualities: Hot 3rd degree

Typical dosage: 25–50 ml per week

Arnica montana

Common names: Arnica

Family: Asteraceae

Part used: Flowerheads

Description: A wound healing effect was attributed to Arnica in a manual of Tabernaemontanus as early as 1613. During the medieval age, Arnica was used as a medical plant for haematoma, injuries, varicosities, phlebitis, gout, rheumatism, indigestion and cardiovascular disease. In Germany, arnica has a long use in cases of injury and as consequences of accidents, e. g. haematoma, distortions (dislocation, sprains), contusions (bruises), against oedema due to fracture, for systematic treatment of rheumatic muscle and joint complaints, against furunculosis, inflammations caused by insect bites and superficial phlebitis, and to treat inflammations of the oral and throat region such as gingivitis and aphthuous ulcers.

Constituents: Helenalin and related sesquiterpene lactones, flavones, flavonols, triterpenoids, phenolic acids, polysaccharides.

Primary actions: Anti-inflammatory, Wound healing/Vulnerary.

All actions: Analgesic, Anti-inflammatory, Anti-inflammatory (musculoskeletal), Antimicrobial, Antiseptic, Counter-irritant, Venotonic, Wound healing/Vulnerary.

Indications:

- Alopecia neurotica, Bruises (topically), Chilblains; unbroken (topically), Sprains (topically), Varicose veins (topically), Venous insufficiency.
- **BHP:** Topically for bruises, sprains, unbroken chilblains and alopecia neurotica. Specific indication: sprains and bruises as a topical application.
- **Commission E:** Injuries and consequences of accidents, e.g., hematomas, dislocations, contusions, oedema due to fracture, rheumatic muscle and joint problems. Also inflammation of oral and throat mucous membranes, furunculosis,

insect bite inflammation, superficial phlebitis.

- **ESCOP:** Externally for the treatment of bruises, sprains, inflammation caused by insect bites, gingivitis and aphthous ulcers, symptomatic treatment of rheumatic complaints.
- **WHO:** As a topical counter-irritant for treatment of pain and inflammation resulting from minor injuries and accidents, including bruises, ecchymoses, haematomas and petechiae. Treatment of inflammation of the oral mucous membranes, insect bites and superficial phlebitis.

Cautions: Not for internal use (except homeopathic preparations). Do not use on open wounds, near eyes or mouth, apply only to unbroken skin and withdraw if any sign of dermatitis. Do not use for prolonged periods.

Contraindications: Contraindicated during pregnancy or lactation. Allergy to Arnica or other members of Compositae (Asteraceae).

Qualities: Cool

Typical dosage: external use only

Artemisia absinthium

Common names: Wormwood, absinthe

Family: Asteraceae

Part used: Leaves and flowering tops

Description: Used by the Egyptians as an antiseptic, a stimulant and tonic, and as a remedy for fevers and menstrual pains (Ebers Papyrus). Hippocrates recommended it as a cure for jaundice. In the Middle Ages, the plant was used to exterminate tapeworm infestation. Paracelsus considered it as a stomachic, anthelminthic herb which also acts as prophylaxis against sea-sickness. Today used for lack of appetite, dyspepsia, gastro-intestinal spasms, and flatulence. Pharmacological investigations have also identified hepatoprotective and antimalarial properties.

Constituents: Sesquiterpene lactones (absinthin), essential oil (thujones)

Primary actions: Anthelmintic, Bitter tonic, Hepatoprotective.

All actions: Anthelmintic, Antiparasitic, Antipyretic, Bitter tonic, Hepatoprotective.

Indications:

- Anorexia, Dyspepsia, Dyspepsia; flatulent, Indigestion, Intestinal worms, Malaria.
- **BHP:** Nematode infestation, anorexia, atonic dyspepsia. Specific indication: infestation with pin or round worms.
- **ESCOP:** Anorexia, e.g. after illness, dyspeptic complaints.

Cautions: Should not be taken continuously for periods of more than 3–4 weeks. Caution in patients with underlying defects in hepatic haem synthesis.

Contraindications: Contraindicated during pregnancy and lactation; in gastric and duodenal ulcers; in known sensitivity to wormwood or the

Asteraceae (Compositae) family

Qualities: Cool, dry 1/2 degree, warm 1/2 degree

Typical dosage: 5–20 ml per week

Artemisia annua

Common names: Sweet Annie, Chinese wormwood, qing hao

Family: Asteraceae

Part used: Aerial parts

Description: Artemisinin and its semisynthetic analogue artesunate, are used in combination with standard antimalarial amodiaquine. The therapy is known as artemisinin or artesunate (a semi-synthetic derivative of artemisinin) Combination Therapy and it is the first-line treatment of uncomplicated malaria. Extract of *A. annua*, artemisinin and its derivatives also have athelmintic, antiviral, immunomodulatory and anticancer properties.

Constituents: Sesquiterpene lactone (artemisinin), essential oil, flavonoids. Artesunate is the semisynthetic derivative of artemisinin.

Primary actions: Anticancer, Antiparasitic, Bitter tonic.

All actions: Anthelmintic, Anti-inflammatory, Anti-inflammatory (musculoskeletal), Anticancer, Antiparasitic, Antiviral (systemically), Bitter tonic, Digestive tonic, Febrifuge, Immunomodulator.

Indications:

- Cancer; including prevention/supportive treatment, Colitis, Intestinal worms, Malaria, Osteoarthritis, Parasites, Rheumatoid arthritis.
- **Other uses:** 9 g infusion in 1 L water may contain about 95 mg artemisinin. Infusions and liquid extracts may be useful in anthelmintic, antiviral and antimicrobial therapy.

Cautions: While animal studies indicate that artesunate can have harmful effects on pregnancy, no such effects have been documented in humans. Ongoing studies continue to demonstrate the safety of artemisinin during pregnancy. Considering that severe malaria represents a substantial risk for pregnant women and their foetuses, WHO recommends that pregnant women with severe malaria be treated with artesunate or quinine in the first trimester, and with artesunate preferentially prescribed to quinine in the second and third trimesters

Qualities: Bitter, cold

Typical dosage: 20–50 ml per week. Higher doses may be necessary for SLE and malaria.

Artemisia vulgaris

Common names: Mugwort

Family: Asteraceae

Part used: Aerial parts

Description: Long traditional use for indigestion, stomach ulcers, liver disorders and worms. Mugwort was used to flavour beer before the introduction of hops. Mugwort is also the herb used in moxibustion in TCM. Mugwort essential oil has been employed for the treatment of diabetes and epilepsy, and in combination for psychoneurosis, depression, irritability, insomnia, and anxiety stress.

Constituents: Essential oil (0.1 and 1.4%), mainly composed of β-pinene, α-pinene, camphor, and 1,8-cineole. Also contains sesquiterpene lactones, flavonol glycosides, coumarins.

Primary actions: Anthelmintic, Bitter tonic, Emmenagogue.

All actions: Anthelmintic, Antibacterial, Antifungal, Antifungal (topically), Bitter tonic, Cholagogue, Digestive tonic, Emmenagogue, Stomachic.

Indications:

- Anorexia, Dyspepsia; nervous, Gastrointestinal tract infestation, Intestinal worms.
- **BHP:** Delayed or irregular menstruation, anorexia, nervous dyspepsia, thread worm and round worm infestation. Specific indications: functional amenorrhoea, dysmenorrhoea.

Contraindications: During pregnancy

Qualities: Dry 2nd degree, hot 2nd degree

Typical dosage: 15–30 ml per week

Asclepias tuberosa

Common names: Pleurisy root, butterfly weed

Family: Asclepiadaceae

Part used: Root

Description: Asclepias was one of the most common of the indigenous medicines in North America and considered one of the best expectorants in the *Ecclectic Materia Medica*: 'Asclepias may be indicated even though the patient be freely perspiring'. It was thought to be very effectual in intercostal neuralgia and rheumatism, as well as in pericardial pains.

Constituents: Cardiac glycosides, flavonols, flavonol glycosides, phytosterols and triterpenes.

Primary actions: Antiseptic (respiratory tract), Diaphoretic, Expectorant (general).

All actions: Antipyretic, Antiseptic (respiratory tract), Antispasmodic (respiratory tract), Diaphoretic, Expectorant (general), Expectorant (stimulating).

Indications:

- Asthma, Asthma; bronchial, Bronchitis, Cough, Emphysema, Influenza, Pertusis, Pleurisy.
- **BHP:** Bronchitis, pneumonitis, pleurisy and influenza. Specific indication: pleurisy.

Qualities: Cold, dry

Typical dosage: 10–20 ml per week

Asparagus racemosus

Common names: Shatavari (Sanskrit), satavari (Hindi), satmuli (Bengali)

Family: Asparagaceae

Part used: Root

Description: Shatavari is both a general tonic and a female reproductive tonic. Urinary herb where its soothing and antispasmodic properties are employed in the treatment of cystitis and urinary stones, and by extension also for rheumatic pain where the diuretic action improves the excretion of inflammatory products. Shatavari is also used for dysentery, tumours, inflammatory disorders, neuropathy, nervous conditions, bronchitis, hyperacidity, infectious diseases, conjunctivitis and chronic fever. The high level of steroidal saponins may be responsible for the oestrogenic effect of shatavari and explain its traditional use as a reproductive tonic.

Constituents: The word asparagus originates from the Greek word for stalk or shoot. The genus Aspargaus has recently been moved from the subfamily Aspragae in the Liliaceous family to a newly created family Asparagaceae. The Asparagaceae genus, containing some 300 species, is considered to be of medical importance because of the presence of sapogenins and saponins. Shatavari contains 8–9% steroidal saponins, known as shatavarin I, immunoside, asparagin A, shatavarins IV–X (Hayes et al. 2008). The major saponins in the roots are shatavarin I and especially shatavarin IV (44%). Shatavari also contains isoflavones including 8-methoxy-5,6,4'- trihydroxyisoflavone 7-O-beta-D-glucopyranoside(Saxena and Chourasia 2001), phytosterols (0.8%), polyphenols (1.7%), alkaloids, including the non-hepatotoxic pyrrolizidine alkaloid asparagamine A, and flavonoids (Visavadiya and Narasimhacharya 2007, Potduang et al. 2008).

Primary actions: Adaptogen, Antispasmodic/Spasmolytic, Reproductive tonic.

All actions: Adaptogen, Anti-inflammatory, Antibacterial, Anticancer, Antidepressant, Antidiarrhoeal, Antiprotozoal, Antispasmodic/Spasmolytic, Antitussive, Anxiolytic, Cardiotonic, Demulcent, Diuretic, Galactagogue, Gastroprotective, Hepatoprotective, Hypoglycaemic, Immunomodulator, Neuroprotective, Reproductive tonic, Sexual tonic.

Indications:

- Calculi; kidney and bladder, Cancer; including prevention/supportive treatment, Cardiac debility, Cough, Diarrhoea, Dysentery, Dyslipidaemia, Dyspepsia, Fatigue, Fluid retention, Gall stones (cholelithiasis), Infertility, Inflammation; gastrointestinal tract, Lactation; poor, Memory and concentration; poor, Menopausal symptoms, Reproductive dysfunction, Rheumatism, Sexual weakness, Stress, Ulcer; gastrointestinal.

- **Other uses:** In Western herbal medicine, shatavari is often seen as a female reproductive tonic and shatavari does indeed mean to 'possess a hundred husbands'. However, it is equally considered a great general tonic. Withania is sometimes also seen as a 'female' female tonic by Western herbalists, perhaps due to the fact that it is less stimulating than Korean ginseng (Panax ginseng). However, in Ayurvedic medicine, shatavari is the main rejuvenative tonic for the female, as is Withania for the male. Shatavari is, however, used for sexual debility and infertility in both sexes. It is also used for menopausal symptoms and to increase lactation (Thakur et al. 1989, Frawley and Lad 1986).

- In Ayurvedic medicine, Shatavari is a significant urinary herb where its soothing and antispasmodic properties are employed in the treatment of cystitis and urinary stones, and by extension also for rheumatic pain where the diuretic action improves the excretion of inflammatory products. Shatavari is also used for dysentery, tumours, inflammatory disorders, neuropathy, nervous conditions, bronchitis, hyperacidity, infectious diseases, conjunctivitis and chronic fever.

- Shatavari be a good subsitute for *Chamaelirium luteum* (false unicorn root), which is an endangered species.

Cautions: The high saponin content may cause upper digestive tract irritations.

Toxicity

The LD50 is >1g/kg. No toxic effects or mortality were observed with doses ranging from 50mg/kg to 1g/kg for four weeks. Acute and subacute (15–30 days administration) toxicity studies did not detect any changes in vital organ function tests (Rege et al. 1999).

Teratogenicity

A methanolic extract of shatavari roots (1000 mg/kg/day for 60 days) has been shown to have teratological effects such as increased resorption of foetuses and gross malformations e.g. swelling in legs and intrauterine growth retardation with a small placental size in Charles Foster rats. Pups born to a mother exposed to shatavari roots for the full duration of gestation showed evidence of higher rate of resorption and therefore smaller litter size. The live pups showed significant decrease in body weight and length and delay of various developmental parameters when compared to respective control groups (Goel et al. 2006). The dosage used would be equivalent to around 70 g or 140 ml of an 1:2 liquid extract per day for a human adult. This is more than 16 times the recommended dosage.

Another study examining the teratogenicity of a formulation containing shatavari did not find any signs of teratogenicity with the dosage used. Rats received 3 g/kg of the product once a day orally from day 0 of gestation till day 21 of lactation or just during gestation. No adverse effects was observed on pregnancy and growth of the foetus (Muralidhar et al.

1993). The daily dose of the formulation was 3 g/kg body weight, which would be equivalent to 210 g for a 70 kg human. It is difficult to calculate the amount of shatavari in the formulation from the ingredients list, but it could be as high as 2–3% which would equate to about 5 g which is not to dissimilar to the recommended dosage of shatavari 1:2 extract.

Contraindications: Use with caution in pregnancy.

Drug interactions: Shatavari has weak oestrogenic activity. Coadministration is unlikely to affect the efficacy of oral contraceptives or postmenopausal hormone therapy.

Qualities: Bittersweet, cooling, drying. Energetically, shatavari is sweet and bitter and it is particularly balancing to the Pitta Dosha (a body type used in Ayurveda in diagnosis and treatment).

Typical dosage: 30–60 ml per week

References online phytotherapydeskreference.com

Astragalus membranaceus

Common names: Astragalus, milk vetch, huang qi (Chinese), ogi (Japanese)

Family: Fabaceae

Part used: Root

Description: Traditional information regarding astragalus is likely to be from the use of decoctions in TCM formulations. Decoctions and hydroethanolic extracts contain polysaccharides, saponins and isoflavones. Pharmacological examinations are mostly based on studies with purified extractions rich in polysaccharides. Injectable astragalus polysaccharides i.p. may help relieve chemotherapy-induced side effects including myelosuppression, fatigue, mucositis, pain, nausea and vomiting, as well as loss of appetite and reduced body weight. Astragalus polysaccharides may exert immunostimulatory activities by stimulating B-lymphocytes, activating T-lymphocytes, inducing cytokine production, and activating macrophages and natural killer cells. Astragalus and its polysaccharides may improve compliance of radiotherapy and/or chemotherapy and quality of life during therapy.

Constituents: Triterpenoid saponins (astragalosides), flavonoids, isoflavonoids, polysaccharides.

Primary actions: Adaptogen, Anticancer, Immunomodulator.

All actions: Adaptogen, Antihypertensive, Antioxidant, Antiviral (systemically), Cardiotonic, Chemoprotective, Diuretic, Immunomodulator, Nrf2-pathway activator, Renal tonic, Tonic, Wound healing/Vulnerary.

Indications:

* Arteriosclerosis, Atherosclerosis, Autoimmune disease, Cancer; including prevention/supportive treatment, Cardiovascular disease prevention, Chemotherapy; to minimise the side effects of, Chronic fatigue syndrome, Congestive heart failure, Convalescence, Debility, Exhaustion, Fatigue, Hepatitis, Hypertension, Immune deficiency, Infection; bacterial, Infection; gastrointestinal system, Infection; systemic, Infection; to improve resistance to, Infection; viral, Longevity, Menopausal symptoms, Nephritis, Night sweats, Palpitations, Post-viral syndromes, Sweating; excessive, Ulcer; gastrointestinal, Wounds.

* **WHO:** As adjunctive therapy in the treatment of colds and influenza. Used to enhance the immune system and to increase stamina and endurance. Treatment of chronic diarrhoea, oedema, abnormal uterine bleeding, diabetes mellitus, and as a cardiotonic agent.

Cautions: Do not administer during acute infection, pregnancy or lactation without professional supervision.

Contraindications: None known

Drug interactions: May have beneficial effects in reducing adverse effects in patients receiving chemotherapy. May reduce chronic paracetamol-induced hepatotoxicity.

Qualities: Sweet and slightly warm

Typical dosage: 30–60 ml per week

Atractylodes macrocephala

Synonym or related species: Atractylodes ovata

Common names: Atractylodes, bai zhu

Family: Asteraceae

Part used: Root

Description: Used as a tonic agent in various ethno-medical systems in East Asia, especially in China, for the treatment of gastrointestinal dysfunction, cancer, osteoporosis, obesity, and foetal irritability.

Constituents: Atractylol, atractylon (essential oil)

Primary actions: Adaptogen, Anticancer, Digestive tonic.

All actions: Adaptogen, Anti-inflammatory, Anticancer, Antidiarrhoeal, Antioedematous, Antiosteoporotic, Bitter tonic, Digestive tonic, Diuretic, Neuroprotective.

Indications:

* Anorexia, Cancer; including prevention/supportive treatment, Chronic fatigue syndrome, Convalescence, Diarrhoea, Exhaustion, Gastrointestinal tract infestation, Indigestion, Night blindness, Stress, Weight loss; to assist.

Contraindications: None known

Qualities: Sweet, bitter and warm

Typical dosage: 25–50 ml per week

Avena sativa (green)

Common names: Oats, green oats, oat straw

Family: Poaceae

Part used: Aerial parts; herbal tincture made from dried, leaf and stem

Description: Considered a nervine tonic with sedative and mood enhancing properties.

Constituents: Beta-glucan (soluble fibre), triterpenoid saponins (avenacosides), alkaloids (avenine, trigonelline), sterol (avenasterol), flavonoids, starch, phytates and coumarins. Nutrients such as silicic acid, calcium, potassium, phosphorous, iron, manganese, zinc, vitamins A, B-complex, C, E and K, and amino acids.

Primary actions: Nervine tonic, Sedative.

All actions: Antidepressant, Antipruritic, Emollient, Nervine tonic, Sedative, Tonic.

Indications:

- Anxiety, Convalescence, Depression, Eczema (topically), Exhaustion, Herpes (topically), Herpes simplex, Insomnia, Nervous exhaustion, Nervous tension, Neurasthenia, Shingles, Stress.

- **Commission E:** Topical use in baths for inflammatory and seborrhaeic skin diseases, especially with itching.

- **Other uses:** Dry skin, itching, eczema (topically or in bath), neurasthenia, shingles, herpes zoster, herpes simplex, exhaustion, convalescence, stress, nervous tension, anxiety, insomnia and depression.

Cautions: Patients with coeliac disease should be able to tolerate moderate amounts of oats in the diet (both short and long-term studies found no adverse immunological effects). Considered less stimulating and tonifying than oats seed.

Contraindications: None known

Qualities: Sweet, warm

Typical dosage: 20–40 ml per week

Avena sativa (seed)

Common names: Oats, groats, oatmeal

Family: Poaceae

Part used: Seed; herbal tincture made from dehusked and rolled starchy endosperm

Description: Native to the Mediterranean region including southern Europe and northern Africa, but now cultivated in many parts of the world. Since classical times it has been grown as staple food and as important feed for stock. Considered a nervine tonic.

Constituents: Beta-glucan (soluble fibre), triterpenoid saponins (avenacosides), alkaloids (avenine, trigonelline), sterol (avenasterol), flavonoids, starch, phytates, protein (including gluten) and coumarins. Nutrients such as silicic acid, calcium, potassium, phosphorous, iron, manganese, zinc, vitamins A, B-complex, C, E and K, and amino acids.

Primary actions: Emollient, Nervine tonic, Nutritive.

All actions: Antidepressant, Antihypertensive, Antipruritic, Blood sugar regulator, Emollient, Nervine tonic, Nutritive, Tonic.

Indications:

- Anxiety, Convalescence, Depression, Dyslipidaemia, Eczema (topically), Exhaustion, Hypertension, Hypoglycaemia, Insomnia, Nervous exhaustion, Nervous tension, Neuralgia, Stress.

- **BHP:** Depression, melancholia, menopausal neurasthenia, and general debility. Specific indication: depressive states.

- **Other uses:** Dry skin, itch, eczema (topically).

Cautions: Patients with coeliac disease should be able to tolerate moderate amounts of oats in the diet (both short and long-term studies found no adverse immunological effects). Considered to be more stimulating and tonifying than green oats.

Contraindications: Avoid dietary oats in cases of intestinal obstruction.

Qualities: Sweet, warm

Typical dosage: 20–40 ml per week

Bacopa monnieri

Synonym or related species: Herpestis monniera

Common names: Bacopa, brahmi

Family: Scrophulariaceae

Part used: Whole plant (mainly leaves and stems)

Description: Brahmi refers to the Hindu creator god, Brahma. Bacopa is classified in Ayurvedic medicine as a *medhyarasayana*, a medicine used to improve memory and intellect (*medhya*). A number of small trials have examined bacopa in the treatment of stress, mood, anxiety, depression, cognitive function, memory, attention-deficit hyperactivity disorder (ADHD) and Alzheimer's disease.

Constituents: Saponins (bacosides), alkaloids (brahmine, herpestine and flavonoids).

Primary actions: Anxiolytic, Neuroprotective, Nootropic.

All actions: Adaptogen, Antiepileptic, Antioxidant, Anxiolytic, Nervine tonic, Nootropic, Sedative.

Indications:

- Alzheimer's disease, Anxiety, Chronic fatigue syndrome, Convalescence, Debility, Dementia, Epilepsy, Memory and concentration; poor, Mental exhaustion, Nerve damage, Nervous exhaustion, Neurasthenia, Stroke; recovery after.

- **Other uses:** Anxiety, nervous exhaustion, mental exhaustion, debility, poor memory, poor concentration, ADHD, nerve damage, neurasthenia, any nervous injury causing deficit and/or requiring rehabilitation (e.g., stroke, epilepsy). Used in Ayurvedic medicine to enhance intellect.

Cautions: Studies suggest 12 weeks continual use required before cognitive benefits apparent. May cause irritation of the gastric mucous membranes and reflux due to high saponin content.

Contraindications: None known

Qualities: Astringent, cold, turning sweet
Typical dosage: 40–90 ml per week

Ballota nigra

Common names: Black horehound
Family: Lamiaceae
Part used: Flowering tops
Description: Traditonal medicine for tenseness, restlessness and irritability with difficulty in falling asleep, and for the relief of mild spasmodic gastric complaints. A small, open study of 28 patients with general anxiety found that about two-thirds responded to the therapy. Patients with sleep disorders had the most improvement. Out of 10 patients taking benzodiazepines prior to the study, 3 discontinued and 4 reduced their dose by half.

Constituents: Diterpenoid lactones (ballotenol, ballotinonone), flavonoid glycosides, phenylpropanoids, traces of essential oil (humulene, pinene).

Primary actions: Antiemetic, Antimicrobial, Sedative.

All actions: Antibacterial, Antiemetic, Antifungal, Antimicrobial, Antispasmodic/Spasmolytic, Anxiolytic, Hypoglycaemic, Sedative.

Indications:

- Anxiety, Dyspepsia; nervous, Insomnia, Morning sickness, Nausea.
- **BHP:** Nausea, vomiting, nervous dyspepsia. Specific indication: vomiting of central origin.
- **ESCOP:** Tenseness, restlessness and irritability with difficulty in falling asleep and for the relief of mild spasmodic gastric complaints

Contraindications: None known
Qualities: Bitter, cold
Typical dosage: 10–20 ml per week

Baptisia tinctoria

Common names: Wild indigo
Family: Fabaceae
Part used: Root
Description: Traditional herb for the common cold and influenza. A key ingredient in the German product Esberitox with *Echinacea pallida, E. purpurea* and *Thuja occidentalis* for rhinosinusitis.

Constituents: Arabinogalactan-proteins with immunostimulant activities. Alkaloids including baptitoxine, glycosides: baptisin, and baptin.

Primary actions: Antiseptic, Antiviral (systemically), Immunomodulator.

All actions: Analgesic, Antimicrobial, Antipyretic, Anxiolytic, Immunomodulator, Lymphatic, Sedative.

Indications:

- Common cold, Fever, Furunculosis, Gingivitis, Infection; throat, Laryngitis, Leucorrhoea and vaginitis (douche), Lymphadenitis, Pharyngitis, Stomatitis, Tonsillitis, Tracheitis, Ulcer; mouth.
- **BHP:** Tonsillitis, pharyngitis, acute catarrhal infection, lymphadenitis, furunculosis, aphthous ulcers, stomatitis, gingivitis, fevers. Topically for indolent ulcers, sore nipples, leucorrhoea (douche). Specific indication: infection of the upper respiratory tract.

Contraindications: None known
Qualities: Bitter, cold
Typical dosage: 15–40 ml per week

Berberis aquifolium

Synonym or related species: Mahonia aquifolium, Mahonia repens, Berberis repens
Common names: Oregon grape, mountain grape
Family: Berberidaceae
Part used: Rhizome, root
Description: Berberine-containing plants have been traditionally used in various parts of the world for the treatment of inflammatory disorders, skin diseases, wound healing, reducing fevers, affections of the eyes, treatment of tumors, digestive and respiratory diseases and microbial pathologies. *B aquifolium* has been shown to have an antiproliferative effect on human keratinocytes and is a major herb for psoriasis.

Constituents: Alkaloids (berberine, berbamine, oxyacanthine), tannins, resin, minerals.

Primary actions: Anti-inflammatory, Antipsoriatic, Lipogenesis- and lipoxygenation-inhibitor.

All actions: Anti-inflammatory, Anti-inflammatory (GIT), Antidiarrhoeal, Antiemetic, Antifungal, Antimicrobial, Antipsoriatic, Bitter tonic, Cholagogue, Hepatotonic, Immunomodulator, Lipogenesis- and lipoxygenation-inhibitor.

Indications:

- Acne (topically), Dermatitis, Diarrhoea, Dyspepsia, Eczema, Gall stones (cholelithiasis), Gallbladder disorders, Gastrointestinal catarrh, Gout, Infection; skin, Psoriasis, Urticaria.
- **BHP:** Cutaneous disease, gastritis, leucorrhoea. Specific indications: psoriasis, eczema, catarrhal gastritis with cholecystitis.

Cautions: Topical use may cause skin reactions or exacerbate chronic skin conditions.

Contraindications: Contraindicated during pregnancy and lactation.

Drug interactions: Pretreatment and coadministration of berberine may lower the oral bioavailability of ciprofloxacin.(Hwang et al., 2012).

Itraconazole and berberine are mutually antagonistic and should not be combined. Use either itraconazole or berberine (or berberine-containing herbal extracts) but not together. The use of berberine is especially relevant since itraconazole is toxic and prone to be associatd with fungal resistance. The incidence of Aspergillus fumigatus infections has become more frequent as a consequence of widespread immunosuppression. At present, the number of available antifungal agents in clinical use is limited, and most of them, such as itraconazole, are toxic and show resistance. Berberine is a plant alkaloid used in the clinic mainly for alimentary infections. Berberine has antifungal effects agains Aspergillus fumigatus, possibly via inhibition of the ergosterol biosynthesis pathway in a similar way to he antifungal drug, itraconazole. The two drugs were found to be mutually antagonistic and should not be combined clinically (Lei et al., 2011).

References:

Hwang, Y. H., Cho, W. K., Jang, D., Ha, J. H., Jung, K., Yun, H. I. and Ma, J. Y. 2012. Effects of berberine and hwangryunhaedok-tang on oral bioavailability and pharmacokinetics of ciprofloxacin in rats. Evid Based Complement Alternat Med, 2012, 673132. Lei, G., Dan, H., Jinhua, L., Wei, Y., Song, G. and Li, W. 2011. Berberine and itraconazole are not synergistic in vitro against Aspergillus fumigatus isolated from clinical patients. Molecules, 16, 9218-33.

Potdar, D. (2012). Phytochemical and Pharmacological applications of Berberis Aristata. Fitoterapia.

Qualities: Warm

Typical dosage: 20–50 ml per week

Berberis aristata

Common names: Daruharidra, daruhaldi, darvi, chitra, Indian barberry

Family: Berberidaceae

Part used: Root

Description: Berberine-containing plants have been traditionally used in different parts of the world for the treatment of inflammatory disorders, skin diseases, wound healing, reducing fevers, affections of the eyes, treatment of tumors, digestive and respiratory diseases and microbial pathologies. Indian barbarry has a very high content of berberine. In Yunani medicine, *B. asiatica* has multiple uses, such as for the treatment of asthma, eye sores, jaundice, skin pigmentation, and toothache, as well as the elimination of inflammation and swelling, and for drying ulcers. Monograph included in the British Pharmacopoeia. The clinically tested hypercholesterolemic product, Berberol K (PharmExtracta, Italy), contains 500 mg berberine from *B. aristata*, 105 mg silymarin and 10 mg monacolins (K and Ka from MPK20 from *Monascus purpureus* fermented red yeast rice standardised extract (natural statin).

Constituents: Berberine is the main constituent.

Primary actions: Anticancer, Antihyperlipidemic, Antimicrobial.

All actions: Antibacterial, Anticancer, Antihyperlipidemic, Antimicrobial, Antioxidant, Antipyretic, Hepatoprotective.

Indications:

- Diabetes, Diarrhoea, Haemorrhoids, Hepatitis, Infection; fungal, Infection; gastrointestinal system, Infection; genitourinary tract, Infection; protozoal, Infection; respiratory tract, Infection; skin, Jaundice, Malaria, Osteoporosis, Sinusitis, Urinary tract infecton, Wounds.

- **Other uses:** Diarrhoea, haemorrhoids, gynaecological disorders, HIV-AIDS, osteoporosis, diabetes, eye and ear infections, wound healing, jaundice, skin diseases and malarial fever (Potdar et al., 2012).

Drug interactions: Pretreatment and coadministration of berberine may lower the oral bioavailability of ciprofloxacin. (Hwang et al., 2012). Itraconazole and berberine are mutually antagonistic and should not be combined. Use either itraconazole or berberine (or berberine-containing herbal extracts) but not together. The use of berberine is especially relevant since itraconazole is toxic and prone to fungal resistance. The incidence of Aspergillus fumigatus infections has become more frequent as a consequence of widespread immunosuppression. At present, the number of available antifungal agents in clinical use is limited, and most of them, such as itraconazole, are toxic and show resistance. Berberine is a plant alkaloid used in the clinic mainly for alimentary infections. Berberine has antifungal effects against Aspergillus fumigatus, possibly via inhibition of the ergosterol biosynthesis pathway in a similar way to he antifungal drug, itraconazole. The two drugs were found to be mutually antagonistic and should not be combined clinically (Lei et al., 2011).

References:

Hwang, Y. H., Cho, W. K., Jang, D., Ha, J. H., Jung, K., Yun, H. I. and Ma, J. Y. 2012. Effects of berberine and hwangryunhaedok-tang on oral bioavailability and pharmacokinetics of ciprofloxacin in rats. Evid Based Complement Alternat Med, 2012, 673132. Lei, G., Dan, H., Jinhua, L., Wei, Y., Song, G. and Li, W. 2011. Berberine and itraconazole are not synergistic in vitro against Aspergillus fumigatus isolated from clinical patients. Molecules, 16, 9218-33.

Potdar, D. (2012). Phytochemical and Pharmacological applications of Berberis Aristata. Fitoterapia.

Typical dosage: 20–40 ml per week (1:2)

Berberis vulgaris

Common names: Barberry

Family: Berberidaceae

Part used: Stem bark, root bark, root

Description: Berberine-containing plants have been traditionally used in different parts of the world for the treatment of inflammatory disorders, skin diseases, wound healing, reducing fevers, affections of eyes, treatment of tumors, digestive and respiratory diseases and microbial pathologies. Indian barbarry has a higher content of berberine.

Constituents: Alkaloids (berberine, oxyacanthine, palmatine, berbamine), chelidonic acids, tannins, wax, resin

Primary actions: Antihyperlipidemic, Bitter tonic, Choleretic.

All actions: Anti-inflammatory, Anti-inflammatory (GIT), Antibacterial, Antiemetic, Antimicrobial, Antiparasitic, Antipyretic, Antiseptic (GIT), Bitter tonic, Cholagogue, Choleretic, Cytoprotective, Depurative/Alterative, Digestive tonic, Hepatotonic, Spleen tonic.

Indications:

- Acne, Arthritis, Boils, Cholecystitis, Eczema, Gall stones (cholelithiasis), Gallbladder disorders, Gastrointestinal catarrh, Gout, Jaundice, Psoriasis, Urticaria.

- **BHP:** Cholecystitis, cholelithiasis, jaundice, leishmaniasis, and malaria. Specific indication: gallstones

Cautions: Use with caution in ileus or liver cancer, septic cholecystitis, acute or chronic hepatocellular disease, unconjugated hyperbilirubinaemia or intestinal spasm.

Contraindications: Contraindicated during pregnancy, lactation, and in jaundiced neonates

Drug interactions: Itraconazole and berberine are mutually antagonistic and should not be combined. Use either itraconazole or berberine (or berberine-containing herbal extracts) but not together. The use of berberine is especially relevant since itraconazole is toxic and prone to be associated with fungal resistance. The incidence of *Aspergillus fumigatus* infections has become more frequent as a consequence of widespread immunosuppression. At present, the number of available antifungal agents in clinical use is limited, and most of them, such as itraconazole, are toxic and show resistance. Berberine is a plant alkaloid used in the clinic mainly for alimentary infections. Berberine has antifungal effects agains Aspergillus fumigatus, possibly via inhibition of the ergosterol biosynthesis pathway in a similar way to he antifungal drug, itraconazole. The two drugs were found to be mutually antagonistic and should not be combined clinically (Lei et al., 2011).

References:

Lei, G., Dan, H., Jinhua, L., Wei, Y., Song, G. and Li, W. 2011. Berberine and itraconazole are not synergistic in vitro against Aspergillus fumigatus isolated from clinical patients. Molecules, 16, 9218-33.

Pretreatment and coadministration of berberine may lower the oral bioavailability of ciprofloxacin.

Hwang, Y. H., Cho, W. K., Jang, D., Ha, J. H., Jung, K., Yun, H. I. & Ma, J. Y. 2012. Effects of berberine and hwangryunhaedok-tang on oral bioavailability and pharmacokinetics of ciprofloxacin in rats. Evid Based Complement Alternat Med, 2012, 673132.

Qualities: Bitter, cold, dry

Typical dosage: 20–40 ml per week

Betula pendula

Synonym or related species: Betula alba, Betula verrucosa

Common names: Silver birch

Family: Betulaceae

Part used: Leaves, bark, leaf buds

Description: Used to increase the amount of urine to achieve flushing of the urinary tract in case of bacterial and inflammatory diseases of the lower urinary tract. Adjuvant treatment of rheumatic complaints.

Constituents: Volatile oil (betulin – camphor-like), flavonoids, flavones, phenolics, steroidal saponins, salicin, resins, tannins.

Primary actions: Anti-inflammatory, Antirheumatic, Diuretic.

All actions: Anti-inflammatory, Anti-inflammatory (urinary), Antioedematous, Antirheumatic, Cholagogue, Diuretic.

Indications:

- Arthritis, Gout.

- **ESCOP:** Irrigation of the urinary tract, especially in cases of inflammation and renal gravel, and as an adjuvant in the treatment of bacterial infections of the urinary tract.

- **Other uses:** Urinary tract infection, urinary lithiasis, kidney and bladder calculi, gout, oedema.

Cautions: When oedema is present and caused by impaired heart and kidney function.

Contraindications: Do not administer to patients with salicylate sensitivities.

Qualities: Cold, dry

Typical dosage: 10–25 ml per week

Bidens tripartita

Common names: Burr marigold, water agrimony, gui zhen cao, longbacao

Family: Asteraceae

Part used: Above ground parts

Description: Used in Western and Eastern traditional medicines. Once esteemed for its styptic properties, use has waned in Western herbal medicine. Good substitute for *Arctostaphylos uva-ursi* in urinary tract infections. Indications are related to its astringent properties which are said to tighten, shrink and tonify structural cells (mucous membrane tonic). Other notable actions are diaphoretic and antimicrobial (local and systemic).

Constituents: Tannins, flavonoids and related compounds including isocoreopsin and isookanin, ployacetylenes, volatile oils including eugenol.

Primary actions: Antidiabetic, Antimicrobial, Antiseptic (urinary).

All actions: Anti-inflammatory, Antibacterial,

Antidiabetic, Antidiarrhoeal, Antimicrobial, Antiseptic, Astringent, Bitter tonic, Blood tonic, Carminative, Diaphoretic, Galactagogue, Hepatoprotective, Immunomodulator, Mucous membrane tonic, Neuroprotective, Styptic/Haemostatic, Wound healing/Vulnerary.

Indications:

- Acne, Common cold, Dysentery, Gastritis, Gout, Haemorrhoids, Infection; gastrointestinal system, Infection; respiratory tract, Infection; skin, Infection; throat, Infection; urinary tract, Influenza, Leucorrhoea and vaginitis (douche), Rhinitis, Ulcer; gastrointestinal.
- **Other uses:** Topically for psoriais and bleeding.

Cautions: As with all herbs high in tannins, long-term use is not recommended.

Qualities: Neutral, clears heat

Typical dosage: 40–80 ml per week

Bistorta officinalis

Synonym or related species: Persicaria bistorta, Polygonum bistorta

Common names: Bistort, common bistort, European bistort or meadow bistort

Family: Polygonaceae

Part used: Root

Description: Bistort is strongly astringent and has traditionally been used as a styptic for both internal and external bleeding, including haemorrhages in stomach and uterus. It has also been used in the treatment of diarrhoea and dysentery.

Constituents: Tannins (oligomeric proanthocyanidins, galloyl and catechol tannins) 15–36%, silicic acid, starch.

Primary actions: Anticatarrhal, Antidiarrhoeal, Astringent.

All actions: Anti-inflammatory, Anticatarrhal, Antidiarrhoeal, Astringent, Styptic/Haemostatic.

Indications:

- Catarrh; naso-pharyngeal congestion, Colitis, Diarrhoea, Dysentery, Gingivitis, Haemorrhoids (topically), Leucorrhoea and vaginitis (douche), Pharyngitis, Sore throat (gargle), Stomatitis, Ulcer (topically), Ulcer; mouth.
- **BHP:** Diarrhoea, dysentery, nasal catarrh, cystitis, mucous colitis, pharyngitis (gargle), stomatitis (mouthwash), leucorrhoea (douche), anal fissure (ointment). Specific indications: diarrhoea in children.
- **Other uses:** Diarrhoea, childhood diarrhoea, dysentery, colitis, naso-pharyngeal catarrh, sore throat, pharyngitis (gargle), mouth ulcer, stomatitis, gingivitis, tooth ache (topically), haemorrhoids (topically), leucorrhoea and vaginitis (douche), ulcer, wounds (topically).

Contraindications: None known

Qualities: Cold, dry

Typical dosage: 20–30 ml per week

Boswellia serrata

Common names: Boswellia, olibanum, frankincense

Family: Burseraceae

Part used: Gum resin

Description: Extracts rich in resins have been found to inhibit the synthesis of pro-inflammatory mediators, including leukotrienes. Animal and in vitro studies suggest possible efficacy for inflammatory conditions such as inflammatory bowel disease, rheumatoid arthritis, and osteoarthritis.

Constituents: Boswellia serrata: oils, terpenoids, sugars, volatile oils, m- and p-camphorene and cernbrenol (serratol). B. carterii contains more aliphatic octyl acetate (responsible for the strong smell when burning), verticilla-4-7,11-triene, incesole acetate, incensole. B. carterii and B. serrata contain the active pentacyclic triterpene acids a- and fl-boswellic acid, 11-keto-β-boswellic acid, acetyl-11-keto-β-boswellic acid, acetyl-11-dien-β-boswellic acid, acetyl-a- boswellic acid and acetyl-fl-boswellic acid. Acetyl-11-keto β-boswellic acid (AKBA) is the major constituent.

Primary actions: Analgesic, Anti-inflammatory, Anticancer.

All actions: Analgesic, Anti-inflammatory, Anti-inflammatory (GIT), Anti-inflammatory (musculoskeletal), Antiasthmatic, Cytoprotective.

Indications:

- Arthritis, Asthma, Cancer; including prevention and supportive treatment, Crohn's disease, Rheumatoid arthritis, Ulcerative colitis.

Cautions: The most common adverse effects in trials have been nausea, urticaria and acid reflux. Allergic contact dermatitis has been associated with the use of a cream containing boswellia extract in one case report; caution in patients with known allergy tendency.

Contraindications: Avoid in individuals with a known allergy to boswellia, its constituents, or members in the family Burseraveae.

Qualities: Frankincense has dual energetics of being both heating and cooling. It is heating due to its stimulation of blood circulation and cooling due to its anti-inflammatory effects. It is bitter, pungent, astringent and sweet.

Typical dosage: 300–400 mg extract standardised to 20–40% boswellic acid, three times daily. Ideally standardised to 3-O-acetyl-11-keto-beta-boswellic acid (AKBA).

Bryonia dioica

Common names: Bryony

Family: Cucurbitaceae

Part used: Root

Description: Bryonia alba is a relatively little known

medicinal plant from eastern and northern Europe. It is traditionally used for bronchitis, pleurisy, rheumatic conditions, and myalgia. It was not considered an adaptogen until Alexander Panossian translated early Russian research on adaptogens and conducted further research.

Constituents: Bryonin (alkaloid), cucurbitacins, glycosides.

Primary actions: Adaptogen, Antipyretic, Expectorant (relaxing).

All actions: Adaptogen, Antipyretic, Antirheumatic, Cathartic, Diaphoretic, Emetic, Expectorant (relaxing).

Indications:

- Bronchitis, Cancer; including prevention/ supportive treatment, Chronic fatigue syndrome, Fatigue, Myalgia, Pleurisy, Stress.
- **BHP:** Bronchitis, pleurisy, rheumatic diseases (low dosage). Topically for myalgia, pleurodynia. Specific indications: rheumatic pains, lumbago.
- **Other uses:** Bronchitis, pleurisy, rheumatic. conditions, myalgia

Contraindications: During pregnancy

Qualities: Cool, moist

Typical dosage: 8–25 ml per week

Bupleurum falcatum

Common names: Sickle-leaved hare's ear

Family: Apiaceae

Part used: Root

Description: Bupleurum is one of the most frequently prescribed herbs in traditional Chinese medicine for the treatment of inflammatory diseases and autoimmune diseases. The two most important formulations are Major Bupleurum Combination (dai-saiko-to in Kampo medicine) and Minor Bupleurum Combination (Sho-saiko-to or TJ-9 in Kampo medicine). Much of the clinical research on bupleurum is as an ingredient in one of these formulations. TJ-9 is used in the treatment of chronic hepatitis, malaria, gastrointestinal disorders, fever and acute influenza. Sho-saiko-to has been shown in vivo to have antitumour and antimetastatic effects on melanomas and to reduce the incidence of hepatocellular carcinoma in a five-year study.

Constituents: Triterpenoid saponins (saikosides, saikosaponins), fatty acids, polyacetylenic compounds, polysaccharides.

Primary actions: Anti-inflammatory, Hepatoprotective, Hepatotonic.

All actions: Anti-inflammatory, Antipyretic, Antitussive, Bitter tonic, Digestive tonic, Hepatoprotective, Hepatotonic, Renal tonic, Tonic.

Indications:

- Autoimmune disease, Calculi; kidney and bladder, Cancer; including prevention/ supportive treatment, Hypoglycaemia, Infection; gastrointestinal system, Menstrual irregularity, Organ prolapse, Splenic enlargement, Ulcer; gastrointestinal.
- **WHO:** Treatment of fever, pain, and inflammation associated with influenza, and the common cold. As an analgesic for the treatment of distending pain in the chest and hypochondriac regions, and for amenorrhoea. Extracts have been used for the treatment of chronic hepatitis, nephrotic syndrome, and autoimmune diseases.
- **Other uses:** Acute infection, auto-immune disease or suppression including cancer treatment, hypoglycaemia, kidney disorders, acute or chronic liver disease, splenic enlargement, menstrual irregularity, organ prolapse, gastrointestinal ulcer.

Cautions: May (rarely) cause loose stool, nausea, flatulence, irritation of the gastric mucous membranes and reflux. Causes sedation when used in large doses, therefore caution when operating a motor vehicle or hazardous machinery. Due to high saponin content, use with caution in patients with coeliac disease, fat malabsorption, pre-existing cholestasis, deficiencies in vitamins A, D, E and K, upper digestive tract irritations, and topically on open wounds.

Contraindications: Contraindicated during pregnancy and lactation

Drug interactions: Avoid with sedatives or CNS depressants (including alcohol).

Qualities: Bitter, cold

Typical dosage: 25–60 ml per week

Calendula officinalis

Common names: Calendula, marigold

Family: Asteraceae

Part used: Flowers

Description: Calendula is mainly used in wound healing and the treatment of infections of wounds and mucous membranes. Oral administrations may be indicated in unresolved infection or erosion of the upper digestive tract, particularly where there is evidence of bleeding into the gut during gastritis and duodenal ulcers. Pharmacological studies have also demonstrated hepatoprotective, hypoglycaemic, cardioprotective, and neuroprotective activities in vivo.

Constituents: Triterpenoid saponins (oleanolic acid and flavonols), carotenoids, bitter principles including calendin, essential oil, sterols, flavonoids, mucilage, resin. Carotenoid content determines flower colour: carotene in orange flowers, xanthophyll in yellow.

Primary actions: Anti-inflammatory, Antimicrobial, Wound healing/Vulnerary.

All actions: Anti-inflammatory, Anti-inflammatory (GIT), Antifungal (topically), Antihyperlipidemic, Antiseptic, Antiseptic (GIT), Antiseptic (topically), Astringent, Choleretic, Emmenagogue, Lymphatic, Styptic/Haemostatic, Wound healing/Vulnerary.

Indications:

- Acne, Acne (topically), Arrhythmia, Benign breast disease, Boils, Boils (poultice), Burns (topically), Candidiasis, Cholecystitis, Dysmenorrhoea; spasmodic, Eczema, Eczema (topically), Gastritis, Glands; swollen, Haemorrhoids (topically), Herpes simplex, Hypertension, Infection; gastrointestinal system, Infection; skin, Inflammation; gastrointestinal tract, Menopausal symptoms, Menstrual irregularity, Mumps, Pruritus, Pruritus ani (topically), Psoriasis, Radiation; side effects of, Sore throat (gargle), Ulcer; gastrointestinal, Ulcer; mouth, Varicose veins (topically), Wounds (topically).

- **BHP:** Gastric and duodenal ulcers, amenorrhoea, dysmenorrhoea, and epistaxis. Topically for leg ulcers, varicose veins, haemorrhoids, eczema, proctitis. Specific indications; enlarged or inflamed lymphatic nodes, sebaceous cysts, duodenal ulcers, acute and chronic inflammatory skin conditions.

- **Commission E:** Internal and topical use for inflammation of oral and pharyngeal mucosa, externally for poorly healing wounds skin and mucous membrane inflammations such as pharyngitis, dermatitis, leg ulcers, bruises, boils and rashes.

- **ESCOP:** Symptomatic treatment of minor inflammations of the skin and mucosa, as an aid to the healing of minor wounds.

- **WHO:** External treatment of superficial cuts, minor inflammations of the skin and oral mucosa, wounds and ulcus cruris.

Cautions: Consider infusion rather than alcohol-based tincture for abraded tissues. Do not administer during pregnancy or lactation without professional supervision.

Contraindications: Known sensitivity to members of the Compositae (Asteraceae) family

Qualities: Cooling potential, dry

Typical dosage: 10–30 ml per week

Camellia sinensis

Synonym or related species: Thea sinensis

Common names: Green tea (green, black or oolong according to processing)

Family: Theaceae

Part used: Young leaves

Description: Green and oolong teas have been popular beverages in Asia for thousands of years; black tea is preferred in many other countries. Black, green, and oolong tea are all prepared from the one plant by steaming, rolling, drying and/or fermenting (green tea leaves are steamed and unfermented, oolong semi-fermented, black fermented and dried). Fermentation changes infusion colour (yellowish green to reddish brown) as well as chemical composition (oxidation of polyphenols,

caffeine content). Variation in caffeine content further influenced by varied growing as well as processing methods.

Constituents: Phenolics (phenolic acids, gallotannins, flavonol glycosides, flavan-type phenolics), triterpene saponins, amino acids including L-theanine, caffeine (alkaloid), and carotenoids. The gallotannins of interests (catechins) are Epicatechin (EC), epicatechin (EGC), epicatechin-3-galate (ECg), and Epigallocatechin-3-gallate (ECGg). EGCG is the most abundant and researched catechin in tea. Black tea is dominated by theaflavins.

Primary actions: Astringent, Chemoprotective, Diuretic.

All actions: Antiandrogenic, Antibacterial, Anticancer, Antihyperlipidemic, Antihyperuricaemic, Antimicrobial, Antioxidant, Antiviral (systemically), Astringent, Chemoprotective, Cytoprotective, Digestive tonic, Diuretic.

Indications:

- Atherosclerosis, Cancer; including prevention/supportive treatment, Cardiovascular disease prevention.

- **Other uses:** Atherosclerosis, prevention of cancer, hypercholesterolaemia.

Cautions: Tannins can bind to iron, thus reducing absorption. Separate intake by at least two hours. Caffeine content may cause CNS stimulation and diuresis if consumed in large amounts.

Contraindications: None known

Drug interactions: Experimental studies suggest that green tea polyphenols or green tea extract may increase or decrease the bioavailability of cancer drugs 5-FU, irinotecan and sunitinib. Avoid concomitant administration.

May increase blood levels of tacrolimus (case report of increased levels in a patient with reduced ability to metabolise drugs via CYP3A4) (Vischini, Niscola et al. 2011). May increase bioavailability of statins (case report). May reduce bioavailability of sunitinib (case report). May interact with warfarin, decreasing INR (case report).

Co-administration of EGCG reduces the systemic exposure of rosuvastatin by 19%, and pretreatment of EGCG can eliminate that effect of co-administration of EGCG (Kim et al., 2017).

References:

Kim TE, Ha N, Kim Y, Kim H, Lee JW, Jeon JY, et al. (2017) Effect of epigallocatechin-3-gallate, major ingredient of green tea, on the pharmacokinetics of rosuvastatin in healthy volunteers. Drug Des Devel Ther 11:1409-1416

Vischini G. Et al. Increased plasma levels of tacrolimus after ingestion of green tea. Am J Kidney Dis. 2011 Aug;58(2):329.

Typical dosage: 20–40 ml per week

Capsella bursa-pastoris

Common names: Shepherd's purse

Family: Brassicaceae

Part used: Whole herb

Description: Traditional medicine from Europe to the Middle East and Asia. Also eaten as a food. Main use is menorrhagia once the cause has been established. It has drying and cooling properties and can be used for infection with *Trillium erectum* and *Hydrastis canadensis*. Also used for erratic cycles and dysfunctional bleeding at menarche.

Constituents: Flavonoids (rutin, diosmin, hesperidin), amino acids (proline), monoterpenoids (camphor), glucosinolates, amines (acetylcholine, choline, tyramine) and saponins.

Primary actions: Antihaemorrhagic (uterine), Antipyretic, Oxytocic.

All actions: Anti-inflammatory, Antihaemorrhagic (uterine), Antipyretic, Diuretic, Oxytocic.

Indications:

- Catarrhal deafness, Cystitis, Dysmenorrhoea, Menopause, Menorrhagia, Metrorrhagia, Nose bleeds, Uterine bleeding; dysfunctional.
- **BHP:** Menorrhagia, haematuria, diarrhoea, and acute catarrhal cystitis. Specific indication: uterine haemorrhage.
- **Commission E:** Symptomatic use for mild menorrhagia and metrorrhagia, topical application for nosebleeds, superficial skin wounds and bruising.

Qualities: Cold, dry

Typical dosage: 20–40 ml per week

Capsicum spp.

Synonym or related species: C. minimum, C. frutescens, C. annum

Common names: Chilli, capsicum, pepper, paprika, cayenne

Family: Solanaceae

Part used: Fruit and seeds

Description: Topical capsaicin is an established treatment option for various painful conditions. Capsaicin has been documented to increase thermogenesis through stimulation of catecholamine secretion and subsequent sympathetic nervous system (SNS) activation. However, the effects are variable in magnitude and duration. Clinical trials have examined capsicum various conditions including topical cream for chronic soft tissue pain, nasal spray for sinusitis, and orally for IBS, appetite regulation, increasing thermogenesis, blood sugar and lipids regulation, and resting energy expenditure.

Constituents: Alkaloids (capsaicin, dihydrocapsaicin etc), flavonoids, carotenoids, volatile oil, vitamins A and C, minerals. Seeds contain steroidal saponins (capsicidins).

Primary actions: Analgesic, Carminative, Counter irritant.

All actions: Analgesic, Antipyretic, Antiseptic, Carminative, Counter-irritant, Decongestant, Diaphoretic.

Indications:

- Arthritis, Circulation; peripheral; impaired, Diabetic foot pain, Digestive complaints, Digestive weakness, Hypochlorhydria, Intermittent claudication, Myalgia, Neuralgia, Neuralgia (topically), Weight loss; to assist.
- **BHP:** Flatulent dyspepsia in absence of inflammation, colic, insufficiency of peripheral circulation, chronic laryngitis (gargle). Externally for neuralgia, rhematic pains, unbroken chilblains. Specific indications: atony of the digestive organs, topically for lumbago, unbroken chilblains.
- **Commission E:** Painful muscle spasms, arthritis, rheumatism, neuralgia, lumbago, chilblains.

Cautions: Occasional hypersensitivity. May cause painful irritation of mucous membranes even in very low concentrations – avoid contact, especially eyes. Do not apply to injured skin.

Contraindications: None known

Qualities: Dry 3rd degree, warm 3rd degree

Typical dosage: 1–3 ml per week

Carica papaya

Common names: Paw paw, papaya

Family: Caricaceae

Part used: Leaf; Fruit, seed, and latex also used

Description: The fruits, leaves, barks, roots, flowers, seeds and latex have been traditionally used for a variety of conditions. Paw paw leaves have been used to treat malaria and Dengue fever, asthma, beriberi, fever, abortion, infectious wounds, jaundice, gonorrhoea, urinary complaints and worms. Papain is used for inflammation and as a meat tenderiser. Although in vitro and in vivo studies have shown that papaya extracts and papaya-associated phytochemicals possess anticancer, anti-inflammatory and immunomodulatory properties, clinical studies are lacking.

Constituents: The leaf contains tannins, saponins, flavonoids, cardiac glycosides, triterpenoids and alkaloids including carpaine, pseudocarpaine and dehydrocarpaine.

The paw paw/papaya proteolytic enzymes known as papain are present in the paw paw leaves, fruit and latex.

Primary actions: Digestive tonic, Immunomodulator, Wound healing/Vulnerary.

All actions: Anti-inflammatory, Anticancer, Antihypertensive, Digestive tonic, Gastroprotective, Hepatoprotective, Wound healing/Vulnerary.

Indications:

- Acne, Asthma, Cancer; including prevention/ supportive treatment, Diabetes, Eczema, Fever, Gingivitis, Hypertension, Indigestion, Infection; gastrointestinal system, Infection; skin, Malaria, Ulcer; gastrointestinal.

Cautions: May have antifertility and abortive actions.

Typical dosage: 15–30 ml per week

Cassia senna

Common names: Senna pod

Family: Fabaceae

Part used: Dried leaves and pods (fruit)

Description: Senna is a laxative, mainly used for short-term relief of constipation. Gum chewing enhances colonoscopy bowel preparation quality. It is a physiologically sound, safe, and inexpensive part of the colonoscopy bowel preparation. Gum chewing could be advised in addition to high-dose senna containing bowel preparation.

Constituents: Dianthorone glycosides, anthraquinone glycosides, flavonoids, mucin, sugars

Primary actions: Laxative.

All actions: Antirheumatic, Antispasmodic (uterus), Emmenagogue, Partus praeparator, Uterine tonic.

Indications:

- Constipation.
- **BHP:** Constipation, conditions in which easy defecation is desirable (anal fissure, haemorrhoids).
- **Commission E:** Constipation.
- **ESCOP:** For short-term use in cases of occasional constipation.
- **WHO:** Short-term use for occasional constipation.

Cautions: Should not be used for more than 1–2 weeks. Excessive or chronic use or abuse may cause electrolyte imbalance including potassium deficiency, albuminuria and hematuria. Adverse effects include diarrhoea, fluid loss, colic, and possible hepatic reactions.

Contraindications: Not recommended during lactation or for children under 10 years. Nausea and vomiting, intestinal obstruction and stenosis, atony, irritation of the bowel, inflammatory colon diseases, appendicitis, abdominal pain of unknown origin, severe dehydration states with water and electrolyte depletion, or chronic constipation.

Drug interactions: Do not administer concurrently with digoxin. Potassium deficiency may potentiate cardiac glycosides and affect anti-arrhythmic medications, and can be exacerbated by simultaneous ingestion with thiazide diuretics, cardiac glycosides (e.g. digoxin), corticosteroids or licorice root.

Qualities: Dry 1st degree, hot 2nd degree

Typical dosage: 10–40 ml per week

Caulophyllum thalictroides

Common names: Blue cohosh

Family: Berberidaceae

Part used: Root

Description: Traditionally used by Native Americans for the preparation of the uterus for labour (partus praeparator), for period pain and inflammation.

Primary actions: Anti-inflammatory, Uterine tonic.

All actions: Anti-inflammatory, Bitter tonic, Uterine tonic.

Indications:

- Amenorrhoea, Childbirth recovery, Dysmenorrhoea, Endometriosis, Menstrual irregularity, Rheumatism.
- **BHP:** Amenorrhoea, threatened miscarriage, false labour pains, dysmenorrhoea, and rheumatic pains. Specific indication: conditions associated with uterine atony.

Cautions: There are three case reports that blue cohosh taken at the time of delivery caused: 1) perinatal stroke, 2) acute myocardial infarction, congestive heart failure and shock and 3) severe multi-organ hypoxic injury. There is one case report that blue cohosh possesses abortifacient properties. There is in vitro evidence that blue cohosh may have teratogenic, embryotoxic and oxytoxic effects. The use of blue cohosh can therefore not be recommended during pregnancy or during breast feeding.

Contraindications: Do not administer during pregnancy or lactation, and to women trying to conceive (contains teratogenic alkaloids).

Drug interactions: In vitro study indicates that blue cohosh may pose a risk of drug–drug interactions if taken with other drugs metabolised by CYP450 enzymes CYP 2C19, 3A4, 2D6, and 1A2.

Qualities: Hot

Typical dosage: 10–20 ml per week

Centaurium erythraea

Synonym or related species: Erythraea centaurium, Centaurium umbellatum

Common names: Centaury

Family: Gentianaceae

Part used: Flowering dried aerial parts

Description: Traditionally used for loss of appetite and indigestion with mild cramps in the gastrointestinal tract (dyspepsia). Pharmacological and preclinical investigations suggest possible use in hypertension, diabetes, NAFLD and gastric ulcers.

Constituents: Bitter secoiridoid glycosides (swertiamarin, gentiopicrin), centauroside, flavonoids, xanthone derivatives, phenolics, triterpenes, sterols.

Primary actions: Anti-inflammatory, Antidiabetic, Antipyretic.

All actions: Adaptogen, Analgesic, Antidiabetic, Antifibrotic, Antihypertensive, Antipyretic, Connective tissue regenerator, Diuretic, Fibrinolytic, Gastroprotective, Hepatoprotective, Nervine tonic, Vasodilator, Venotonic, Wound healing/Vulnerary.

Indications:

- Anorexia, Diabetes, Digestive complaints, Dyspepsia, Fever, Hypertension, Non-alcoholic fatty liver disease (NAFLD), Ulcer; gastrointestinal.
- **BHP:** Anorexia, dyspepsia. Specific indication: anorexia, especially in children with gastric or hepatic weakness.
- **ESCOP:** Dyspeptic complaints, lack of appetite.
- **Other uses:** Nausea in pregnancy.

Contraindications: Not normally indicated in patients with stomach or duodenal ulcers, although this may need to be revised.

Qualities: Cold, pungent

Typical dosage: 20–40 ml per week

Centella asiatica

Synonym or related species: Centella coriacea, Hydrocotyle asiatica, Hydrocotyle lunata

Common names: Gotu kola, brahmi, Indian pennywort

Family: Apiaceae

Part used: Dried whole plant

Description: Traditionally used for wound healing, and for the treatment of leprosy, lupus, varicose ulcers, eczema, psoriasis, diarrhoea, fever, amenorrhea, diseases of the female genitourinary tract and also for relieving anxiety and improving cognition.

Constituents: Triterpenes (asiatic acid, madecassic acid), triterpenoid ester glycosides (asiaticoside, brahminoside), volatile oil.

Primary actions: Antinociceptive, Connective tissue regenerator, Venotonic.

All actions: Adaptogen, Antifibrotic, Antinociceptive, Connective tissue regenerator, Depurative/Alterative, Nervine tonic, Venotonic, Wound healing/Vulnerary.

Indications:

- Arthritis, Capillary fragility, Cellulitis, Chronic fatigue syndrome, Connective tissue disorders, Convalescence, Endometriosis, Memory and concentration; poor, Night cramps, Radiation; side effects of, Scleroderma, Surgery; recovery, Varicose veins, Varicose veins (topically), Venous insufficiency.
- **BHP:** Rheumatic condition, cutaneous affections. Topically for indolent wounds, leprous ulcers, cicatrisation after surgery.
- **WHO:** Treatment of wounds, burns, and ulcerous skin ailments, and prevention of keloid and hypertrophic scars. Extracts have been employed to treat second- and third-degree burns and

stress-induced stomach and duodenal ulcers, and topically to accelerate healing in cases of chronic post-surgical and post-trauma wounds.

- **Other uses:** Damaged skin and other soft tissues after surgery.

Contraindications: Allergy to gotu kola or plants of the Apiaceae family

Qualities: Bitter, cold

Typical dosage: 20–40 ml per week

Chamaelirium luteum

Synonym or related species: Helonias dioica, H. luteum

Common names: False unicorn root, helonias

Family: Liliaceae

Part used: Rhizome and root

Description: At risk due to unsustainable wild crafting; use should be restricted until cultivation occurs. Shatavari (Asparagus racemosus) may prove to be a suitable substitute.

Constituents: Steroidal saponins (diosgenin, chamaelirin, helonin), starch, calcium oxalate, oleoresin

Primary actions: Hypothalamic-pituitary-ovarian (HPO) regulator, Menstrual cycle regulator, Uterine tonic.

All actions: Anthelmintic, Digestive tonic, Diuretic, Hypothalamic-pituitary-ovarian (HPO) regulator, Menstrual cycle regulator, Selective oestrogen receptor modulator (SERM), Uterine tonic.

Indications:

- Adenomyosis, Amenorrhoea, Cystic hyperplasia, Digestive complaints, Digestive weakness, Dysmenorrhoea, Endometriosis, Fibroids, Infertility, Inflammation; pelvic, Leucorrhoea, Menopausal symptoms, Menstrual irregularity, Miscarriage; repeated, Miscarriage; threatened, Morning sickness, Ovulation; eratic, Ovulation; painful, Polycystic ovarian syndrome, Pregnancy; to prepare uterus for labour, Premenstrual syndrome, Prolapse; uterine, Uterine bleeding; dysfunctional, Weight loss; to assist.
- **BHP:** Amenorrhoea, ovarian dysmenorrhoea, leucorrhoea, reported to be useful in vomiting of pregnancy and threatened miscarriage. Specific indication: amenorrhoea.

Contraindications: None known

Qualities: Sweet, warm

Typical dosage: 15–40 ml per week

Chelidonium majus

Common names: Greater celandine

Family: Papaveraceae

Part used: Flowering dried aerial parts

Description: Dioscorides recommended chelidonium

as a cholagogue for liver disease, jaundice and pain. Polish common name of 'glistnik' translates as roundworm herb. Generally used for mild to moderate spasms of the upper gastrointestinal tract, minor gallbladder disorders, dyspeptic complaints such as bloating and flatulence.

Constituents: Alkaloids – protopine, berberine, coptisine, chelidonine, sanguinarine and chelerythrine complexed by chelidonic acid

Primary actions: Anthelmintic, Bitter tonic, Cholagogue.

All actions: Anthelmintic, Antiemetic, Bitter tonic, Cholagogue, Hepatotonic, Laxative.

Indications:

• Cholecystitis, Gall stones (cholelithiasis), Warts (topically).

• **BHP:** Cholecystitis

• **ESCOP:** Symptomatic treatment of mild to moderate spasms of the upper gastrointestinal tract, minor gallbladder disorders, dyspeptic complaints such as bloating and flatulence.

Cautions: Excessive intake may cause nausea or gastrointestinal symptoms. May cause liver damage in susceptible individuals if used in high dose. Use with caution in patients with acute or chronic hepatocellular disease, septic cholecystitis, intestinal spasm, ileus or liver cancer, or unconjugated hyperbilirubinaemia. Recommended for short-term use only; discontinue if liver damage arises.

The Australian regulator, the TGA, has made an Interim Decision in relation to *Sanguinaria canadensis* (bloodroot) due to safety issues concerning the use of 'black salve'. A delegate of the TGA previously made an application to the Advisory Committee of Medicine Scheduling to make *Sanguinaria canadensis* a Schedule 10 substance when containing 0.01% or more of sanguinarine. S10 are substances of such danger to health as to warrant prohibition of sale, supply and use. This decision is not expected to affect medicines currently listed on the ARTG, including other herbs with sanguinarine as a component such as Greater Celandine (*Chelidonium majus*), or homoeopathic listings of *S. canadensis*, but will make ineligible any and all supply, in Australia, of black salve or similar topical preparations or any preparations of blood root with more than 0.01% sanguinarine.

Source: Interim decision-sanguinarine: https://www.tga.gov.au/book-page/13-interim-decision-relation-sanguinarine

Contraindications: Contraindicated during pregnancy and lactation, and in the case of biliary obstructions, existing or previous liver disease

Qualities: Dry 3rd degree, hot 3rd degree

Typical dosage: 5–15 ml per week

Chionanthus virginicus

Common names: Fringe tree, old man's beard

Family: Oleaceae

Part used: Dried root bark

Description: The bark was described by Cook (The Physiomedical Dispensatory 1869) as a rather bitter tonic, with an excess of relaxing properties, but stimulating qualities pretty well marked. It promotes all the secretions slowly, but especially those of the liver, gall-ducts, and kidneys. Fringe tree is a cholagogue with stimulating action on the liver, gallbladder and spleen.

Constituents: Saponins, lignan glycoside (phyllyrin), secoiridoid glucoside (ligustrolide).

Primary actions: Bitter tonic, Cholagogue, Hepatotonic.

All actions: Antiemetic, Bitter tonic, Cholagogue, Hepatotonic.

Indications:

• Cholecystitis, Gall stones (cholelithiasis), Jaundice, Liver insufficiency, Splenic enlargement.

• **BHP:** Hepatic disease, cholecystitis, duodenitis, glycosuria of hepatic or alimentary origin, splenic enlargement and portal hypertension. Specific indication: hepatic disease with icterus and glycosuria.

• **Other uses:** Portal hypertension.

Contraindications: None known

Qualities: Cold, neutral

Typical dosage: 20–40 ml per week

Cinnamomum verum

Synonym or related species: *Cinnamomum zeylanicum, C. cassia, C. aromaticum*

Common names: Cinnamon, cassia bark, rou gui

Family: Lauraceae

Part used: Inner bark, essential oil

Description: In traditional medicine cinnamon is considered a remedy for respiratory, digestive and gynaecological ailments. In vitro and in vivo studies have found antimicrobial, antiparasitc, hypoglycaemia, antihypertensive, antidyslipidaemic, antiulcerogenic, anti-inflammatory, hepatoprotective and wound healing properties.

Constituents: Volatile oil (cinnamaldehyde, eugenol, trans-cinnamic acid), phenolic compounds, condensed tannins, catechins, proanthocyanidins, monoterpenes, sesquiterpenes (pinene), calcium-monotoerpenes oxalate, gum, mucilage, resin, starch, sugars, coumarin.

Primary actions: Antidiabetic, Antihyperlipidemic, Carminative.

All actions: Anti-inflammatory, Antidiabetic, Antidiarrhoeal, Antiemetic, Antihyperlipidemic, Antimicrobial, Carminative, Hepatoprotective.

Indications:

- Colic, Common cold, Diabetes, Diabetes; gestational, Diarrhoea, Dyspepsia, Dyspepsia; flatulent, Flatulence, Inflammatory bowel disease, Influenza, Morning sickness, Nausea.
- **BHP:** Flatulent dyspepsia, anorexia, intestinal colic, infantile diarrhoea, common cold, influenza. Specific indications: flatulent colic, dyspepsia with nausea.
- **Commission E:** Anorexia, dyspeptic complaints such as mild spasticity of gastrointestinal system, bloating, flatulence.
- **ESCOP:** Dyspeptic complaints such as gastrointestinal spasms, bloating and flatulence, loss of appetite, diarrhoea.
- **WHO:** Treatment of dyspeptic conditions such as mild spastic conditions of the gastrointestinal tract, fullness and flatulence, loss of appetite, abdominal pain with diarrhoea, and pain associated with amenorrhoea and dysmenorrhoea.

Contraindications: Patients with known allergy to cinnamon, cinnamon bark oil, cinnamaldehyde or Peru balsam. Should not be used during pregnancy, or in cases of fever of unknown origin, stomach or duodenal ulcers.

Drug interactions: Co-administration of cinnamon/ ginger with dabigatran should be avoided (case report). The American Heart Association/American College of Cardiology/Heart Rhythm Society recommend that direct-acting oral anticoagulants (DOACs) rather than warfarin in patients with non-valvular atrial fibrillation. A case where self-administration of ginger and cinnamon together with dabigatran in an 80-year-old man caused fatal bleeding. The history of recent combination of herbal products (ginger and cinnamon) with DOACs (dabigatran) and the presence of diffuse haemorrhage of the mucosal membrane of the upper gastrointestinal tract raised the possibility of a herb–drug interaction leading to severe gastrointestinal bleeding (Maardarani et al., 2019).

Reference:

Maadarani O, Bitar Z, Mohsen M (2019) Adding Herbal Products to Direct-Acting Oral Anticoagulants Can Be Fatal. Eur J Case Rep Intern Med 6:001190

Qualities: Dry 2nd degree, warm 2nd degree

Typical dosage: 20–40 ml per week

Citrus reticulata

Common names: Chen pi, mandarin, tangerine

Family: Rutaceae

Part used: Peel

Description: In TCM, chen pi is used for Spleen and Stomach Qi stagnation with symptoms such as nausea and vomiting due to rebellious Stomach Qi, fullness, distention, or bloating in the abdominal or epigastric region, stomach ache, belching, and

poor appetite. Citrus essential oils are used as natural preservatives due to their broad spectrum of biological activities including antimicrobial and antioxidant effects.

Constituents: Dihydroflavonone glycosides narirutin, hespiridin and didymin. Polymethoxylated flavones nobiletin, hepatamethoxoyflavone and tangeretin.

Primary actions: Anticatarrhal, Antiseptic (GIT), Digestive tonic.

All actions: Antibacterial, Anticatarrhal, Antifungal, Antimicrobial, Antiseptic (GIT).

Indications:

- Anorexia, Cough, Digestive complaints, Digestive weakness, Gastrointestinal catarrh, Morning sickness, Nausea.

Contraindications: None known

Qualities: Warm

Typical dosage: 25–50 ml per week

Cnicus benedictus

Synonym or related species: Centaurea benedicta

Common names: Blessed or holy thistle

Family: Asteraceae

Part used: Aerial parts

Description: Aromatic bitter for stimulation of appetite and increasing gastric juice secretion. A polyphenolic- and ursolic-rich extract shown to have anti-inflammatory and antidiabetic activities.

Constituents: Sesquiterpene lactone glycosides, phenolic acids, principally the chlorogenic acid and sinapic acid, ursolic acid, genistin, and isorhamnetin, alkaloids, cnicin, benedictin, mucilage, polyacetylene, triterpenoide, lignans, flavonoids, tannin, phytosterines, and volatile oils.

Primary actions: Anti-inflammatory, Antiseptic, Bitter tonic.

All actions: Anti-inflammatory, Antidepressant, Antifungal, Antimicrobial, Antiseptic, Bitter tonic, Digestive tonic, Stomachic, Wound healing/Vulnerary.

Indications:

- Anorexia, Diabetes, Dyspepsia; flatulent, Inflammation.
- **BHP:** Loss of appetite, anorexia, flatulent dyspepsia.
- **Commission E:** Loss of appetite, dyspepsia.

Contraindications: None known

Qualities: Dry 2nd degree, hot 2nd degree

Typical dosage: 20–40 ml per week

Codonopsis pilosula

Common names: Dang shen, codonopsis

Family: Campanulaceae

Part used: Root

Description: Used in TCM to replenish qi (vital

energy) deficiency, strengthen the immune system, improve poor gastrointestinal function, gastric ulcer and appetite, and decrease blood pressure. Dang shen is considered a blood tonic, general and immune system tonic. It is also used as a replacement for *Panax ginseng* in traditional formulations due to the high cost of panax.

Constituents: Polyacetylenes, phenylpropanoids, alkaloids, triterpenoids and polysaccharides, essential oil, mucilage, resin, saponins.

Primary actions: Adaptogen, Anti-inflammatory, Immunomodulator.

All actions: Adaptogen, Anti-inflammatory, Antiageing, Anticancer, Antidiabetic, Antidiarrhoeal, Blood sugar regulator, Blood tonic, Gastroprotective, Immunomodulator, Neuroprotective.

Indications:

* Anaemia, Anorexia, Bronchitis, Cancer; including prevention/supportive treatment, Chemotherapy; to minimise the side effects of, Chronic fatigue syndrome, Convalescence, Diabetes, Diabetes; gestational, Digestive complaints, Digestive weakness, Exhaustion, Hepatitis, Hypoglycaemia, Indigestion, Stress.

Contraindications: None known

Qualities: Neutral, sweet

Typical dosage: 30–60 ml per week

Cola spp.

Synonym or related species: C. nitida, C. acuminata (alternative C. vera), C. anomala, C. verticillata

Common names: Kola nut, cola nut

Family: Sterculiaceae

Part used: Seeds (nuts)

Description: The seeds contain caffeine and are chewed as a stimulant; used in the manufacture of soft drinks.

Constituents: Caffeine, alkaloids (xanthines), tannins (catechins), phenolics

Primary actions: Antidepressant, Circulatory stimulant, Stimulant.

All actions: Antidepressant, Circulatory stimulant, Diuretic, Stimulant.

Indications:

* Depression, Exhaustion, Migraine.

* **BHP:** Depressive states, melancholia, atony, exhaustion, dysentery, atonic diarrhoea, anorexia, migraine. Specific indication: depressive states associated with general muscular weakness.

* **Commission E:** Mental and physical fatigue, supportive treatment for depressive states.

Cautions: Contains caffeine. Do not use in excess or for prolonged periods.

Contraindications: Gastric and duodenal ulcers

Qualities: Warm

Typical dosage: 12–25 ml per week

Collinsonia canadensis

Common names: Stone root
Family: Lamiaceae
Part used: Root

Description: The botanical name, *Collinsonia canadensis*, was given to this plant in honour of the English merchant, botanist and Quaker Peter Collinson (1693-1768) whom, it is told, had an affinity for transporting and cultivating North American plants. The most commonly used name, stone root, was given to the plant by the Quakers who were also the first to use the plant commercially. At this time in Europe, the plant was not actually used medicinally, but had been used by Native Americans and early American settlers for a variety of conditions. Most often the leaves of the plant were crushed, and then applied topically to cuts, bruises, ulcers, and ringworm. Stone root was included in the material medica after observing Native American using it as a medicinal plant. By 1854 it was listed in the first edition of King's American Dispensatory.

Stone root seems to have become a forgotten medicinal plant. Searching MedLine for '*Collinsonia canadensis*' brings up one result about a new flavonoid isolated from the leaf and stem. 'Stone root' does not produce any studies at all. However, stone root was a key herb for both the Eclectics and the Physiomedicalist, and it seems worthwhile to further explore the uses of this medicinal plant in spite of the lack of scientific evidence for its actions.

Constituents: Early (1885) investigations of stone root found it to contain resin, starch, tannin, wax in all parts of the plant, mucilage in the root, and volatile oil in the leaves. The therapeutic constituent or constituents of stone root have never been determined. The old Eclectic concentration (or resinoid) quickly became obsolete in the practice of modern Eclectics who favoured a 1:1 liquid extract.

Stone root is reported to contain about 0.05% essential oil consisting mainly of the sesquiterpenes germacrene-D and caryophyllene, the monoterpenes limonene and alpha- and beta-pinenes and the phenylpropanoi, elemicin (one of the notable constituents in nutmeg). Caryophyllene is a constituent of many essential oils, in particular, clove and black pepper. Several biological activities are attributed to beta-caryophyllene, such as anti-inflammatory, antibiotic, antioxidant, anticarcinogenic and local anaesthetic activities. Germacrenes and pinenes are typically produced in a number plant species for their antimicrobial and insecticidal properties. Monoterpenes including limonene have anticarcionogenic activities by inducing phase II hepatic metabolising enzymes. Limonen increases the levels of liver enzymes Glutathione S-transferase (GST) involved in detoxifying carcinogens. Limonene has been shown to reduce hepatocarcinogenesis by inhibiting cell proliferation and enhancing apoptosis. Stone root also contains caffeic acid derivative

43

including rosmaric acid. It is proposed that the reported activities of stone root are due to the essential oil and rosmaric acid. It is difficult to attribute the reported actions of stone root to these constituents as they are found in quite low concentrations in root. The leaf contains flavones including 2,5-dihydroxy-6,7-dimethoxyflavanone, baicalein-6,7-dimethyl ether, norwogenin-7,8-dimethyl ether, and tectochrysin (5-hydroxy-7-methoxyflavone).

Primary actions: Astringent, Depurative/Alterative, Venotonic.

All actions: Astringent, Depurative/Alterative, Diaphoretic, Diuretic, Stomachic, Venotonic.

Indications:

- Constipation, Dysentery, Gastritis, Haemorrhoids (topically), Incontinence, Laryngitis.

Contraindications: No scientific information. Considered safe to use during pregnancy by the early herbalists.

Typical dosage: 20–80 ml per week

Commiphora myrrha

Synonym or related species: Commiphora molmol
Common names: Myrrh
Family: Burseraceae
Part used: Resin

Description: Myrrh has been used throughout history in incense and as a perfume. Since biblical times it has been used for the treatment of wounds. The first attempts to identify content compounds were almost 100 years ago. Myrrh is perhaps best known for its historical role in many religious traditions as an ingredient in anointing oils, incense and an embalming ointment. It was also used as a highly valued perfume. Myrrh has a long history of use as an antiseptic and astringent, and used to treat problems of the mouth, gum and throat and as a digestive tonic. Myrrh was a common ingredient in tooth powders and for parasites.

Constituents: Gum myrrh contains D-galactose, L-arabinose, and 4-methyl D-glucuronic acid. Extraction with 90% aqueous alcohol largely removes the resins and the crude polysaccharides are obtained. After hydrolysis at least 15 aminoacids were detected and in fractions D-galactose, L-arabinose, and 4-methyl D-glucuronic acid (in proportions 4:1:3) were identified. Hydrolysis of purified polysaccharides of gum myrrh gave high yields of a mixture of neutral sugars and acidic oligosaccharides. The sesquiterpen commiferin has also been isolated. Myrrh essenatial oil contains mainly curzerene, fuarnoeudesma-1,3-diene and beta-elemene.

Primary actions: Anti-inflammatory, Antiseptic, Astringent.

All actions: Analgesic, Anti-inflammatory, Antiparasitic, Antiseptic, Astringent, Cytoprotective, Hepatoprotective, Nrf2-pathway activator.

Indications:

- Acne, Acne (topically), Gingivitis, Haemorrhoids (topically), Irritable bowel syndrome, Migraine, Ovarian hyperstimulation syndrome, Parasites, Periodontitis, Pharyngitis, Rosacea, papulepostular, Schistosomiasis, Tonsillitis, Trichomoniasis vaginalis, Ulcer; gastrointestinal, Ulcer; mouth, Wounds (topically).

- **BHP:** Gargle to treat pharyngitis and tonsillitis. Mouthwash for gingivitis and ulcers. External application for sinusitis and minor skin inflammations.

- **Commission E:** Topical treatment of mild inflammation of the oral and pharyngeal mucosa.

- **ESCOP:** Topical treatment of gingivitis, stomatitis (aphthous ulcers), minor skin inflammations, minor wounds and abrasions, supportive treatment for pharyngitis, tonsillitis.

- **WHO:** Topical treatment of mild inflammations of the oral and pharyngeal mucosa. As a gargle or mouth rinse for the treatment of aphthous ulcers, pharyngitis, tonsillitis, common cold and gingivitis.

- **Other uses:** As an emmenagogue, expectorant and antidote for poisons, and to inhibit blood coagulation. Treatment of menopausal symptoms, arthritic pain, diarrhoea, fatigue, headache, jaundice and indigestion, and applied topically for treatment of burns and haemorrhoids.

Cautions: The irritant potentials of essential oil and seven sesquiterpenoids compounds newly isolated from the oleo-gum-resin of *Commiphora myrrha* were investigated by open mouse ear assay. The essential oil, curzerenone, furanodiene-6-one and furanoeudesma-1,3-diene showed potent and persistent irritant effects while others possess least irritant potentials.

Contraindications: A case of a 32-year-old pregnant woman with a history of infertility and recurrent miscarriages. She used large amounts of myrrh for two months, since a traditional healer told her that her current pregnancy would progress safely by its use. However, her pregnancy was complicated with an acute abdominal pain. Her symptom was relieved as soon as she stopped taking myrrh. It was assumed that myrrh acted as a uterine stimulant causing acute abdominal pain. Scientific studies should be carried out to evaluate the safety of myrrh intake during pregnancy.

Drug interactions: Antagonism of the anticoagulant effect of warfarin caused by the use of Commiphora molmol as a herbal medication.

Typical dosage: 10–30 ml per week

Convallaria majalis

Common names: Lily of the valley
Family: Liliaceae
Description: 'It without doubt strengthens the brain and renovates a weak memory. The distilled water dropped into the eyes helps inflammations thereof. The spirit of the flowers, distilled in wine, restoreth

lost speech, helps the palsy, and is exceedingly good in the apoplexy, comforteth the heart and vital spirits.'
– *Culpepper, Complete Herbal, 1653.*

Priest & Priest described Lily of the valley as a cardiac tonic and ganglionic trophorestorative: increases coronary circulation and myocardial action. Suitable for all cardiac disturbances. They recommended combining with *Leonurus cardiaca* in congestive heart failure and echinacea/phytolacca in endocarditis.

Convallaria may increase cardiac output without increasing the demand for oxygen for the heart muscle. The positive ionotropic effect strengthens the heart's contractions and reduces its workload.

Convallaria is indigenous to the cool temperate regions of the northern regions of Europe.

Part used: Leaves

Constituents: Cardiac glycosides (0.1–0.5%). The main glycosides are convallatoxin (4–40%), convalloside (4–24%), convallatoxol (10–20%), desglucocheirotoxin (3–15%) andlokundjoside (1–25%). Other constituents include saponins, flavonoids and asparagin. The cardenolides (cardiac glycosides) exert their action mainly by inhibition of the membranous Na,K-adenosine triphosphatase (ATPase) in the cardiac muscle: increases intracellular calcium and enhances cardiac contractility. The action is similar to digoxin found in Digitalis. Standardised convallaria powder contains 0.2–0.3% cardiac glycosides. The recommended daily oral dose for a mono-preparation containing the natural cardenolide fraction of convallaria corresponds to a total glycoside content of 3.6 to 7.2 mg.

Primary actions: Cardiotonic, diuretic, antiarrhythmic

Indications:

- Arrhythmia, congestive heart failure, cardiac oedema, cardia asthma, dyspnoea, orthopnoea, endocarditis, mitral insufficiency, bradycardia

- **BHP:** Arrhythmia, congestive heart failure, cardiac oedema, cardia asthma. Specific indications: Congestive heart failure with dropsy. Combines well with *Leonurus cardiaca* and *Selenicereus grandiflorus* in heart disease.

Cautions: Toxicity signs include nausea, vomiting, violent purging, cardiac arrhythmias, increased blood pressure, restlessness, trembling, mental confusion, extreme weakness, depression, collapse of circulation.

Pregnancy/Lactation: Not recommended in pregnancy or lactation

Contraindications: Potassium deficiency.

Drug interactions: Do not use with potassium depleting drugs such as diuretics, quinidine, anthraquinone glycoside containing botanicals and corticosteroids.

Dosages: Fluid extract 10–20 ml per week
Tincture 1:5, 0.5–1 ml three times daily

Coptis chinensis

Synonym or related species: C. japanica

Common names: Huang lian (China), makino (Japan)

Family: Ranunculaceae

Part used: Rhizome

Description: Traditionally used to treat bacillary dysentery, diabetes, pertussis, sore throat, aphtha, and eczema in TCM. The common name, *huang lian* (yellow thread), refers to the intense yellow colour of the rhizome. Coptis rhizome contains about 10 mg/g berberine. A 1:2 extract may thus contains about 5 mg/ml berberine.

Constituents: 128 chemical constituents have been isolated and identified. Alkaloids are the characteristic components, together with organic acids, coumarins, phenylpropanoids and quinones. Berberine is the most important active constituent and the primary toxic component.

Primary actions: Antibacterial, Anticancer, Antihyperlipidemic.

All actions: Anti-inflammatory, Antiarrhythmic, Antibacterial, Antidiabetic, Antidiarrhoeal, Antifungal, Antihyperlipidemic, Antihypertensive, Antiobesity, Antiparasitic, Antiviral (systemically), Antiviral (topically), Bitter tonic, Cardioprotective, Cholagogue, Renal protective.

Indications:

- Arrhythmia, Atherosclerosis, Cancer; including prevention/supportive treatment, Candidiasis, Cardiovascular disease prevention, Common cold, Diabetes, Diabetic neuropathy, Dysentery, Dyslipidaemia, Gastrointestinal tract dysbiosis, Hypertension, Influenza, Irritable bowel syndrome, Metabolic syndrome, Non-alcoholic fatty liver disease (NAFLD), Obesity, Psoriasis.

Cautions: Acute toxicity study showed that the oral medial lethal dose (LD50) of the coptis rhizome was greater than 7000mg/kg body weight in mice. LD50 values of four alkaloids (berberine, coptisine, palmatine and epiberberine) were determined as 713.57, 852.12, 1533.68 and 1360mg/kg, respectively. An Ames test, a mouse micronucleus test, and a mouse sperm abnormality test provided negative results. To determine the no-observed-adverse effect level (NOAEL) and the toxicity of coptis, rats received repeated oral administration of coptis rhizome for 13 weeks. No mortality or remarkable clinical signs were observed during this 13-week study. The NOAEL of coptis rhizome was determined as 667mg/kg/day for male rats and 2000mg/kg/day for female rats. The currently recommended doses of coptis alkaloids and coptis consumption are relatively safe.

Contraindications: Berberine-containing plants are best avoided during pregnancy and lactation.

Drug interactions: Itraconazole and berberine are mutually antagonistic and should not be combined.

Use either itraconazole or berberine (or berberine-containing herbal extracts) but not together. The use of berberine is especially relevant since itraconazole is toxic and prone to be associated with fungal resistance. The incidence of *Aspergillus fumigatus* infections has become more frequent as a consequence of widespread immunosuppression. At present, the number of available antifungal agents in clinical use is limited, and most of them, such as itraconazole, are toxic and show resistance. Berberine is a plant alkaloid used in the clinic mainly for alimentary infections. Berberine has antifungal effects against *Aspergillus fumigatus*, possibly via inhibition of the ergosterol biosynthesis pathway in a similar way to the antifungal drug, itraconazole. The two drugs were found to be mutually antagonistic and should not be combined clinically (Lei et al., 2011).

References:

Lei, G., Dan, H., Jinhua, L., Wei, Y., Song, G. & Li, W. 2011. Berberine and itraconazole are not synergistic in vitro against Aspergillus fumigatus isolated from clinical patients. Molecules, 16, 9218-33.

Hwang, Y. H., Cho, W. K., Jang, D., Ha, J. H., Jung, K., Yun, H. I. & Ma, J. Y. 2012. Effects of berberine and hwangryunhaedok-tang on oral bioavailability and pharmacokinetics of ciprofloxacin in rats. Evid Based Complement Alternat Med, 2012, 673132.

Qualities: Clears heat, dries dampness

Typical dosage: 20–50 ml per week

Cordyceps militaris

Synonym or related species: C. sinensis and many other related species

Common names: Cordyceps, orange catapillar fungus, dong chong xia cao (China), hyakurakusou (Japan)

Family: Clavicipitaceae

Part used: Mycelium

Description: Cordyceps militaris, Cordyceps guangdongensis and Isaria cicadae are well recognised and commercialised cordyceps fungi in China.

C. militaris has been increasingly viewed as a substitute for Chinese cordyceps in traditional Chinese medicine and health foods because of their similar chemical profiles and medicinal properties.

However, natural Cordyceps militaris is very rare and expensive, a commercial cordyceps is produced from artificially cultivated fungal fruiting bodies (intracellular polysaccharides) or mycelia fermentation broths (extracellular polysaccharides).

The approved indications in China include invigorating the kidney, nourishing the lung, and for the treatment of cough, asthma, phlegm, spontaneous perspiration, susceptibility to cold, fatigue, dizziness, and tinnitus.

Constituents: Many bioactive components of cordyceps have been extracted, such as cordycepin, cordycepic acid, ergosterol, polysaccharides, nucleosides and peptides. Cordycepin is considered to be the main active compound.

Primary actions: Anticancer, Immunomodulator, Neuroprotective.

All actions: Anti-inflammatory, Antiageing, Antibacterial, Anticancer, Antifungal, Antihyperlipidemic, Antimicrobial, Antiparasitic, Antiviral (systemically), Hypoglycaemic, Immunomodulator, Male tonic, Neuroprotective, Sexual tonic.

Indications:

• Asthma, Bronchitis, Cancer; including prevention/supportive treatment, Dyslipidaemia, Hepatitis, Immune deficiency, Inflammation; kidney and bladder, Liver cirrhosis, Renal insufficiency, Reproductive dysfunction.

Cautions: Human and animal model toxicity profile have indicated that the fungus is safe up to 80 g/kg in mice for 7 days and 10 g/kg in rabbits for an extended period of 3 months with no evidence of adverse effects on the liver, blood or kidney function.

Typical dosage: 20–40 ml per week

Corydalis ambigua

Synonym or related species: Corydalis yanhusuo

Common names: Corydalis

Family: Papaveraceae

Part used: Rhizome

Description: The Chinese corydalis, Yan hu suo, is classified as a blood vitaliser in TCM. Considered to be the second most effective pain reliever after opium. Dehydrocorybulbine and DL-Tetrahydropalmatine (THP) have been found to be antinociceptive in inflammatory and neuropathic pain models.

Constituents: Alkaloids (corydalis L, dl-tetrahydropalmatin (THP), dehydrocorybulbine, papaveraceae type alkaloids). Levo-tetrahydropalmatine (l-THP) in the genera Stephania and Corydalis and has been approved and used in China for a number of clinical indications under the drug name Rotundine. The pharmacological profile of l-THP, which includes antagonism of dopamine D1 and D2 receptors and actions at dopamine D3, alpha adrenergic and serotonin receptors, suggests that it may have utility for treating cocaine addiction.

Primary actions: Antiarrhythmic, Cardioprotective, Sedative.

All actions: Analgesic, Anodyne, Antiarrhythmic, Antispasmodic (muscles), Bitter tonic, Cardioprotective, Hypnotic, Sedative.

Indications:

• Arrhythmia, Blood stasis, Dysmenorrhoea, Endometriosis, Headache, Insomnia, Myocardial ischaemia, Visceral pain.

Contraindications: Do not use during pregnancy.

Qualities: Bitter, slightly acrid and warm

Typical dosage: 30–60 ml per week

Crataegus monogyna

Synonym or related species: Crataegus oxyacantha

Common names: Hawthorn

Family: Rosaceae

Part used: Fruit, leaves

Description: Hawthorn has a long history of use, confirmed safety and clinical evidence to support its cardiovascular benefits, especially cardiotonic activity.

Hawthorn has been extensively studied in Germany. A review on hawthorn preparations used in cardiology found that hawthorn can be employed for indications for which digitalis is not yet indicated. The European Pharmacopoeia monograph is based on a combination extract of leaf and flower defined as a minimum 1.5% of total flavonoids, expressed as hyperoside (dried drug).

There is a lack of evidence for cardioactivity for the fruit extract. Use in chronic, mild heart failure is related to crataegus' ability to increase myocardial contractility (positive inotropic action) while also causing vasorelaxation.

Constituents: Flavonoids (flavones and flavonoles) mainly in form of glycosides (e.g., vitexin, Vitexin-2, rhamnoside, isovitexin, hyperoside, quercetin; flavan compounds (e.g., (+)-catechin, (-)-epicatechin, oligo- and polymeric procyanidins); triterpenic acids (e.g., crataegolic acid, urolic acid, oleanic acid); amines (e.g., phenethylamine, acetylcoline, ethylamine); organic acids (e.g., caffeic acid, chlorogenic acid); and other constituents (e.g., purine derivatives, minerals).

Primary actions: Cardioprotective, Cardiotonic, Vasodilator.

All actions: Antiarrhythmic, Antihyperlipidemic, Antihypertensive, Antioxidant, Antiplatelet, Cardioprotective, Cardiotonic, Vasodilator.

Indications:

- Angina pectoris, Arteriosclerosis, Cardiovascular disease prevention, Hypertension, Tachycardia.

- **BHP:** Cardiac failure or earlier myocardial weakness, hypertension, arteriosclerosis, Buerger's disease, paroxysmal tachycardia. Specific indication: hypertension with myocardial weakness, angina pectoris.

- **ESCOP:** Used for declining cardiac performance and function.

- **WHO:** Treatment of chronic congestive heart failure. Support of cardiac and circulatory functions.

- **Other uses:** Prevention of the development of aging-related endothelial dysfunction. Cardiac hypertrophy is an adaptive enlargement of the myocardium in response to diverse pathophysiological stimuli such as hypertension, valvular disease or myocardial infarction. Crataegus has been shown in vivo to lower the pathological effects of hypertension.

Cautions: Do not administer during lactation without professional advice.

Contraindications: Do not administer during pregnancy due to possible uterine activity.

Drug interactions: In various clinical trials (patients received three or more concomitant drugs according to current treatment guidelines, especially ACE-inhibitors, AT-II-antagonists, beta-blockers, diuretics, spironolactone, and digitalis) adverse drug interactions were not seen.

Lack of additive response with digoxin coadministration in vivo. Synergistic effect with digoxin and antihypertensives is possible.

Qualities: Cold 1st degree, dry

Typical dosage: 20–40 ml per week

Crateva magna

Synonym or related species: Crataeva religiosa, C. nurvala

Common names: Varuna

Family: Capparidaceae

Part used: Bark

Description: Used in Ayurvedic Medicine for urinary disorders. Crataeva produced hypertonic curves in dog cystometric studies and increased bladder tone and bladder capacity in humans in cases of hypotonic bladder due to prostatic hypertrophy. Crataeva demonstrated beneficial effects on neurogenic bladder and significantly decreased residual urine volume, normalising the tone of the urinary bladder.

Crataeva has also been shown to be effective in the treatment of urinary calculi and infection.

Constituents: Flavonoids, glucosinolates, lupeol (plant sterol), saponins, tannin

Primary actions: Anti-inflammatory (urinary), Antilithic, Bladder tonic.

All actions: Anti-inflammatory, Anti-inflammatory (urinary), Antilithic, Antiseptic (urinary), Bladder tonic.

Indications:

- Benign prostatic hyperplasia, Bladder; atonic, Calculi; kidney and bladder, Cystitis, Incontinence, Urethritis.

Cautions: Do not use during pregnancy or lactation without professional supervision.

Contraindications: None known

Qualities: Cool

Typical dosage: 40–90 ml per week

Crocus sativus

Common names: Saffron
Family: Iridaceae
Part used: Stigmas

Description: Saffron is the common name for the stigmas from the flowers of *Crocus sativus*. Saffron is exclusively obtained from cultivation. The word saffron derives from the Arab word *zafaran*, meaning yellow, and it was mentioned as far back as 1500 B.C. Further derivations come from the Old French *safran*, Medieval Latin *safranum*, and Middle English *safroun*.

Saffron is widely used as a spice in rice dishes and fish recipes in Mediterranean countries and the Middle East. In Europe, much saffron went into the production of various alcoholic bitters, and was used as a dye in baking cakes and pastry. The use of an adaptogen is documented in Indian Ayurvedic medicine. Significant anti-stress effects and anxiolytic properties have been evidenced in animal experiments and human studies.

Constituents: Saffron contains 0.4 to 1.3% of essential oil with pinene, 1,8-cineol and safranal as the major component. Safranal is responsible for the typical aroma of saffron. Fresh Crocus flowers do not strongly smell of safranal. This compound is only formed in the course of the drying process from the bitter terpene glucoside picrocrocin by cleavage of glucose and water.

The picrocorin content of fresh saffron can be up to 4%, whereas this constituent is usually not present in well-stored saffron. In addition the stigmas contains hydroxysafranal, 2-phenylethanol, the isophoron 3,5,5-trimethylcyclohexenon and various other isophorons.

Primary actions: Antidepressant, Chemoprotective, Neuroprotective.

All actions: Adaptogen, Anti-inflammatory, Antiacetylcholinesterase, Antiallergic, Anticancer, Anticonvulsant, Antidepressant, Antiepileptic, Antihyperlipidemic, Antihypertensive, Antimicrobial, Antioxidant, Antitussive, Anxiolytic, Chemoprotective, Cytoprotective, Decongestant, Immunomodulator, Neuroprotective.

Indications:

- Age-related macular degeneration, Anaemia, Asthma, Cough, Depression, Dyslipidaemia, Dysmenorrhoea, Erectile dysfunction, Fever, Infertility, Libido; low, Liver congestion, Memory and concentration; poor, Menstrual irregularity, Muscular tension, Nervous exhaustion, Nervous tension, Premenstrual syndrome, Rheumatism.

Cautions: Daily doses of up to 1.5 g are thought to be safe. According to the monograph of the German Commission E high doses (5 g and above) are toxic, with a lethal dose of approximately 20 g. With the ingestion of 5 g adverse effects such as purpura, thrombocytopenia and hypothrombinaemia were supposedly observed. Further adverse effects of high saffron doses (for abortive uses in doses > 10 g) vomiting, uterus bleeding, bloody diarrhea, haematuria, bleedings of the gastrointestinal mucosas as well as vertigo and dizziness were reported. The coloured constituents may accumulate in sclera, skin or mucosas, and may thus mimic icteric complaints.

Contraindications: Known allergy to saffron.

Typical dosage: 10–25 ml per week

Cryptolepis sanguinolenta

Common names: Yellow dye root, delboi
Family: Apocynaceae
Part used: Root

Description: Traditionally, the roots and aerial parts are used in the treatment of various diseases such as malaria, bacterial respiratory diseases, hypertension, and diarrhea, and as a cicatrizant.

Constituents: Alkaloids including indoloquinoline cryptolepine, isocryptolepine and cryptosanguinolentine. Also tannins and anthocyanosides.

Primary actions: Anti-inflammatory, Antibacterial, Antimicrobial.

All actions: Anti-inflammatory, Antibacterial, Anticancer, Antidiabetic, Antihypertensive, Antiparasitic, Antipyretic, Vasodilator, Vasoprotective.

Indications:

- Diabetes, Diarrhoea, Fever, Gastroenteritis, Gastrointestinal amoebiasis, Hepatitis, Hypertension, Infection; genitourinary tract, Infection; respiratory tract, Insomnia, Malaria, Parasites.

Cautions: Cryptolepsis may reduce fertility in both sexes. Shown to have reproductive toxic effects in rodent studies.

Contraindications: Pregnancy

Drug interactions: Avoid with CNS depressants or sedatives.

Typical dosage: 30–100 ml per week

Curcuma longa

Synonym or related species: Curcuma domestica, Curcuma rotunda
Common names: Turmeric
Family: Zingiberaceae
Part used: Rhizome

Description: The active compounds, collectively known as curcuminoids, of this Indian curry spice have attracted great interest in recent decades because it contains bioactive curcuminoids with anticancer, antibiotic, anti-inflammatory, and antiaging agent as suggested by several in vitro and in vivo studies, and clinical trials. Several curcumin formulations have been developed to enhance the poor bioavailability of curcumin. Notably Meriva, Theracumin, C3 Complex and Longvida.

Constituents: Curcuminoids including curcumin, demethoxycurcumin, and bisdemethoxycurcumin.

Primary actions: Anti-inflammatory, Anticancer, Antihyperlipidemic.

All actions: Anti-inflammatory, Anti-inflammatory (musculoskeletal), Antiangina, Antiasthmatic, Antihyperlipidemic, Antioxidant, Antiplatelet, Chemoprotective, Choleretic, Cytoprotective, Hepatoprotective, Neuroprotective.

Indications:

- Alzheimer's disease, Arthritis, Asthma, Atherosclerosis, Cancer; including prevention/ supportive treatment, Cardiovascular disease prevention, Cholecystitis, Dementia, Digestive complaints, Digestive weakness, Eczema, Endometriosis, Liver insufficiency, Psoriasis.

- **ESCOP:** Symptomatic treatment of mild digestive disturbances and minor biliary dysfunction

- **WHO:** Principally for the treatment of acid, flatulent, or atonic dyspepsia. Treatment of peptic ulcers, and pain and inflammation due to rheumatoid arthritis and of amenorrhoea, dysmenorrhoea, diarrhoea, epilepsy, pain, and skin diseases

- **Other uses:** Curcumin is also used intravenously, mostly as an adjuvant cancer therapy.

Cautions: Turmeric may cause iron deficiency by reducing iron absorption in the gut. Turmeric inhibits iron absorption by 20%–90% in humans in a dose-dependent manner. Curcumin binds ferric iron (Fe^{3+}) to form a ferric-curcumin complex.

Curcumin has been shown to suppress the expression of liver hepcidin and ferritin, and reduced iron concentrations in the liver and spleen by over 50%.

Curcumin represses the synthesis of hepcidin, one of thepeptides involved in iron balance, and has the potential to induce iron deficiency in the setting of prior subclinical iron deficiency (Smith et al., 2019)

Contraindications: Obstruction of the biliary tract. Hypersensitivity to turmeric.

Drug interactions: Curcumin is a safe and tolerable adjunct to FOLFOX chemotherapy in patients with metastatic colorectal cancer (Howells et al., 2019).

May descrease blood levels of talinolol (clinical study).

Qualities: Pungent, warm

Typical dosage: 40–80 ml per week

References:

Howells LM, Iwuji COO, Irving GRB, et al. Curcumin Combined with FOLFOX Chemotherapy Is Safe and Tolerable in Patients with Metastatic Colorectal Cancer in a Randomized Phase IIa Trial. J Nutr. 2019;149(7):1133-1139.

Smith T J, Ashar B H 2019 Iron Deficiency Anemia Due to High-dose Turmeric. Cureus11(1): e3858.

Cynara scolymus

Common names: Globe artichoke

Family: Asteraceae

Part used: Leaves

Description: Artichoke leaf has been used as a choleretic and diuretic in traditional European medicine since Roman times. Artichoke leaf is considered choleretic (bile-increasing), hepatoprotective, cholesterol-reducing, and diuretic. Clinical studies have examined its effects in hypercholesterolaemia, metabolic syndrome, NAFLD, hypertension, chronic hepatitis, functional dyspepsia and alcoholic hangovers.

Constituents: Coumarin, cynaropicrin (bitter sesquiterpene lactones), luteolin derivatives (flavonoids), plant phenolic acid derivatives.

Primary actions: Antihyperlipidemic, Digestive tonic, Hepatoprotective.

All actions: Antihyperlipidemic, Bitter tonic, Choleretic, Digestive tonic, Diuretic, Hepatoprotective, Hepatotonic.

Indications:

- Allergies/Sensitivities, Anorexia, Arteriosclerosis, Atherosclerosis, Diabetes, Diabetes; gestational, Digestive complaints, Digestive weakness, Gall stones (cholelithiasis), Gallbladder disorders, Liver insufficiency, Weight loss; to assist.

- **Commission E:** The German Commission E approved artichoke leaf for dyspeptic problems.

- **ESCOP:** Stomach ache, nausea, vomiting, feeling of fullness, flatulence and hepatobiliary disturbances. Use as an adjuvant to a low fat diet in the treatment of mild to moderate hyperlipidaemia.

Cautions: Use with caution in patients with acute or severe hepatocellular disease (e.g., cirrhosis), septic cholecystitis, intestinal spasm, ileus or liver cancer, or unconjugated hyperbilirubinaemia. Flatulence, contact dermatitis, urticaria/angioedema, and feelings of weakness and hunger have been reported.

Contraindications: Not to be used by people with known allergy to globe artichoke or members of the Asteraceae (Compositae) family. Contraindicated in patients with bile duct obstruction.

Qualities: Cold, moist

Typical dosage: 15–30 ml per week

Dioscorea spp.

Common names: Wild yam

Family: Dioscoreaceae

Part used: Rhizome, root

Description: Traditionally used for gastrointestinal disorders including colic, flatulence, and for muscular spasms and cramping associated with menstrual disorders including dysmenorrhoea. Pharmacological and preclinical studies have shown diosgenic to have anticancer, cardiovasucular protective, antihyperlipidaemic, antidiabetic, and neuroprotective activities. A diosgenin-rich yam extract has been shown in an RCT to safely enhance cognitive function in healthy adults.

Constituents: Alkaloids, beta-sitosterol, botogenin, diodenin, dioscin, dioscorin, dioscorine, phytosterol, resin, saponin glycosides, starch, steroidal saponins, stigmasterol, tannin, taraxerol, trillin. The saponin glycosides are considered to be amongst the most active constituents. Once ingested, the normal gut bacteria cleave the glucose molecule, leaving the sapogenin (aglycone) diosgenin (SERM), which is absorbed. The alkaloids are said to be the active constituent responsible for the stomachic action of the herb.

Primary actions: Anti-inflammatory, Antispasmodic/ Spasmolytic, Selective oestrogen receptor modulator (SERM).

All actions: Anti-inflammatory, Anti-inflammatory (GIT), Antirheumatic, Antispasmodic (muscles), Antispasmodic (uterus), Antitussive, Diaphoretic, Diuretic, Nervine tonic, Selective oestrogen receptor modulator (SERM), Stomachic, Styptic/Haemostatic, Venotonic.

Indications:

*   Cholecystitis, Colic, Colic; intestinal, Cystic hyperplasia, Cystitis, Diverticulitis, Dysmenorrhoea, Dysmenorrhoea; spasmodic, Endometriosis, Flatulence, Gallbladder disorders, Intermittent claudication, Menopausal symptoms, Miscarriage; threatened, Morning sickness, Muscular tension, Ovarian and uterine pains, Premenstrual syndrome, Rheumatism, Uterine bleeding; dysfunctional.

Cautions: Mild diarrhoea is sometimes reported; *Dioscorea spp.* should therefore be used cautiously in those who have 'weak digestion' and develop diarrhoea easily. Generally considered safe in all trimesters of pregnancy when consumed in low doses.

Contraindications: None known

Drug interactions: Wild yam has mild oestrogen-like activity. It is very unlikely that it would reduce the effects of oral contraceptives or have an additive effect during HRT.

Qualities: Cold, sweet

Typical dosage: 20–40 ml per week

Dipsacus asper

Common names: Teasel root

Family: Dipsacaceae

Part used: Root

Description: Traditionally uses as a tonic, analgesic and anti-inflammatory agent for the therapy of low back pain, rheumatic arthritis, traumatic hematoma, habitual abortion and bone fractures in traditional Chinese medicine. Teasel root is considered a yang tonic in TCM which acts on the liver and kidneys.

Constituents: Phenolic acids including caffeic acid, cinnamic acid derivatives, vanillic acid and caffeoylquinic acid; iridoid glycosides including loganin, cantleyoside, triplostoside A and sweroside derivaties; furofuran lignans; sterol compounds such as β-sitosterol, campesterol, stigmasterol; triterpenoids such as oleanic acid, akebiasaponin D and other asperosaponins.(Tian, Wang et al. 2007) Triterpenoids with antibacterial and cytotoxic properties.(Yu, Yu et al. 2019)

Primary actions: Anti-inflammatory, Antinociceptive, Tonic.

All actions: Anti-inflammatory, Antifungal, Antihyperlipidemic, Antinociceptive, Blood sugar regulator, Tonic, Wound healing/Vulnerary.

Indications:

*   Diabetes, Hepatic steatosis, Menorrhagia, Osteoarthritis, Osteoporosis, Osteoporosis prevention, Rheumatoid arthritis.

Cautions: Teasel root is traditionally used in pregnancy to control bleeding and prevent miscarriage however its safety in pregnancy has not been medically assessed.

Typical dosage: 15–50 ml per week

Drosera spp.

Synonym or related species: Drosera anglica, D. longifolia, D. rotundifolia

Common names: Sundew

Family: Droseraceae

Part used: Aerial parts

Description: Drosera, commonly known as the sundew, is one of the largest genera of carnivorous plants, with at least 194 species. They lure, capture, and digest insects using stalked mucilaginous glands covering their leaf surfaces. Traditionally used for asthma and bronchitis. Naphthoquinones present in *Drosera spp.* exhibit potent TB activity.

Constituents: Naphtaquinones, plumbagin, flavonoids.

Primary actions: Antiasthmatic, Antispasmodic (respiratory tract), Bronchodilator.

All actions: Antiasthmatic, Antibacterial, Antispasmodic (respiratory tract), Bronchodilator, Demulcent.

Indications:

*   Asthma, Bronchitis, Pertussis.
*   **BHP:** Bronchitis, asthma, pertussis, tracheitis, gastric ulceration. Specific indications: asthma, chronic bronchitis with peptic ulceration or gastritis.

Contraindications: None known

Qualities: Acrid, warm

Typical dosage: 10–20 ml per week

Dulacia inopiflora

Synonym or related species: Ptychopetalum olacoides

Common names: Muira puama

Family: Oleaceae

Part used: Root bark

Description: Nootropic and antidepressant properties in vivo, also claimed to be a possible adaptogen. Shown to attenuates cognitive impairment and neurological degeneration in a mouse Alzheimer model and to improve memory retrieval in young and ageing mice. However, also found to be anxiogenic in a rodent study. (An anxiogenic substance is one that causes anxiety. This effect is in contrast to anxiolytic agents, which inhibits anxiety.) Muira puama is promoted for sexual disorders, increasing sexual desire in healthy people, menstrual disorders, joint pain, and other conditions, but there is no good scientific evidence to support these uses.

Constituents: Volatile oil containing alpha-pinene, alpha-humulene, beta-pinene, beta-caryophyllene, camphene, and camphor. Uncosanoic, tricosanoic, and pentacosanoic acids make up 20% of the constituents of muira puama. Other minor compounds: coumarin, fatty acid esters of sterols, free fatty acids, beta-sitosterol, lupeol and free sterols.

Primary actions: Digestive tonic, Nervine tonic, Nootropic.

All actions: Adaptogen, Antidepressant, Antioxidant, Digestive tonic, Nervine tonic, Nootropic.

Indications:

- Colic; intestinal, Depression, Dysmenorrhoea, Dyspepsia, Sexual weakness, Stress.

- **Other uses:** Historically to prevent sexual disorders, as an aphrodisiac, for dyspepsia, menstrual irregularities, paralysis, and rheumatism. Indigenous tribes in Brazil use the tea for treating neuromuscular problems, rheumatism, influenza, cardiac and gastrointestinal asthenia and to prevent baldness. In Europe, muira puama has a long history as an anti-rheumatic, aphrodisiac, nervine tonic, and in the treatment of gastrointestinal disorders. In Brazil, a herbal medicinal extract named Catuama containing a mixture of *Paullinia cupana* (guarana), *Trichilia catigua* (catuaba), *Ptychopetalum olacoides* (muirapuama) and *Zingiber officinale* (ginger) is used as a stimulant, energy tonic and aphrodisiac.

Contraindications: Not recommended in pregnancy.

Typical dosage: 10–40 ml per week

Echinacea spp.

Common names: Echinacea, coneflower

Family: Asteraceae

Part used: Root, whole plant

Description: Best known for its immunostimulatory and anti-inflammatory properties, used especially the alleviation of cold symptoms. Pharmacological and preclinical studies have also demonstrated antianxiety, antidepression, cytotoxicity, and anticancer properties. *Echinacea angustifolia, Echinacea pallida,* and *Echinacea purpurea* are the main species used in phytotherapy. The root of *E. angustifolia* was the preferred medicine by the early US herbalists, however, fresh plant extract of *E. purpurea* is the dominant medicine used in Europe today, especially for viral infections.

Constituents: Alkylamides, caffeic acid derivatives, polysaccharides and polysaccharides. Dodeca-2E, 4E- dienoic acid isobutylamide induces tingling paresthesia on the tongue by inhibition of background potassium currents and numbing analgesia by blocking voltage-gated sodium channels.This tingling is most notable in *E. angustifolia.*

Primary actions: Anti-inflammatory, Chemoprotective, Immunomodulator.

All actions: Anti-inflammatory, Antidiarrhoeal, Antimicrobial, Antiseptic (GIT), Antiseptic (respiratory tract), Antiseptic (topically), Antiseptic (urinary), Chemoprotective, Immunomodulator, Lymphatic, Sialogogue, Vasodilator, Wound healing/Vulnerary.

Indications:

- Acne, Acne (topically), Boils, Bronchitis, Cancer; including prevention/supportive treatment, Candidiasis, Catarrh; naso-pharyngeal congestion, Chemotherapy; to minimise the side effects of, Chronic fatigue syndrome, Circulation; peripheral; impaired, Common cold, Connective tissue disorders, Cystitis, Diarrhoea, Dysentery, Eczema, Fever, Furunculosis, Gingivitis, Glands; swollen, Hayfever, Herpes simplex, Immune deficiency, Infection; fungal, Infection; gastrointestinal system, Infection; protozoal, Infection; respiratory tract, Infection; skin, Infection; systemic, Infection; throat, Infection; to improve resistance to, Infection; viral, Inflammation; oral cavity, Influenza, Intestinal worms, Irritable bowel syndrome, Pertussis, Pharyngitis, Post-viral syndromes, Psoriasis, Shingles, Sinusitis, Tonsillitis, Tracheitis, Ulcer (topically), Ulcer; gastrointestinal, Ulcer; mouth, Urethritis, Warts, Wounds, Wounds (topically).

- **BHP:** Furunculosis, septicaemia, naso-pharyngeal catarrh, pyorrhoea, and tonsillitis. Specific indications: boils, carbuncles and abscesses.

- **Commission E:** To support and promote the natural powers of resistance of the body, especially to infectious conditions (e.g., influenza, colds) in the upper respiratory tract and urinary tract, as an alternative in influenza, inflammatory and purulent wounds, abscesses, furuncles, indolent leg ulcers, herpes simplex, inflammation of connective tissue, wounds, headaches, metabolic disturbances, as a diaphoretic and an antiseptic.

- **ESCOP:** Internal use: Adjuvant therapy and prophylaxis of recurrent infections of the upper respiratory tract and urogenital tract. External use: As an adjuvant for the treatment of superficial wounds.
- **WHO:** Supportive therapy for colds and infections of the respiratory and urinary tract. Beneficial effects in the treatment of these infections are thought to be due to stimulation of the immune response.

Cautions: Echinacea has been shown to modulate cytokines, which may provoke the inflammatory response in asthmatics. However, echinacea may reduce the frequency of respiratory viral infections, which can aggravate asthma. Use with caution, and within recommended dosage guidelines. Use with caution during lactation, or for children. Adverse effects include digestive upset, skin reactions, unpleasant taste sensation; leucopenia and erythema have been reported.

Contraindications: Contraindicated in transplant patients taking immunosuppressant medication and those with known hypersensitivity to plants of the Compositae (Asteraceae) family.

Drug interactions: May theoretically counter the effects of immune-suppressive medication. However, *E. purpurea* extract has been shown to ameliorate reductions in red and white blood cells induced by cyclosporine (Khattab, Abounasef et al. 2019). May alter anti-HIV medication levels. Clinical significance unknown. Echinacea has no clinically significant effects on P450 CYP enzymes.

Qualities: Acrid, sweet, warm 2nd degree

Typical dosage: 20–40 ml per week. May be increased to 10–20 ml daily in acute conditions.

Eleutherococcus senticosus

Synonym or related species: Acanthopanax senticosus

Common names: Eleuthero, eleutherokokk, Siberian ginseng

Family: Araliaceae

Part used: Root

Description: Extensive use probably only dates back to the mid-1950s. Eleutherococcus was never called 'Siberian ginseng' by the Soviets who called it '*eleutherokokk*'. The adopted common name gaining some traction in English is *eleuthero* – it should never be referred to as *Siberian* ginseng, just the way withania should not be referred to as *Indian* ginseng. Eleuthero is of course an adaptogen, which can be simply defined as any product of botanical origin that enabled the body to counteract negative effects of 'stress'. Contrary to common belief, eleuthero is not contraindicated in hypertension nor in acute infections.

Constituents: Eleutherosides including eleutherosides B (syringin) and E (syringaresinol) that

are also used to identify eleuthero. Other ingredients are acanthosides, phytosterols, triterpene saponins, dihydrodehydrodiconiferyl alcohol monopyranose, glycosides, 5-O-caffeoylquinic acid isomers, glucopyranosides, and lignans.

Primary actions: Adaptogen, Anticancer, Immunomodulator.

All actions: Adaptogen, Anticancer, Hepatoprotective, Immunomodulator, Nootropic, Tonic.

Indications:

- Cancer; including prevention/supportive treatment, Chemotherapy; to minimise the side effects of, Chronic fatigue syndrome, Convalescence, Debility, Exhaustion, Immune deficiency, Infection; systemic, Infection; to improve resistance to, Post-viral syndromes, Stress.
- **Commission E:** Tonic for fatigue and debility, poor stamina and concentration and during convalescence.
- **ESCOP:** Decreased mental and physical capacities such as weakness, exhaustion, tiredness and loss of concentration, as well as during convalescence.
- **WHO:** As a prophylactic and restorative tonic for enhancement of mental and physical capacities in cases of weakness, exhaustion and tiredness, and during convalescence. Treatment of rheumatoid arthritis, insomnia and dream-disturbed sleep.

Contraindications: Should not be used in patients with known allergies to the plants of the Araliaceae family. Often stated to be contraindicated in hypertension or during acute infections with fever although there is no evidence to support this. Furthermore, the majority of studies on the beneficially effects of *Andrographis paniculata* in acute respiratory conditions are actually based on a combination product with eleuthero.

Qualities: Warm

Typical dosage: 20–55 ml per week

Elymus repens

Synonym or related species: Agropyron repens, Elytrigia repens, Triticum repens

Common names: Couch grass

Family: Poaceae

Part used: Rhizome

Description: Agropyron repens has been used traditionally since ancient times. Its name was mentioned in the publications of Dioskurides, Plinius, Tabermontanus-Bauhinus 1588 and Matthiolus 1626, according to Madaus (1938). Mainly used for urinary disorder including irritable condition of bladder and to promote urination and for related conditions such as gout and rheumatism.

Constituents: Couch grass contains 3–8% triticin

(similar to inulin), which yields fructose upon hydrolysis. The drug also contains 3–4% fructose, 2–3% sugar alcohols (mannitol, inositol). The presence of agropyrene has been disputed. Furthermore, small amounts of vanillin monoglucoside, vanillic acid, phenolic carboxylic acids, hydroxycinnamic acid alkyl ester, silicic acid and silicates are present. Also polysacharides, flavonoids, tannins, phenolic compounds, essential oil, and anthraquinone.

Primary actions: Anti-inflammatory (urinary), Demulcent, Diuretic.

All actions: Anti-inflammatory (urinary), Antilithic, Demulcent, Diuretic.

Indications:

- Arthritis, Benign prostatic hyperplasia, Cystitis, Gout, Infection; urinary tract, Inflammation; kidney and bladder, Lithuria, Prostatitis, Rheumatism, Urethritis.
- **BHP:** Cystitis, urethritis, prostatitis, benign prostatic hypertrophy, renal calculus, and lithuria. Specific indication: cystitis with irritation or inflammation of the urinary tract.
- **Other uses:** Arthritis, Benign prostatic hyperplasia, kidney and bladder calculi, cystitis, gout, infection of the urinary tract, inflammation of the urinary tract, lithuria, prostatitis, rheumatism, and urethritis.

Cautions: Large amounts of fluid should not be taken in oedema due to impaired cardiac or renal function exists.

Contraindications: None known

Qualities: Cooling, moistening

Typical dosage: 20–40 ml per week

Ephedra sinensis

Common names: Ma-huang

Family: Ephedraceae

Description: Ma-huang is one of the major herbs in TCM formulations for asthma and bronchitis and related respiratory symptoms such as the San'ao decoction. Ephedra is included in the national pharmacopoeias of China, Germany, and Japan.

Ephedra was banned in several countries in the last couple of decades due to adverse events associated with its street use as a weight loss product, CNS stimulant activity and as a performance enhancing drug.

Ephedra is indigenous to northern China and Mongolia. Current controls over ephedra in the United Kingdom restrict doses of more than 600 mg herb (equivalent to 12 mg ephedrine alkaloids) and daily doses of more than 1800 mg herb to pharmacy supply. Below these doses, ephedra products can only be supplied following a one-to-one consultation with a herbalist.

Part used: Aerial parts

Constituents: Ephedra contains 0.5–2% alkaloids, the main active constituents are the alkaloids ephedrine and pseudoephedrine; volatile oil mainly terpenoids; tannins, ephedran glycans and acids. Ephedrine and pseudoephedrine are sympathomimetic agents that have direct and indirect effects on both alpha- and beta-adrenoceptors, as well as stimulating the CNS.

Primary actions: Respiratory spasmolytic, bronchodilating, antiasthmatic

All actions: Smooth muscle relaxant, anti-inflammatory, immunemodulating, CNS stimulant, cardiovascular stimulant, antimicrobial, bronchodilation, vasoconstricting, respiratory spasmolytic, antiasthmatic

Indications:

- Asthma, hay fever, cough, common cold, fever, urticaria, enuresis, narcolepsy, myasthenia gravis, chronic postural hypotension, rheumatism, allergic rhinitis, sinusitis, urticaria,
- **Other Uses:** Ephedrine is an appetite suppressant.
- **BHP Specific Indications:** Asthma, to reduce the frequency and severity of spams. Hay fever. Allergic symptoms. May be used with lobelia, grindelia, *Symplocarpus foetidus* in asthma, and echinacea and *Gnaphalium uliginosum* in hay fever, with equisetum in enuresis.
- **Commission E:** The Commission E approved the internal use of ephedra herb for diseases of the respiratory tract with mild bronchospasms in adults and children over the age of 6. Short-term use only because of tachyphylaxis and danger of addiction.
- **WHO:** The World Health Organization lists the use of ephedra is the treatment hay fever, allergic rhinitis, acute rhinitis, common cold, sinusitis, and as a bronchodilator in treatment of bronchial asthma is supported by clinical evidence.

Cautions: Side effects and adverse events of ephedrine and pseudoephedrine include tachycardia, anxiety, restlessness, insomnia, tremor, dry mouth, hypertension, cardiac arrhythmia, skin rashes, and urinary retention.

Pregnancy/Lactation: Not recommended in pregnancy or lactation.

Contraindications: Ephedra should be avoided in hypertension and cardiovascular disease.

Drug interactions: Avoid with cardiac glycosides or halothane, guanethidine, MAO-inhibitors, secale alkaloid derivatives and oxytocin.

Qualities: Warming, acrid

Dosages: Fluid extract 20-60 ml per week

Liquid extract 1–3 ml three times daily

Tincture (1:4) 6–8 ml three times daily

Epilobium parviflorum

Synonym or related species: Epilobium angustifolia

Common names: Willow herb

Family: Onagraceae

Part used: Aerial parts

Description: The roots and also the aerial parts of *E. angustifolium* and other species were used externally by Native Americans to treat skin infections and rectal bleeding. Infusions from the aerial parts of Epilobium, especially *E. angustifolium*, were recommended by American herbalists in the 19th and 20th centuries as a very effective agent to treat gastrointestinal diseases such as dysentery and diarrhoea of different aetiologies, as well as other bowel and intestinal disorders associated with infection, irritation and inflammation. In Russia, the aerial parts were consumed untreated or fermented as infusion to treat stomach ulceration, gastritis and sleeping disorders. In Europe, epilobium was used for the treatment of wounds, to stop bleeding and for the treatment of female disorders. In the 20th century it is used as a herbal tea in the treatment of benign prostatic hyperplasia and prostatitis as well as bladder and kidney disorders.

Constituents: Flavonoids and ellagitannins, such as oenothein B, are among the compounds considered to be the primary biologically active components. Tannins (4–14%) including oenothein B, oenothein A, tri-, tetra-, and penta-O-galloylglucose. Flavonoids (1–2%) including kaempferol, querceting, and myricetin. Phenolic acids and their derivatives including ellagic acid, valoneic acid dilactone, chlorogenic acid, neochlorogenic acid, coumaroylyquinic acids, feruloylquinic acids, gallic acid, cinnamic acid, protocatechuic acid, caffeic acid, ferulic acid. Steroids (0.4%) and triterpenes (ca. 1.5%): including cholesterol, campesterol, stigmasterol, β-sitosterol, ursolic acid, corosolic acid, oleanolic acid.

Primary actions: Anti-inflammatory, Antihyperprostatic.

All actions: Analgesic, Anti-inflammatory, Antibacterial, Antidiarrhoeal, Antifungal, Antihyperprostatic.

Indications:

*   Benign prostatic hyperplasia, Inflammation; kidney and bladder.

Typical dosage: 20–40 ml per week

Epimedium sagittatum

Common names: Horny goat weed, barrenwort, yin yang huo, Inyokaku

Family: Berbridaceae

Part used: Leaf

Description: Traditional use in TCM for deficient Kidney yang patterns including impotence, fatigue, cold lower back, frequent urination and memory deficits. Common name refers to shepherds noticing increased sexual behaviour when goats were grazing on this herb.

Don't be fooled by the light-hearted common name. This is a serious herbal medicine. The active compound icariin has wide-ranging properties.

Constituents: Flavonoids including icariin, icarisides, epimedin A, B and C. Lignans, phenolic glucosides and sesquiterpenes. Polysaccharides (usually not found in hydroethanol extracts) have immune modulating properties.

Primary actions: Antiosteoporotic, Neuroprotective, Phosphodiesterase-5 inhibitor.

All actions: Anti-inflammatory, Antiageing, Anticancer, Antidepressant, Antinociceptive, Antioxidant, Antiviral (systemically), Aphrodisiac, Cardioprotective, Hepatoprotective, Immunomodulator, Male tonic, Neuroprotective, Phosphodiesterase-5 inhibitor, Sexual tonic, Tonic, Vasodilator.

Indications:

*   Asthma, Atherosclerosis, Benign prostatic hyperplasia, Cardiovascular disease prevention, Dementia, Depression, Erectile dysfunction, Fatigue, Infertility, Menopausal symptoms, Menstrual irregularity, Nephritis, Osteoarthritis, Osteoporosis prevention, Premature ovarian failure, Sexual weakness.

Drug interactions: May interact with other phosphodiesterase-5 inhibitors (sildenafil/viagra). Rat plasma was sampled from each anesthetised rat after pretreatment with three days Epimedium sagittatum extract (0.5 g/kg/day) and intravenous injection with sildenafil (10/30 mg/kg). The pharmacokinetic data demonstrate that the area under the concentration-time curve (AUC) of sildenafil (10 mg/kg) was significantly decreased in groups that received a high dose of Epimedium sagittatum extract. In conclusion, the study demonstrates that there was significant herb–drug interaction of Epimedium sagittatum extract on the pharmacokinetics of sildenafil at low and high daily doses, suggesting co-administration use of Epimedium sagittatum extract and sildenafil in clinical practice should be prevented due to possible herb–drug interactions. (Hsueh, Ho et al. 2016)

Reference:

Hush, T. Et al. Herb-drug interaction of Epimedium extract on the pharmacokinetic of dapoxetine in rats J Chromatogr B Analyt Technol Biomed Life Sci. 2016 Mar 1;1014:64-9.

Qualities: Acrid, sweet, warm

Typical dosage: 20–45 ml per week

Equisetum arvense

Common names: Horsetail

Family: Equisetaceae

Part used: Aerial parts

Description: Traditionally used for bacterial and inflammatory diseases of the lower urinary tract and renal gravel and for the adjuvant treatment of kidney and urinary inflammations and infections. Topically used as compress for superficial wounds.

Constituents: Inorganic minerals including silicic acid, aluminum chloride, potassium chloride and manganese, flavonoids: mostly kaempherol and querceting glycosides (the pharmacopoeial standard is 0.3% flavonoids), small amount of various alkaloids.

Primary actions: Antilithic, Diuretic, Natriuretic.

All actions: Antilithic, Astringent, Diuretic, Natriuretic.

Indications:

- Cystitis with haematuria, Enuresis, Prostatitis, Urethritis.
- **BHP:** Enuresis, prostatic disease, cystitis with haematuria, urethritis. Specific indications: inflammation or benign enlargement of the prostate gland, urinary incontinence, enuresis of children.

Cautions: Large amounts of fluid should not be taken if oedema due to impaired cardiac or renal function exists. Allergic reactions are possible.

Contraindications: None known

Drug interactions: Increases the excretion of urinary potassium and chloride, suggesting that it may act in a similar way to hydrochlorothiazide.

Qualities: Cold, pungent

Typical dosage: 20–40 ml per week

Eschscholzia californica

Common names: Californian poppy

Family: Papaveraceae

Part used: Aerial parts

Description: California poppy is a traditional Native American medicinal plant used for its mild analgesic and sedative properties for the symptomatic treatment of neurotonic disturbances in adults and children; mainly for minor sleep disorders. It is frequently used in conjunction with other herbs such as passionflower or valerian.

Constituents: Alkaloids (six groups, 0.5 to 1.2% total) expressed as californidine, putin and purple-red pigment eschscholtz-xanthin. French pharmacopoeial standard is not less than 0.50% and not more than 1.20% of total alkaloids, expressed as californidine.

Primary actions: Analgesic, Anxiolytic, Hypnotic.

All actions: Analgesic, Antispasmodic/Spasmolytic, Anxiolytic, Diaphoretic, Hypnotic, Sedative.

Indications:

- Anxiety, Dyspepsia; nervous, Hyperactivity, Insomnia, Nervous exhaustion, Nervous tension, Neurasthenia.
- **Commission E:** Reduction in spontaneous motility and prolongation of pentobarbital-induced sleep (in mice) as well as prevention of spasms induced by BaCl2 (isolated jejunum).
- **Other uses:** Combinations of California poppy herb with other components (valerian root, St. John's wort, passionflower herb, lemon balm leaf and others) are traditionally used for several disorders such as reactive, agitated and masked depressions, melancholy, neurasthenia, neuropathy, organ neurosis, vegetative-dystonic disturbances, constitutional lability of the nervous system, as well as a sleep-inducer and sedative tea.

Contraindications: None known

Drug interactions: Avoid concurrent use with sedative pharmaceutical drugs.

Qualities: Bitter, cool

Typical dosage: 20–40 ml per week

Eupatorium perfoliatum

Common names: Boneset, feverwort

Family: Asteraceae

Part used: Aerial parts

Description: Leaves and flowering parts used in Native American traditional medicine as diaphoretic medicine, used mainly for the common cold and fever.

Constituents: Volatile oil, caffeic acid derivatives, flavonoids, sesquiterpene lactones, tannins, polysaccharides.

Primary actions: Anti-inflammatory, Antipyretic, Diaphoretic.

All actions: Anti-inflammatory, Antipyretic, Antirheumatic, Diaphoretic.

Indications:

- Arthritis, Bronchitis, Catarrh; naso-pharyngeal congestion, Gout, Influenza.
- **BHP:** Influenza, acute bronchitis, nasopharyngeal catarrh. Specific indications: influenza with deep aching and congestion of the respiratory mucosa.

Contraindications: None known

Qualities: Cold, dry

Typical dosage: 0.7–2 g per day

Euphorbia hirta

Synonym or related species: Chamaesyce hirta, Euphorbia pilulifera

Common names: Euphorbia

Family: Euphorbiaceae

Part used: Aerial parts

Description: Traditionally used to treat respiratory conditions including asthma and bronchitis; intestinal disorders including dysentery and intestinal amoebiasis. Pharmacological research has demonstrated anti-inflammatory, antirheumatic, anthelmintic, antidiarrhoeal, antidiabetic, and antimicrobial activities.

Constituents: Alkaloids, beta-sterol, flavonoids, tannin, triterpenoids, glycoside.

Primary actions: Antiasthmatic, Bronchodilator, Expectorant (relaxing).

All actions: Anthelmintic, Antiasthmatic, Antimicrobial, Antiparasitic, Antispasmodic (respiratory tract), Bronchodilator, Expectorant (relaxing).

Indications:

- Asthma, Bronchitis, Cough, Dysentery, Emphysema, Gastrointestinal amoebiasis, Gastrointestinal tract dysbiosis, Gastrointestinal tract infestation, Pertussis.
- **BHP:** Asthma, bronchitis, upper respiratory catarrh, intestinal amoebiasis, laryngeal spasm. Specific indication: bronchitic asthma.

Cautions: While lower dosage range is recommended, oral administration of *E. hirta* extract for 90 days does not cause sub-chronic toxicity.

Contraindications: None known

Qualities: Acrid, bitter, cool

Typical dosage: 5–15 ml per week

Euphrasia officinalis

Synonym or related species: Euphrasia rostkoviana

Common names: Eyebright

Family: Scrophulariaceae

Part used: Aerial parts

Description: Traditional herbal medicinal product for symptomatic treatment and prevention of conjunctivitis of any etiology (allergic, irritative, infectious), common cold. The common name refers to the symptoms of conjunctivitis.

Constituents: Flavonoids including apigenin, luteolin, kaempferol, rhamnetin, quercetin; polyphenol, phenolic acids including caffeic, coumaric and chlorogenic acids, and their derivatives, hydroxycinnamic derivatives, tannins and iridoids, notably aucubin.

Primary actions: Anti-inflammatory, Anticatarrhal, Astringent.

All actions: Anti-inflammatory, Anticatarrhal, Astringent, Mucous membrane tonic.

Indications:

- Catarrh; naso-pharyngeal congestion, Common cold, Conjunctivitis (locally as eye lotion), Hayfever, Sinusitis.
- **BHP:** Nasal catarrh, sinusitis, conjunctivitis (locally as eye lotion). Specific indication: conjunctivitis.

Contraindications: None known

Qualities: Dry 1st degree, hot 1st degree

Typical dosage: 20–40 ml per week

Eutrochium purpureum

Synonym or related species: Eupatorium purpureum

Common names: Gravel root, purple or sweet Joe Pye weed

Family: Asteraceae

Part used: Root

Description: Mainly used for disorders of the urogenital system including urinary and renal calculi and gravel. Also used for irritable bladder and incontinence including nocturnal enuresis.

Constituents: Essential oil, euparin (yellow flavonoid), resin.

All actions: Antilithic, Antirheumatic, Diuretic.

Indications:

- Cystitis, Dysuria, Gout, Influenza, Prostatitis, Psoriasis, Rheumatism, Urethritis.
- **BHP:** Urinary calculus, cystitis, dysuria, urethritis, prostatitis, rheumatism, gout. Specific indication: renal or vesicular calculi.

Contraindications: None known

Qualities: Cooling potential, dry

Typical dosage: 15–30 ml per week

Filipendula ulmaria

Common names: Meadowsweet

Family: Rosaceae

Part used: Aerial parts

Description: Contrary to popular belief, acetylsalicylic acid (aspirin) was eventually synthesised from compounds in meadowsweet, not willow bark. Mostly used in gastrointestianal and urological disorders. Meadowsweet extract has recently been shown in rodent studies to inhibit breast carcinogenesis, prevent or ameliorate cisplatin side effects, and to inhibit radiation carcinogenesis.

Constituents: Phenolic glycosides, essential oil, tannins, mucilage and flavonoids. Contains 0.2% essential oil consisting of 75% salicylaldehyde, 3% phenylethyl alcohol, 2% benzyl alcohol, 2% anisaldehyde, and 1.3% methyl salicylate.

Primary actions: Antacid, Anti-inflammatory, Antirheumatic.

All actions: Antacid, Anti-inflammatory, Anti-inflammatory (GIT), Antidiarrhoeal, Antirheumatic, Antiseptic (urinary), Astringent, Diaphoretic, Diuretic, Gastroprotective, Stomachic.

Indications:

- Calculi; kidney and bladder, Cystitis, Diarrhoea, Dyspepsia, Dyspepsia; nervous, Flatulence, Gastric reflux, Gastritis, Gastrointestinal catarrh, Gout, Hyperchlorhydria, Indigestion, Inflammation; gastrointestinal tract, Inflammatory bowel disease, Irritable bowel syndrome, Rheumatism, Ulcer;

gastrointestinal, Wounds.

BHP: Atonic dyspepsia with heartburn and hyperacidity, acute catarrhal cystitis, rheumatic muscle and joint pains, diarrhoea of children. Specific indication: peptic ulcer (prophylaxis and treatment).

ESCOP: As supportive therapy for common cold. It is also used to enhance the renal elimination of water, although published scientific evidence does not adequately support this indication.

Contraindications: Due to the presence of salicylates it should not be used in cases of hypersensitivity to salicylates. Contraindicated in constipation, iron deficiency anaemia, and malnutrition, due to high tannin content.

Drug interactions: Suspend use of concentrated extracts one week before major surgery. Increased bleeding may occur due to anticoagulant activity; observe patients taking warfarin concurrently.

Qualities: Cold, dry

Typical dosage: 15–30 ml per week

Foeniculum vulgare

Synonym or related species: Anethum foeniculum

Common names: Fennel

Family: Apiaceae

Part used: Seed

Description: Traditionally used for dyspeptic complaints such as mild, spasmodic gastrointestinal ailments, bloating and flatulence and catarrh of the upper respiratory tract.

Constituents: Anethole (essential oil), bergapten (5-methoxypsoralen), camphene, coumarin, fenchone, fixed oil, kaempferol, limonene, phellandrene (essential oil), pinene (essential oil), protein, quercetin glucosides, resin, rutin, sterols, tannin.

Primary actions: Aromatic, Carminative, Galactagogue.

All actions: Anti-inflammatory, Antimicrobial, Aromatic, Carminative, Diuretic, Galactagogue, Selective oestrogen receptor modulator (SERM).

Indications:

• Anorexia, Colic; childhood, Colic; intestinal, Dyspepsia; flatulent, Indigestion, Inflammatory bowel disease, Lactation; poor, Pharyngitis.

• **BHP:** Flatulent dyspepsia, anorexia, flatulent colic in children. Topically for conjunctivitis, blepharitis, pharyngitis. Specific indication: flatulence in infants.

• **ESCOP:** Dyspeptic complaints such as mild, spasmodic gastrointestinal ailments, bloating and flatulence. Catarrh of the upper respiratory tract.

• **WHO:** Symptomatic treatment of dyspepsia, bloating and flatulence. As an expectorant for mild inflammation of the upper respiratory tract. Treatment of pain in scrotal hernia and dysmenorrhoea.

Cautions: Aqueous infusions of fennel may be used at the recommended dosage during pregnancy, under professional supervision. The pure essential oil from the fruits may cause inflammation, and has an irritant action on the gastrointestinal tract.

Contraindications: Persons with known sensitivity to anethole and plants in the Apiacaeae family should avoid the use of fennel. Preparations containing essential oils or alcoholic extracts should not be used during pregnancy and lactation. Pure essential oils should not be given to infants and young children owing to the danger of laryngeal spasm, dyspnoea and CNS excitation.

Qualities: Dry, warm

Typical dosage: 20–40 ml per week

Fucus vesiculosus

Common names: Bladderwrack

Family: Phaeophyceae

Part used: Aerial parts

Description: Traditionally used as a source of iodine. Brown macroalgae, particularly those from Fucus genus, are a rich and balanced source of bioactive nutrients and phytochemicals, including fucoidan.

Constituents: Dietary fibres (fucoidans, laminarins, and/or alginates), phlorotannins, and fucoxanthin, and some minerals, including iodine.

Primary actions: Antiobesity, Antirheumatic, Thyroid stimulant.

All actions: Anti-inflammatory, Anticancer, Antidiabetic, Antiobesity, Antirheumatic, Thyroid stimulant.

Indications:

• Cancer; including prevention/supportive treatment, Diabetes, Metabolic syndrome, Rheumatism, Rheumatoid arthritis, Thyroid gland; impaired, Weight loss; to assist.

• **BHP:** Myxoedema, lymphadenoid goitre, obesity, rheumatism and rheumatoid arthritis internally and/or the juice applied topically. Specific indication: obesity associated with hypothyroidism.

Cautions: Iodine can cross the placenta, therefore should not be taken in high and prolonged doses during pregnancy. Do not use during pregnancy or lactation without professional advice. Use with caution in patients with underlying thyroid disorders other than low thyroid function or conditions resulting from iodine deficiency. Monitor patient thyroid hormone levels, particularly if using long-term.

Contraindications: Not recommended in patients with hyperthyroidism, cardiac problems associated with hyperthyroidism or a known sensitivity to iodine.

Drug interactions: May theoretically increase effect of hyperthyroid medication. Avoid with carbimazole (antithyroid medication), including neo-mercazole, thyroid replacement therapies (e.g. thyroxine), lithium carbonate and iodine-containing medication (e.g. amiodarone, benziodarone).

Qualities: Cold 1st degree, moist

Typical dosage: 30–60 ml per week

Fumaria officinalis

Common names: Fumitory

Family: Fumariaceae

Part used: Aerial parts

Description: Traditionally used to increase bile flow for the relief of symptoms of indigestion such as sensation of fullness, flatulence and slow digestion. Also used for diabetes, hypertension and cardiac disorders.

Constituents: Fumitory contains seven alkaloids, the principal one being fumarine. Alkaloids, caffeic acid, chlorogenic acid, flavonoids, fumaric acid, fumarine, potassium, quercetin glycosides, tannic acid.

Primary actions: Choleretic, Digestive tonic, Diuretic.

All actions: Choleretic, Diuretic, Hepatoprotective, Laxative, Stomachic, Tonic.

Indications:

- Digestive complaints, Digestive weakness, Eczema, Gallbladder disorders, Liver insufficiency.
- **BHP:** Cutaneous eruptions, as eye lotion for conjunctivitis. Specific indication: chronic eczema.
- **Commission E:** Spastic discomfort in the area of the gall bladder and bile ducts, as well as the gastrointestinal tract.
- **Other uses:** A clinical trial examined *Curcuma xanthorriza* 60 mg daily and 1500 mg fumitory for IBS. Neither fumitory nor curcuma showed any therapeutic benefit over placebo in patients with IBS.

Contraindications: None known

Qualities: Cold 1st degree, dry

Typical dosage: 10–30 ml per week

Galega officinalis

Common names: Goat's rue

Family: Fabaceae

Part used: Aerial parts

Description: The hypoglycemic effect of goat's rue was investigated in 1927, however, the literature data concerning the sugar-lowering effects of the herb and seeds are controversial. Galegine's blood glucose-lowering activity was the foundation for the discovery of metformin. Two small studies found that a galactogogue combination of *Galega officinalis* and silymarin improved breastfeeding to preterm neonates after discharge and for the first three months of life.

Constituents: Alkaloids (0.1–0.2%), including derivatives of guanidine galegine and hydroxyl-

4-galegine; derivatives of quinazoline – peganine and 2-3-oxy-quinazolone-4, glycoside galuteolin, flavonoids (kaempferol, quercetin, rutin), tannins, hydroxycinnamic acids, saponins, bitters, pectins.

All actions: Antidiabetic, Galactagogue, Hypoglycaemic.

Indications:

- Diabetes, Fluid retention, Lactation; poor.
- **BHP:** Diabetes mellitus.

Contraindications: None known

Drug interactions: Caution with people taking insulin or oral hypoglycaemic drugs due to possible enhanced reduction of blood glucose.

Qualities: Cool, dry

Typical dosage: 30–60 ml per week

Galium aparine

Common names: Clivers, cleavers

Family: Rubiaceae

Part used: Aerial parts

Description: Written up as a remedy for chronic ulcers in the British Medical Journal 1883. Galium is a traditional alterative for chronic skin disorders including acne, eczema, urticaria and psoriasis, asthma, gout, and lymphadenopathy.

Constituents: Iridoids, including monotropein, 10-desacetylasperulosidic acid and asperulosidic acid; p-hydroxybenzoic acid; hydroxycinnamic acid derivatives including 3-O-caffeoylquinic, 5-O-caffeoylquinic, 3,4-O-dicaffeoylquinic, 3,5-O-dicaffeoylquinic, 4,5-O-dicaffeoylquinic acids and caffeic acid derivatives; flavonoids, including rutin, quercetin 3-O-rhamnoglucoside-7-O-glucoside, and isorhamnetin 3-O-glucorhamnoside.

Actions: Astringent, Diuretic, Lymphatic.

Indications:

- Acne, Asthma, Eczema, Glands; swollen, Gout, Lymphadenopathy, Mumps, Osteoarthritis, Psoriasis, Urticaria.
- **BHP:** Dysuria, lymphadenitis, psoriasis. Specific indication: enlarged lymph nodes.

Contraindications: None known

Qualities: Cold, pungent

Typical dosage: 30–50 ml per week

Ganoderma lucidum

Common names: Reishi, lingzhi

Family: Ganodermataceae

Part used: Fruiting body

Description: Reishi has been used as a medicine for over 2000 years as documented in ancient scripts. Chinese physicians readily employ it to support immune resistance in patients treated with chemotherapy and/or radiation treatment for various forms of cancer. Reishi is also used for its hepatoprotective, antihyperlipidaemic, and hypoglycemic properties and is considered to have marked positive effects on sleep and mental well-being. Considered a qi tonic in TCM.

Constituents: The dried and whole fruiting body of reishi has been reported to contain approximately 400 different bioactive compounds, which mainly include triterpenes, triterpenoids, polysaccharides, sterols, steroids, fatty acids, proteins, peptides, and trace elements, among others. The main bioactive compounds are ganomastenol, ganomastenol B, ganomastenol C, ganomastenol D, ganoderic acids A–Z, ganoderal A–B, ganoderol A–B, epoxyganoderiol A–C, ganoderenic acid A–D, β-1-3, β-1-6 homo D-glucan, acidic glucan, polyglycan, protein bound heteroglucan, arabinoxyoglucan, ganoderan A–C (peptidoglycans), serine, alanine, glycine, threonine, aspartic acid, glutamic acid, proline, valine, other minor amino acids, ergosterol, adenosine, among numerous others.

Primary actions: Anticancer, Hepatoprotective, Immunomodulator.

All actions: Antiandrogenic, Antiatherosclerotic, Anticancer, Antidiabetic, Antihyperlipidemic, Antihypertensive, Antimicrobial, Antiviral (systemically), Expectorant (general), Gastroprotective, Hepatoprotective, Hepatotonic, Immunomodulator, Sedative, Tonic.

Indications:

- Asthma; bronchial, Atherosclerosis, Cancer; including prevention/supportive treatment, Cough, Debility, Diabetes, Dyslipidaemia, Dyspepsia, Fatigue, Hepatitis, Immune deficiency, Infection; gastrointestinal system, Stress.

Contraindications: Reishi and its extracts should be avoided in organ transplant patients receiving immunosuppressive agents or in patients with autoimmune diseases.

Qualities: Sour, bitter, sweet, hot, salty (depending upon strain)

Typical dosage: 1.5–3 g daily.

Gentiana lutea

Synonym or related species: Asterias lutea

Common names: Gentian

Family: Gentianaceae

Part used: Root

Description: Gentian is a key ingredient in apéritifs, liqueurs, and tonics. Best known as a bitter tonic used in digestive disorders and anorexia, pharmacological investigations have also found antiviral, antibacterial, anti-inflammatory, analgesic, hepatoprotective and choleretic activities.

Constituents: Iridoids (loganic acid), secoiridoids (swertiamarin, gentiopicroside, amarogentin, sweroside), xanthones (gentisin, isogentisin) and two xanthone glycosides (gentiosides). Analysis of several commercially available G. lutea samples showed that gentiopicroside is the most dominant compound in the specimens (4.46–9.53%), followed by loganic acid (0.10–0.76%), swertiamarin (0.21–0.45%) and the xanthone glycosides. Gentisin and isogentisin were found in much lower concentrations between 0.02 and 0.11%, respectively. Recent studies indicate that bitters elicit a range of cephalic responses which alter postprandial gastric phase haemodynamics. Gentian and wormwood have been found elicit cephalic responses which facilitate rather than stimulate digestive activity when postprandial hyperaemia is inadequate.

Primary actions: Bitter tonic, Cholagogue, Digestive stimulant.

All actions: Bitter tonic, Cholagogue, Choleretic, Digestive tonic, Sialogogue.

Indications:

- Allergies/Sensitivities, Anorexia, Convalescence, Digestive complaints, Dyspepsia, Flatulence, Halitosis, Hypochlorhydria, Nausea.
- **BHP:** Anorexia, atonic dyspepsia and gastrointestinal atony. Specific indication: dyspepsia with anorexia.
- **Commission E:** Anorexia, eg., after illness, dyspeptic complaints.
- **WHO:** Treatment of digestive complaints, such as dyspepsia, loss of appetite, feeling of distension and flatulence. As an appetite stimulant during convalescence.

Cautions: Overdose may lead to nausea and vomiting.

Contraindications: Contraindicated in gastric or duodenal ulcer, or hyperacidity.

Qualities: Cold, dry

Typical dosage: 5–15 ml per week. For optimal effect, take 15 minutes before meals.

Geranium maculatum

Common names: Cranesbill

Family: Geraniaceae

Part used: Root

Description: 'Geranium is a powerful astringent. Used in an infusion with milk in the second stage of dysentery, diarrhoea, and cholera infantum. Relaxed mucous tissues, with profuse, debilitating discharges; chronic diarrhoea, with mucus discharges; chronic dysentery; diarrhoea, with constant desire to evacuate the bowels; passive haemorrhages.' King's American Dispensary, 1898

Constituents: Tannin

Primary actions: Antidiarrhoeal, Astringent, Wound healing/Vulnerary.

Indications:

- Diarrhoea, Dysentery, Haematemesis, Haemorrhoids, Menorrhagia, Ulcer (topically),

Ulcer; gastrointestinal.

BHP: Diarrhoea, dysentery, haemorrhoids, duodenal ulceration, haematemesis, melaena, menorrhagia, metrorrhagia. Topically for leucorrhoea and indolent ulcers. Specific indications: diarrhoea (particularly in the young and old), peptic ulcer.

Cautions: Because of the tannin content, long-term use should be avoided. Use cautiously in highly inflamed or ulcerated conditions of the gastrointestinal tract.

Contraindications: Contraindicated in constipation and iron-deficiency anaemia.

Qualities: Cold, dry

Typical dosage: 15–35 ml per week

Ginkgo biloba

Common names: Maidenhair

Family: Ginkgoaceae

Part used: Leaves

Description: Revered for its beauty and its longevity, the ginkgo is a living fossil, unchanged for more than 200 million years. It is the oldest tree on earth. Cultivation started in China over 1000 years ago. Wild species native to China are believed to be members of mixed mesophytic forests that at one point covered the hill country along the Yangtze River valley border. The ginkgo has tremendous medicinal, spiritual, and horticultural importance in Chinese culture. First introduced to the Western world by Engelbert Kaempfer who worked for the Dutch East India Company in Japan in 1692. In traditional medicine, the ginkgo seed was used for digestive complaints. The medical use of the leaf was developed in Germany starting in 1965. The first commercially extract, EGb761 was registered in France in 1974.

Constituents: Bilobalides (sesquiterpenes), ginkgoflavonoid glycosides, ginkgolides (diterpener).

Primary actions: Nootropic, Vasoprotective, Venotonic.

All actions: Anti-inflammatory, Antioxidant, Antiplatelet, Cytoprotective, Nootropic, PAF inhibitor, Vasodilator, Venotonic.

Indications:

- Alzheimer's disease, Arteriosclerosis, Atherosclerosis, Benign breast disease, Cataract and diabetic complications, Catarrhal deafness, Cerebrovascular disease, Circulation; peripheral; impaired, Dementia, Depression, Diabetes, Diabetic neuropathy, Diabetic retinopathy, DVT prophylaxis, Dysmenorrhoea, Dysmenorrhoea; congestive, Intermittent claudication, Mastalgia, Memory and concentration; poor, Mental exhaustion, Psoriasis, Raynaud's syndrome, Retinal blood flow disorders, Retinal damage, Senile macular degeneration, Stroke; recovery after, Tinnitus, Venous insufficiency, Vertigo.

- **ESCOP:** Symptomatic treatment of mild to moderate dementia syndromes, cerebral insufficiency and peripheral arterial occlusive disease. For the treatment of neurosensory disturbances such as dizziness, vertigo and tinnitus. Used to enhance cognitive performance.

- **WHO:** Symptomatic treatment of mild to moderate cerebrovascular insufficiency (demential syndromes in primary degenerative dementia, vascular dementia, and mixed forms of both) with the following symptoms: memory deficit, disturbance in concentration, depressive emotional condition, dizziness, tinnitus, and headache. To improve pain-free walking distance in people with peripheral arterial occlusive disease such as intermittent claudication, Raynaud disease, acrocyanosis, and post-phlebitis syndrome. To treat inner ear disorders such as tinnitus and vertigo of vascular and involutive origin.

Drug interactions: Antiplatelet activity may theoretically potentiate antiplatelet or anticoagulant medication, however, clinical studies and meta-analysis found no increased risk of increased bleeding (no effect on INR, haemorrhage, or bruising. May decrease efficacy of anticonvulsant medication (case report) and HIV non-nucleoside transcriptase (case report). May potentiate the efficiency of antipsychotic medication for schizophrenia. May increase blood levels of talinolol. May enhance hypoglycaemic activity of metformin, pioglitazone and glipizide. Effect on benzodiazepines unlikely to be clinically significant. May interact with nifedipine (headaches, dizziness and hot flushes reported). Interaction with statins and other cholesterol-lowering drugs unlikely to be clinically significant.

Sodium aescinate

Avoid: A case of a 58-year-old man with phalangeal fractures suffered from acute kidney injury that was most likely induced by the drug interaction between sodium aescinate and ginkgo biloba extract due to the protein-binding and metabolic characteristics of these drugs (Ji, Zhang et al. 2017).

Ginkgo may accelerate the metabolism of atorvastatin (in vivo study). The clinical dose of atorvastatin may be decreased when co-administered with ginkgo (Ren et al., 2019).

Ginkgo may increase the plasma concentration of losartan and decrease the concentration of its metabolite EXP3174 through inhibiting the metabolism of losartan (Dong et al., 2018).

References:

Dong B, Yuan S, Hu J, Yan Y (2018) Effects of Ginkgo leaf tablets on the pharmacokinetics of losartan and its metabolite EXP3174 in rats and its mechanism. Pharm Biol 56:333-336

Ji H, Zhang G, Yue F, Zhou X (2017) Adverse event due to a likely interaction between sodium aescinate and ginkgo biloba extract: a case report. J Clin Pharm Ther 42:237-238

Ren Y, Li H, Liu X (2019) Effects of Ginkgo leaf tablets on the pharmacokinetics of atorvastatin in rats. Pharm Biol 57:403-406

Qualities: Cooling

Typical dosage: 20 ml per week (standardised extract). Double dose for severe dementia or Alzheimer's disease. 120–240 mg of 50:1 extract standardised to 24% ginkgo flavones.

Glechoma hederacea

Synonym or related species: Nepeta hederacea

Common names: Ground ivy

Family: Lamiaceae

Part used: Aerial parts

Description: Traditional anticatarrhal for upper respiratory tract infections and for inflammatory disorders. Not be confused with *Hedera helix* (English ivy) which also has anticatarrhal and expectorant properties. In mice, ground ivy inhibited the release of interferon-gamma and lipopolysaccharide-stimulated macrophages, decreasing the release of nitric oxide in a dose-dependent manner. A hot water extract significantly decreased the LPS-induced mRNA expression of iNOS, COX-2, TNF-α, IL-6, and IL-1β in RAW264.7 macrophages, and reduced the LPS-induced protein expression of iNOS and COX-2 in RAW264.7 macrophages. These results show that the hot water extracts have significcnat antioxidant and anti-inflammatory properties. In traditional Chinese medicine, *Glechoma hederacea* is frequently prescribed to patients with cholelithiasis, dropsy, abscess, diabetes, inflammation, and jaundice.

Constituents: Essential oil, glechomine (bitter principle), tannin, triterpenoids, such as ursolic acid and oleanic acid. Rosmarinic acid, chlorogenic acid, caffeic acid, rutin, genistin, and ferulic acid were the most abundant phytochemicals in a hot water extract. Ursolic acid and oleanolic acid shown to inhibits 12-O-tetradecanoylphorbol-13-acetate (TPA)-induced activation of Epstein Barr virus. These constituents also inhibit in vivo TPA tumor promotion in mouse skin.

Primary actions: Anticatarrhal, Antidiarrhoeal, Astringent.

All actions: Anti-inflammatory, Antidiarrhoeal, Astringent, Diuretic, Hepatoprotective, Stomachic, Wound healing/Vulnerary.

Indications:

- Bronchitis, Cystitis, Diarrhoea, Gastritis, Haemorrhoids.
- **BHP:** Chronic diarrhoea, pharyngitis (gargle), leucorrhoea and boils (topically). Specific indications: leucorrhoea and vaginitis (douche)

Contraindications: None known

Qualities: Pungent, warm

Typical dosage: 20–40 ml per week

Glycine max

Common names: Soy, soy germ, soy isoflavones (genistein), phyto-oestrogens, tofu (bean curd)

Family: Fabaceae

Part used: Bean

Description: Phyto-oestrogens exert oestrogenic and antioestrogenic effects depending on the status of the hormonal system. Isoflavones should no longer be considered phyto-oestrogens, as they do not act as simple oestrogen agonists; today they are considered as selective oestrogen receptor modulators (SERMs).

Soy isoflavones inhibit lipid oxidation, stimulate hormone binding globulin, inhibit aromatase, inhibit 5-alpha reductase, inhibit 17 beta-hydroxysteroid-dehydrogenase, reduce proliferation (via inhibition of tyrosine kinase, vascular endothelial growth factor (VEGF) and NFkappaB), angiogensis (inhibits VEGF) and stimulate apoptosis of cancer cells.

Constituents: Soy contains carbohydrates, proteins and lipids (15% saturated fat, 61% polyunsaturated fat, and 24% monounsaturated fat; no cholesterol). The nutritional profile of soy germ is similar to whole soy; however, several nutrients are found in higher quantities than in whole soybeans, such as tocopherols, oligosaccharides, phytosterols and slightly more protein and isoflavones. The high level of oligosaccharides in soy germ acts as a prebiotic.

The main isoflavones are genistein and daidzein. Soybean contains micronutrients including isoflavones, phytate, soyaponins, phytosterol, vitamins and minerals.

All actions: Antihyperlipidemic, Antioxidant, Chemoprotective, Selective oestrogen receptor modulator (SERM).

Indications:

- Allergies/Sensitivities, Arteriosclerosis, Atherosclerosis, Cancer; including prevention/supportive treatment, Crohn's disease, Diarrhoea, Digestive complaints, Hypertension, Menopausal symptoms, Migraine, Obesity, Osteoarthritis, Osteoporosis prevention, Rheumatoid arthritis, Weight loss; to assist.

- **Commission E:** For moderate disturbances of fat metabolism, especially hypercholesterolaemia, if dietary and other non-medical interventions are not sufficient.

- **Other uses:** The effects are likely to be more significant if the soy intake is started early in life. Many of the effects are seen in population studies where the soy intake was initiated in childhood. As soy has direct anti-cancer properties including pro-apoptotic and pro-differentiating activity and wholefood soybased foods including tofu and soymilk as well as soygerm or soy extracts can be used for all cancers including oestrogen-sensitive prostate cancer.

Cautions: Avoid use of soy isoflavone supplements during pregnancy and lactation.

Contraindications: Isolated isoflavones are not recommended for women or men with a personal or family history of cancer, particularly prostate cancer and oestrogen-positive tumours, respectively. Avoid if allergic to soy.

Drug interactions: Soy isoflavones act as selective oestrogen receptor beta (ER-β) agonists. This favours a normalisation of cell proliferation at the breast, the uterus and the prostate; a reduction of hot flushes; health benefits for the cardiovascular system, dyslipidaemia and an improvement of bone mineral modelling. Coadministration with oestrogens may provide additive effects and may reduce drug-adverse effects.

Typical dosage: Used as a food. Soygerm and isolated flavanoid extracts available. Soy extract equivalent to 50 mg isoflavones daily.

Glycyrrhiza spp.

Synonym or related species: G. glabra, G. uralensis

Common names: Licorice, Liquorice, Gan Cao

Family: Fabaceae

Part used: Root

Description: Liquorice is a great flavour modifier and sweetener for strong tasting liquid herbal extracts but also a great medicinal plant.

Constituents: Bitter principles, coumarin, flavonoids, glycyrrhizin (triterpene saponin), liquiritin, polysaccharides, sterols.

Primary actions: Anti-inflammatory, Expectorant (general), Taste improver.

All actions: Adaptogen, Aldose reductase inhibitor, Anti-inflammatory, Anti-inflammatory (GIT), Anti-inflammatory (urinary), Antiandrogenic, Antiasthmatic, Antihyperprolactinaemic, Antiseptic (urinary), Antispasmodic (muscles), Antispasmodic (respiratory tract), Antispasmodic (uterus), Antitussive, Antiviral (topically), Blood sugar regulator, Choleretic, Cytoprotective, Demulcent, Expectorant (relaxing), Gastroprotective, Hepatoprotective, Laxative, Selective oestrogen receptor modulator (SERM), Taste improver.

Indications:

- Acne (topically), Addison's disease, Androgen excess, Asthma, Bronchitis, Chronic fatigue syndrome, Constipation, Convalescence, Cough, Eczema, Emphysema, Endometriosis, Flavouring, Gastritis, Gout, Hepatitis, Herpes (topically), Infertility, Inflammation; respiratory tract, Irritable bowel syndrome, Ovarian cyst, Polycystic ovarian syndrome, Psoriasis, Sore throat (gargle), Stress, Tracheitis, Ulcer; gastrointestinal.

- **BHP:** Bronchial catarrh, bronchitis, chronic gastritis, peptic ulcer, colic and primary adrenocortical insufficiency. Specific indication: gastric or duodenal ulcer, Addison's disease.

- **ESCOP:** Adjuvant therapy of gastric and duodenal ulcers and gastritis. As an expectorant to treat coughs and bronchial catarrh.

- **WHO:** As a demulcent in the treatment of sore throats, and as an expectorant in the treatment of coughs and bronchial catarrh. Also in the prophylaxis and treatment of gastric and duodenal ulcers, and dyspepsia. As an anti-inflammatory agent in the treatment of allergic reactions, rheumatism and arthritis, to prevent liver toxicity, and to treat tuberculosis and adrenocorticoid insufficiency.

Cautions: Large doses over a long period may result in depletion of potassium levels in the body (especially the high grade licorice which contains a higher amount of glycyrrhizin) and reduce sodium excretion, causing water accumulation, swelling of the hands and feet and possible raised blood pressure. Do not administer during lactation or with corticosteroid treatment without medical supervision. In rare cases, myoglobinuria and myopathy can occur. Use with caution in men with a history of impotence, infertility or decreased libido, as it may reduce testosterone levels. Caution in the elderly and those with cardiac, renal or hepatic disease.

Contraindications: Do not administer during pregnancy, cardiovascular related disorders such as hypertension, congestive heart failure and fluid retention, renal disorders, cholestatic or inflammatory liver disorders, hypokalaemia, hypotonia, anorexia nervosa and severe obesity.

Drug interactions: Oral contraceptives may increase the risk of licorice-induced side effects including hypokalaemia, fluid retention and hypertension.

Avoid with betablockers and other hypotensive medication (Enalapril, Peridopril, Atenolol, amlodipine). Long-term use may elevate blood pressure, reducing drug efficacy. Licorice may increase potassium excretion, therefore avoid with digoxin (Lanoxin, Sigmaxin), potassium depletion may increase digoxin toxicity. Avoid with thiazide (potassium-depleting diuretics including Accuretic and Amizide).

A constituent of licorice has demonstrated potentiation of chemotherapy medication (paclitaxel, vinblastine).

Liquiritigenin inhibits aromatase, reducing the conversion of androgens to oestrogens and has been shown to have a weak oestrogen-like effect by binding to the oestrogen receptor beta (ER-β).

May decrease metabolism and therefore potentiate the effect of cortisone and prednisolone (Cortate, Presolone, Solone): use with caution to avoid corticosteroid excess.

Glycyrrhiza and glycyrrhetinic acid may slow the metabolism of warfarin via inhibition of CYP3A4 potentially increase bleeding time (Song et al., 2020).

Reference: Song J, Dai H, Zhang H, Liu Y, Zhang W (2020) Influence of glycyrrhetinic acid on the pharmacokinetics of warfarin in rats. Xenobiotica 50:602-605

Grindelia camporum

Qualities: Moist, neutral

Typical dosage: 20–40 ml per week

Synonym or related species: Grindelia robusta

Common names: Gum weed

Family: Asteraceae

Part used: Aerial parts

Description: 'Traditionally used for asthmatic breathing, with soreness and raw feeling in the chest; cough, harsh and dry; breathing labored, with a dusky coloration of the face in plethoric individuals.' – *King's American Dispensatory*, 1898. What a description from the masters of yesteryear!

Constituents: Essential oil containing borneol (15.2%), alpha pinene (10.3%), trans-pinocarveol (7.0%), bornyl acetate (4.5%), limonene (4.3%); flavonoids and hydroxycinnamic acids, grindelin (saponin), grindeline (bitter alkaloid), resin. Diosmetin-7-O-glucuronide-3'-O-pentoside-apigenin-7-O-glucuronide-4'-O-pentoside, apigenin-7-O-glucuronide+diosmetin-7-O-glucuronide and 3,5-dicaffeoylquinic acid+3,4-dicaffeoylquinic acid are the major flavonoid compounds.

Primary actions: Antiasthmatic, Anticatarrhal, Antifungal.

All actions: Anti-inflammatory, Antiasthmatic, Antifungal, Antispasmodic (respiratory tract), Expectorant (stimulating).

Indications:

- Asthma, Bronchitis, Pertussis, Tachycardia.
- **BHP:** Asthma and bronchitis, upper respiratory catarrh, whooping cough, cystitis. Specific indication: bronchial asthma associated with tachycardia.

Cautions: Large doses have been reported to cause irritation to the kidneys. Contact dermatitis has been reported as an adverse reaction.

Contraindications: None known

Qualities: Pungent, warm

Typical dosage: 10–20 ml per week

Guaiacum officinale

Synonym or related species: Guaiacum sanctum

Common names: Guaiacum

Family: Zygophyllaceae

Part used: Resin

Description: Guaiacum is used to treat chronic rheumatism and gout, relieving the pain and inflammation between the attacks, and lessening their recurrence if doses are continued. Reumalex (a herbal medicine containing 100 mg dried White Willow bark, 40 mg dried Guaiacum Resin, 35 mg dried *Actaea racemosa*, 25 mg, dry extract of sarsparilla 4:1 and 17 mg dry extract of *Populus*

spp. 7:1) equivalent to 20–40mg/day salicylic acid was found in a small, randomised controlled clinical trial to exert a mild analgesic effect in 82 patients with arthritic pain compared to placebo. Guaiacum powder can be used for tonsillitis.

Constituents: Resin acids and triterpenoid saponins. Main ingredients are α- and β-guaiaconic acid, guaiaretic acid, guaiacic acid, guaiacsapnoic acid, and guaiacsaponin.

Primary actions: Anti-inflammatory, Antirheumatic, Diuretic.

All actions: Anti-inflammatory, Antirheumatic, Diaphoretic, Diuretic, Hepatoprotective.

Indications:

- Arthritis, Gout, Rheumatism, Rheumatoid arthritis.
- **BHP:** Rheumatoid arthritis, sub-acute and chronic rheumatism, prophylactically for gout. Specific indications: chronic rheumatism, rheumatoid arthritis.

Cautions: Guaiacum is a threatened species. Use sparingly or find a suitable alternative.

Contraindications: None known

Qualities: Bitter, cool

Typical dosage: 5–15 ml per week

Gymnema sylvestre

Common names: Gumar, meshashringi

Family: Asclepiadaceae

Part used: Leaves

Description: Gumar means 'sugar destroyer' in Hindi. Gymnemic acid has anti-obesity and antidiabetic properties, decreases body weight and also inhibits glucose absorption. Several components extracted from gymnema prevent the accumulation of triglycerides in muscle and liver, and also decrease fatty acid accumulation in the circulation. May be beneficial in both type 1 and 2 diabetes. Chewing a small leaf or applying a few drops of an extract to the tongue will anesthetise the sweet taste buds for several hours. Great party trick!

Constituents: Damarene and triterpene saponins, flavonol glycosides, quercitol, lapel, anthraquinone, sterols including gurmarin, gymnemic acid and gymnemasaponins.

Primary actions: Antidiabetic, Hypoglycaemic, Pancreatic trophorestorative.

All actions: Anti-inflammatory, Anticancer, Antihyperlipidemic, Antimicrobial, Appetite inhibitor, Astringent, Blood sugar regulator, Hepatoprotective, Hypoglycaemic, Pancreatic trophorestorative.

Indications:

- Cataract and diabetic complications, Diabetic neuropathy, Diabetic retinopathy, Hypoglycaemia, Metabolic syndrome, Obesity, Sweet cravings, Weight loss; to assist.
- **Other uses:** In Ayurveda, gymnema is prescribed

for the treatment of dyspepsia, constipation, jaundice, haemorrhoids, renal calculi, cardiopathy, asthma, bronchitis, amenorrhea.

Cautions: May cause irritation of the gastric mucous membranes and reflux.

Contraindications: None known

Drug interactions: May potentiate the blood glucose-lowering effects of insulin and hypoglycaemic agents; use with caution. Concomitant administration of *G. sylvestre* extract improved the clinical outcome of treatment with glimepiride in a diabatic rat model (Kamble et al., 2016).

Reference: Kamble B, Gupta A, Moothedath I, Khatal L, Janrao S, Jadhav A, et al. (2016) Effects of Gymnema sylvestre extract on the pharmacokinetics and pharmacodynamics of glimepiride in streptozotocin induced diabetic rats. Chem Biol Interact 245:30-38

Qualities: Cold 1/2 degree

Typical dosage: 30–75 ml per week

Gynostemma pentaphyllum

Common names: Jiaogulan, xiancao

Family: Cucurbitaceae

Part used: Leaf

Description: Used in traditional Chinese and Japanese medicine. Xiancao means 'immortality herb'. Key indications are elevated uric acid and dyslipidaemia in diabetics with non-alcoholic fatty liver disease (NAFLD) and to help with glycaemic control. AMPK-activator: AMP-activated protein kinase (AMPK) is an energy sensor and master regulator of cellular metabolism. Collectively, activation of AMPK in skeletal muscle, liver, and adipose tissue results may contribute to the prevention or treatment of T2D, i.e., decreased circulating glucose, reduced plasma lipid, and ectopic fat accumulation, as well as enhanced insulin sensitivity.

Constituents: Saponins, known as gypenosides. Of these gypensoides, eight are identical to ginsenosides in *Panax ginseng*, three also occur in *Panax quinquefolius*, and five also in *Gynosemma pentaphyllum*. A sweet tasting variety has the highest level of the gypenosides. The saponins damulin A and B have been found to stimulate AMP-activated protein kinase (AMPK) in vitro. Also contains flavonoids.

Primary actions: Adaptogen, AMPK-activator, Anti-inflammatory.

All actions: Adaptogen, AMPK-activator, Anti-inflammatory, Antihypertensive, Immunomodulator, Tonic.

Indications:

•   Bronchitis, Chronic fatigue syndrome, Diabetes, Dyslipidaemia, Fatigue, Hypertension, Indigestion,

Leukopenia, Metabolic syndrome, Non-alcoholic fatty liver disease (NAFLD), Obesity, Renal insufficiency, Rheumatism.

Drug interactions: May work synergistically with metformin in glucose control.

Qualities: Has been described as bitter and cold, but also sweet and warming depending on the variety.

Typical dosage: 20–40 ml per week

Hamamelis virginiana

Common names: Witch hazel

Family: Hamamelidaceae

Part used: Leaves

Description: Consistent scientific data supporting the efficacy of hamamelis preparations are still limited. Some controlled clinical trials have showed positive outcomes but of weak statistical interpretation. The beneficial effect of hamamelis is primarily supported by traditional use. Diluted ethanol preparations of hamamelis distillate with virtually no tannin content and only a small amount of the essential oil of witch hazel have been widely used in many eye cleansing products.

Constituents: Bitter principles, condensed tannins, essential oil, flavonoids, galotannins, procyanidins, resin

Primary actions: Anti-inflammatory, Astringent, Venotonic.

All actions: Anti-inflammatory, Antidiarrhoeal, Antiseptic (GIT), Astringent, Venotonic.

Indications:

•   Colitis, Diarrhoea, Haemorrhoids, Haemorrhoids (topically).

•   **BHP:** Diarrhoea, mucus colitis, haematemesis, haemoptysis, haemorrhoids. Locally for bruises, inflamed swellings, haemorrhoids. Specific indications: colitis and haemorrhoids.

•   **Commission E:** Minor skin injuries, local inflammation of skin mucous membranes, haemorrhoids and for varicose veins.

•   **ESCOP:** Internal use: Symptomatic treatment of complaints related to varicose veins and haemorrhoids. External use: Bruises, sprains and minor injuries of the skin. Local inflammations of the skin and mucosa, haemorrhoids. Symptom relief for neurodermitis atopica.

•   **WHO:** Topically for minor skin lesions, bruises and sprains, local inflammation of the skin and mucous membranes, haemorrhoids and varicose veins.

Cautions: Do not administer during pregnancy or lactation or to children without professional supervision. Allergic contact dermatitis may occur in sensitive individuals.

Contraindications: None known

Qualities: Cold

Typical dosage: 20–40 ml per week

Handroanthus impetiginosus

Synonym or related species: *Tabebuia impetiginosa*

Common names: Pau d'arco, lapacho (Spanish)

Family: Bignoniaceae

Part used: Dried inner bark

Description: Lapacho was promoted as a cure for cancer in the late 1960s. Traditionally, lapacho is widely used as a decoction prepared from the inner bark of the tree to treat bacterial and fungal infections, fever, syphilis, malaria and protozoal infections, as well as stomach and bladder disorders.

Constituents: Naphthoquinones including lapachol, α-lapachone and β-lapachone with antineoplastic and anti-inflammatory properties.

Primary actions: Anti-inflammatory, Anticancer, Antimicrobial.

All actions: Anthelmintic, Anti-inflammatory, Anticancer, Antifungal, Antimicrobial, Antiviral (systemically).

Indications:

- Allergies/Sensitivities, Cancer; including prevention/supportive treatment, Candidiasis, Gastrointestinal tract dysbiosis, Hypertension, Immune deficiency, Migraine.

- **Other uses:** Orasol Plus™, a Lapacho-based medication, has been shown to ameliorate radiotherapy-induced oral mucositis. Tabetri™ (ethanol extract) has been shown in a mouse model to protect against the development of atopic dermatitis through the inhibition of mRNA expression of T helper 2-specific cytokines and other proinflammatory cytokines. The product has also been shown to reduce inflammation by targeting the nuclear factor-kappa B (NF-κB) and activator protein-1 (AP-1) signaling pathways in macrophages and chondrocytes. In an animal model, Tabetri™ significantly ameliorated OA symptoms and reduced the serum levels of inflammatory mediators and proinflammatory cytokines without any toxicity. β-Lapachone has been shown to be neuroprotective in a mouse mode of Parkinson's disease.

Cautions: Impetiginosa has been associated with interference in the biological cycle of Vitamin K in the body. Caution in patients with allergic profile, as may cause contact dermatitis.

Contraindications: Contraindicated during pregnancy and in patients taking anticoagulant medication.

Drug interactions: Do not use concurrently with anticoagulant medication.

Qualities: Bitter, cold

Typical dosage: 20–50 ml per week

Harpagophytum procumbens

Synonym or related species: *Harpagophytum zeyheri*

Common names: Devil's claw

Family: Pedaliaceae

Part used: Root

Description: Devil's claw has been used in traditional African medicine to treat a variety of disorders including diabetes, hardening of the arteries, lumbago, gastrointestinal disturbances, menstrual difficulties, neuralgia, headache, heartburn and gout. The common name is derived from the unusual appearance of its fruits, which appear to be covered in small hooks. *Harpagophytum*: a direct translation of 'grapple plant' into Greek, and *procumbens*, meaning prostrate. The hooks on the fruits can become entangled in animals' fur and hooves, thus aiding in the dispersal of the seeds. In Southern Africa grazing animals can be injured if they tread on the sharp 'claws' of the fruit, or may even starve if the fruit becomes caught in their mouth.

Constituents: Devil's claw contains 0.5–3% iridoid glucosides primarily the bitter tasting harpagoside, and the slightly sweetly tasting harpagide, as well as 8-(4-coumaroyl)-harpagide, procumbide, its 6'-4'-coumaroyl ester and procumboside. The European Pharmacopoeia prescribes no less than 1.2% harpagoside. Devil's claw also contains sugars including stachyose, raffinose and monosacchararides; as well as flavonol glycosides including verbascoside and isoacteoside; triterpenes, mainly oleanic acid, phytosterols, mainly beta-sitosterol, stigmasterol and their glycosides.

Primary actions: Analgesic, Anti-inflammatory, Bitter tonic.

All actions: Analgesic, Anti-inflammatory, Anti-inflammatory (musculoskeletal), Antiarrhythmic, Antidiarrhoeal, Bitter tonic, Digestive tonic, Vasodilator.

Indications:

- Anorexia, Anxiety, Arrhythmia, Arthritis, Cardiovascular disease prevention, Diarrhoea, Digestive weakness, Gout, Hypertension, Migraine, Myocardial ischaemia, Neuralgia, Osteoarthritis, Rheumatism, Rheumatoid arthritis.

- **BHP:** Rheumatism, arthritis, gout, myalgia, fibrositis, lumbago, pleurodynia. Specific indication: rheumatic disease.

- **Commission E:** Loss of appetite, dyspepsia, degenerative disorders of the locomotive system.

- **ESCOP:** Symptomatic treatment of painful osteoarthritis, relief of lower back pain, loss of appetite and dyspepsia.

- **WHO:** Treatment of pain associated with rheumatic conditions. Treatment of loss of appetite and dyspeptic complaints; supportive treatment of degenerative rheumatism, painful arthrosis and tendonitis.

Cautions: Mild and infrequent gastrointestinal symptoms and allergic reactions of the skin, eyes and respiratory passages have been reported in clinical trials.

Contraindications: Gastric and duodenal ulcers and cases of known hypersensitivity to the roots. Should not be used during pregnancy and lactation due to oxytocic activity.

Drug interactions: Devil's claw may potentiate the effects of warfarin (rare cases), requiring caution and possible dose adjustments. Suspend use of concentrated extract one week before major surgery to avoid increased risk of bleeding.

Qualities: Cold, pungent

Typical dosage: 20–40 ml per week. Higher doses for anti-inflammatory activity. Administer between meals to reduce damage to active constituents by stomach acids.

Hedera helix

Common names: Ivy leaf, English ivy

Family: Araliaceae

Part used: Leaf

Description: Numerous clinical trials support the use of ivy leaf as an expectorant in case of productive cough associated with acute respiratory infection. Several reviews have concluded that ivy leaf is associated with a statistically significant and clinically relevant reductions in the severity of symptoms associated with cough and acute bronchitis. A systematic review found that it improved respiratory functions of children with chronic bronchial asthma. Traditionally, it was used externally for cellulitis, rheumatism, oedema, erythema/burn. Ivy leaf is not to be confused with ground ivy (*Glenchoma hederacea*).

Constituents: Bidesmosidic triterpene saponins (2.5–6%) with hederagenin, oleanolic acid and bayogenin (2β-hydroxyhederagenin) as aglycones. Small amounts of monodesmosides such as α-hederin and hederagenin-3-*O*-β-D-glucoside. Main saponin is the hederasaponin C (hederacoside C) with other hederasaponins (B, D, E, F, G, H and I). Flavonoids such as quercetin and kaempferol including their derivatives isoquercitrin and astragalin. Caffeic acid derivates and other phenolics such as caffeic acid and dihydroxy-benzoic acid. Coumarin glycoside scopolin, polyacetylenes falcarinone, falcarinol and 11,12-dihydrofalcarinol. Phytosterols as stigmasterol, sitosterol, cholesterol, campesterol, α-spinasterol and a volatile oil (in the fresh leaves 0.1–0.3%) consists of methylethyl ketone, methyl isobutyl ketone, trans-hexanal, germacrene D, β-caryphyllene, sabinene, α- and β-pinene.

Primary actions: Anticatarrhal, Antispasmodic (respiratory tract), Bronchodilator.

All actions: Antibacterial, Anticatarrhal, Antifungal, Antispasmodic (respiratory tract), Antiviral (systemically), Bronchodilator, Diaphoretic, Febrifuge,

Hepatoprotective, Spasmolytic, Wound healing/Vulnerary.

Indications:

- Asthma; bronchial, Bronchitis, Common cold, Emphysema, Gall stones (cholelithiasis), Hypertension, Infection; respiratory tract, Laryngitis, Rheumatism, Sinusitis, Tonsillitis, Tracheitis.

- **Commission E:** Treatment of catarrh of the respiratory passages and for symptoms of chronic inflammatory bronchial secretions.

- **ESCOP:** Cough, particularly when associated with hypersecretion of viscous mucus; as adjuvant treatment of inflammatory bronchial disease.

Typical dosage: 5–10 ml per week

Hemidesmus indicus

Common names: Anantamul, Indian sarsparilla

Family: Asclepiadaceae

Part used: Root

Description: Widely used in Indian traditional medicine for treating snakebites, scorpion stings, diabetes, urinary diseases, dyspnoea, menorrhagia, oligospermia, anorexia, fever, abdominal colic and pain, dysentery, diarrhoea, cough, rheumatism, headache, inflammation, pyrosis, skin diseases, leprosy, sexually transmitted diseases and cancer.

Constituents: Coumarin, triterpenoid saponins

Primary actions: Anti-inflammatory, Antiallergic, Depurative/Alterative.

All actions: Anti-inflammatory, Antiallergic, Antiatherosclerotic, Anticancer, Antidiabetic, Antimicrobial, Antispasmodic (muscles), Cardioprotective, Depurative/Alterative, Diaphoretic, Gastroprotective, Hepatoprotective, Neuroprotective, Nootropic.

Indications:

- Allergies/Sensitivities, Autoimmune disease, Eczema, Rheumatoid arthritis, Sinusitis.

Contraindications: None known

Qualities: Cool

Typical dosage: 30–60 ml per week

Houttuynia cordata

Common names: Yu Xing Cao, chameleon plant, fish mint

Family: Saururaceae

Part used: Leaves and stems

Description: Used in TCM for lung disorders including abscess, mucus, cough and dyspnoea. Medical research suggests it has systemic antimicrobial and antimycoplasma activities. Whole plant is eaten raw as a medicinal salad for lowering the blood sugar level. Leaf juice is taken for the treatment of cholera, dysentery, curing of blood deficiency and purification of blood. A decoction of this plant is used internally for the treatment of many ailments including cancer, coughs, dysentery, enteritis and fever.

Constituents: Aristolactams, 5,4-dioxoaporphines including cepharadione B and norcepharadione B, oxoaporphines, amides including houttuynamide A, indoles, ionones, flavonoids including quercitrin, rutin, quercetin and isoquercetin, benzenoids including houttuynoside A, and volatile oils.

Primary actions: Anti-inflammatory, Antimicrobial, Immunomodulator.

All actions: Anti-inflammatory, Antiallergic, Antibacterial, Antidiabetic, Antifungal, Antimicrobial, Antiviral (systemically), Immunomodulator.

Indications:

- Acne, Asthma, Boils, Dermatitis, Diabetes, Infection; bacterial, Infection; fungal, Infection; respiratory tract, Infection; urinary tract, Infection; viral, Leucorrhoea.

Drug interactions: Houttuynia cordata ethanol extract improved glucose-lowering effect of metformin in vivo by reduced renal excretion (You et al., 2018).

Reference: You BH, Chin YW, Kim H, Choi HS, Choi YH (2018) Houttuynia cordata extract increased systemic exposure and liver concentrations of metformin through OCTs and MATEs in rats. Phytother Res 32:1004-1013

Qualities: Cooling

Typical dosage: 10–25 ml per week

Humulus lupulus

Common names: Hops

Family: Cannabinaceae

Part used: Strobilus

Description: Hops are a key ingredient in beer brewing. It is also a source of many biologically active molecules. A notable compound, 8-prenylnaringenin structurally belonging to the group of prenylated flavonoids, has been shown to be a potent phytoestrogen.

Constituents: Condensed tannins, geraniol, humulene (essential oil), linalol (essential oil), luparol (essential oil), lupulin (bitter resin compound), myricin (essential oil), phyto-oestrogeni prenylated flavonoids are isoxanthohumol (IX), 8-prenylnaringenin (8-PN), and 6-prenylnaringenin (6-PN).

Primary actions: Bitter tonic, Sedative, Selective oestrogen receptor modulator (SERM).

All actions: Anodyne, Antitussive, Antiviral (topically), Bitter tonic, Galactagogue, Hypnotic, Sedative, Selective oestrogen receptor modulator (SERM).

Indications:

- Anxiety, Colitis, Diabetes, Dysmenorrhoea, Dyspepsia; nervous, Excitability, Insomnia, Menopausal symptoms, Metabolic syndrome, Neuralgia, Polycystic ovarian syndrome, Restlessness, Weight loss; to assist.
- **BHP:** Neuralgia, insomnia, excitability, priapism, mucous colitis. Topically for crural ulcers. Specific indication: restlessness associated with nervous tension headache and/or indigestion.
- **Commission E:** Mood disturbances such as restlessness and anxiety and sleep disorders.
- **ESCOP:** Tenseness, restlessness and sleep disorders.
- **WHO:** As a sedative for the treatment of nervous tension and insomnia. Treatment of dyspepsia and lack of appetite.
- **Other uses:** Isohumulones can improve insulin sensitivity in high fat diet-fed mice with insulin resistance and in patients with type 2 diabetes.

Cautions: Caution during pregnancy and lactation due to possible hormonal effects. May cause drowsiness in high doses. Avoid in cases of insomnia marked by increasing restlessness during the early hours of the morning. Avoid long-term use.

Contraindications: Contraindicated in cases of known allergy to the plant material, and in patients with oestrogen-dependent tumours and depressive illness.

Drug interactions: Avoid concurrent use with sedative medication. Hops contain flavonones including 8-prenylnaringenin with oestrogenic properties. Coadministration may reduce the activity of prescribed oestrogens.

Qualities: Cold, dry

Typical dosage: 10–30 ml per week

Hydrangea arborescens

Common names: Smooth hydrangea, seven bark

Family: Hydrangeaceae

Part used: Root and rhizome

Description: Hydrangea was used by Native American for kidney and bladder stones. The Physicomedicalists of the 19th century used Hydrangea as part of a remedial formula in treating kidney disorders including nephritis. Also used or kidney and bladder stones and for gravel, cystitis, bladder inflammation and urethritis.

Constituents: Glycoside (hydrangin), hydragenol, hydrangeaic acid, flavonoids (quercetin, rutin) saponin, essential oil (kaempferol), resins, gum, starch.

Primary actions: Antilithic, Diuretic.

All actions: Antilithic, Cathartic, Diuretic.

Indications:

- Calculi; kidney and bladder, Cystitis, Prostatitis, Urethritis.
- **BHP:** Urinary calculi with gravel and cystitis.

Typical dosage: 20–80 ml per week

Hydrastis canadensis

Common names: Goldenseal

Family: Ranunculaceae

Part used: Rhizome, root.

Description: Traditional Native American medicine for wounds, ulcers, digestive disorders, cancer, and skin and eye ailments. Considered a 'mucous membrane tonic', goldenseal is mainly used for infections and inflammation of the mucous membranes. There is a lack of clinical trials with goldenseal but the main ingredient, berberine, is well researched. *H. canadensis* is listed as 'Vulnerable' by the IUCN Red List. It is threatened or endangered in many states. Due to the sharp decline in goldenseal populations after the herbal medicine boom of the late 1990s, it is incredibly important for commercial harvest to be restricted to cultivated farms. Consider other berberine-containing herbs such as *Phellodendron amurense* which is also widely available in solid dose forms.

Constituents: Berberine, canadine (isoquinoline alkaloid), hydrastine (isoquinoline alkaloid).

Primary actions: Antimicrobial, Choleretic, Mucous membrane tonic.

All actions: Antimicrobial, Antiparasitic, Antiseptic (topically), Antiviral (systemically), Bitter tonic, Choleretic, Decongestant, Oxytocic, Stomachic, Uterine tonic.

Indications:

- Anorexia, Candidiasis, Catarrh; naso-pharyngeal congestion, Catarrhal deafness, Colitis, Dysmenorrhoea, Eczema, Gastritis, Gastrointestinal catarrh, Gastrointestinal tract dysbiosis, Gastrointestinal tract infestation, Hypochlorhydria, Infection; gastrointestinal system, Pruritus, Pruritus ani (topically), Rhinitis, Sinusitis, Ulcer; gastrointestinal, Wounds (topically).

- **BHP:** Digestive disorders, gastritis, peptic ulceration, colitis and anorexia. Upper respiratory catarrh. Menorrhagia, postpartum haemorrhage, dysmenorrhoea. Topically for eczema, pruritus, otorrhea, catarrhal deafness, tinnitus, conjunctivitis. Specific indication: atonic dyspepsia with hepatic symptoms.

- **WHO:** Treatment of digestive complaints, such as dyspepsia, gastritis, feeling of distension and flatulence.

Contraindications: Contraindicated in pregnancy and lactation, in cases of known allergy to the plant material, in kidney disease (inadequate excretion of alkaloids) hypertension, and in jaundiced neonates.

Drug interactions: Berberine may increase the plasma concentration of cyclosporine; observe during concomitant use.

Itraconazole and berberine are mutually antagonistic and should not be combined. Use either itraconazole or berberine (or berberine-containing herbal extracts) but not together. The use of berberine is especially relevant since itraconazole is toxic and prone to be associated with fungal resistance. The incidence of *Aspergillus fumigatus* infections has become more frequent as a consequence of widespread immunosuppression. At present, the number of available antifungal agents in clinical use is limited, and most of them, such as itraconazole, are toxic and show resistance. Berberine is a plant alkaloid used in the clinic mainly for alimentary infections. Berberine has antifungal effects agains *Aspergillus fumigatus*, possibly via inhibition of the ergosterol biosynthesis pathway in a similar way to the antifungal drug, itraconazole. The two drugs were found to be mutually antagonistic and should not be combined clinically (Lei et al., 2011).

References:

Lei, G., Dan, H., Jinhua, L., Wei, Y., Song, G. & Li, W. 2011. Berberine and itraconazole are not synergistic in vitro against Aspergillus fumigatus isolated from clinical patients. Molecules, 16, 9218-33.

Qualities: Cold

Typical dosage: 15–30 ml per week

Hypericum perforatum

Common names: St John's wort

Family: Clusiaceae

Part used: Aerial parts

Description: Comprehensive reviews and meta-analyses of the clinical trials of St John's wort extracts have been conducted separately by various authors, all coming to the conclusion that St John's wort is superior to placebo, and has a similar effect to pharmaceutical antidepressants. The EU community monograph on St John's wort confirms that it is more effective than placebo and comparable to standard antidepressants in the treatment of mild to moderate depressive episodes. The monograph further states that St John's wort can be used to prevent a relapse of depressive symptoms. The monograph also confirms that products containing less than 1 mg hyperforin does not increase P450 enzyme activity and therefore would not even require a label warning of possible drug interactions.

Constituents: Naphthodianthrones including hypericin and pseudohypericin. Flavonoids including hyperoside, rutin and quercetin, phenolic compound including hyperforin, procyanidins, essential oil and xanthones.

Primary actions: Antidepressant, Antiviral (systemically), Photosensitising.

All actions: Anti-inflammatory, Antidepressant, Antiseptic (topically), Antiviral (topically), Astringent, Nervine tonic, Photosensitising, Relaxant, Wound healing/Vulnerary.

Indications:

- Anorexia, Anxiety, Chronic fatigue syndrome,

Depression, Depression; postnatal, Eczema (topically), Herpes simplex, Infection; viral, Insomnia, Irritability, Menopausal symptoms, Menopause, Nerve damage, Nervous exhaustion, Nervous tension, Neuralgia, Post-viral syndromes, Premenstrual syndrome, Shingles, Wounds, Wounds (topically).

- **BHP:** Excitability, neuralgia, fibrositis, sciatica. Topically for wounds. Specific indication: menopausal neurosis.

- **ESCOP:** Episodes of mild depressive disorders or mild to moderate depressive episodes.

- **WHO:** Symptomatic treatment of mild and moderate depressive episodes (classified as F32.0 and F32.1 in ICD-10). Externally for the treatment of minor cuts, burns and skin ulcers. Topically for viral infections.

Cautions: Do not administer during pregnancy or lactation or to children without medical supervision. Avoid excessive sunlight. Gastrointestinal symptoms may occur.

Contraindications: Not to be used after organ transplants, or by HIV-antibody positive individuals treated with protease-1 inhibitors.

Drug interactions: Some *H. perforatum* preparations enriched in hyperforin induce metabolic pathways involved in the clearance of drugs: such *H. perforatum* preparations have been consistently and reproducibly shown to activate the P-glycoprotein transporter (PGP) and cytochrome (CyP) P450. Within the group of CyP 450 subtypes, the clinically relevant effects are largely restricted to CyP 3A4, a metabolic enzyme responsible for the clearance of more than 50% of all drug substances. There are other subtypes frequently proposed as additional pathways for interactions with *H. perforatum*, mainly CyP 1A2, but other subtypes than CyP 3A4 – especially CyP 1A2 – have never been shown to contribute to a clinically important mechanism of action for herb–drug interactions triggered by *H. perforatum*.

Liquid extracts are generally very low in hyperforin. Traditionally, hypericum is harvested when flowering and hyperforin is typically very low during this time.

However, some dry extracts used in capsules or tablets are enriched in hyperforin by harvesting at different times and concentrating the level of hyperforin during manufacturing.

Preparations high in hyperforin induce the CYP450 enzyme system, and should not be used with indianvir, cyclosporin, oral contraceptives, digoxin, theophylline, HIV protease inhibitors, HIV non-nucleoside reverse transcriptase inhibitors, methadone, antineoplastic drugs, anticonvulsants (phenobarbiton, phenytoin), antidepressants, tacrolimus, omeprazole, midazolam, alprazolam and carbamazepine (Tegretol).

Avoid with anticoagulants warfarin (Coumadin, Marevan) and phenprocoumon. May decrease prothrombin time and international normalised ratio (INR) values; monitor these parameters. Suspend use of concentrated extract one week before general anaesthesia.

Qualities: Cold, pungent

Typical dosage: 10–40 ml per week

Hyssopus officinalis

Common names: Hyssop

Family: Zamiaceae

Part used: Aerial parts

Description: Traditional European and Middle Eastern medicine for upper respiratory illness, asthma, cough, sore throat, intestinal infections, gastrointestinal upset, gallbladder disease, poor appetite, urinary tract infections, dysmenorrhea and to improve circulation. Pharmacological investigations have found it to have antihyperlipidaemic, anti-inflammatory, antiviral, antiproliferative, choleretic activities. Hyssop is also used topically in gargles, medicinal baths, and creams for skin irritation, burns and frostbite. Hyssop oil is used in cooking and as a fragrance in soaps and cosmetics.

Constituents: Pinocamphone, pinene, borneol, geraniol, thujone, camphene, limonene and phellandrene. Terpenoids with known pharmacological actions that are found in hyssop include marrubiin, ursolic acid and oleanolic acid. Other characteristic compounds identified in hyssop are hyssopin (a glucoside), caffeic acid, tannins and resin. The volatile oil of hyssop is composed of camphor, pinacaphone, thujone, isopinocamphone, alpha- and beta-pinene, alpha terpinene, linalool, and bornylacetate.

Primary actions: Antipyretic, Antiviral (systemically), Diaphoretic.

All actions: Anti-inflammatory, Antipyretic, Antiviral (systemically), Carminative, Choleretic, Diaphoretic, Sedative.

Indications:

- Bronchitis, Catarrh; naso-pharyngeal congestion, Fever; childhood.

- **BHP:** Bronchitis, chronic nasal catarrh. Specific indications: bronchitis and the common cold.

Contraindications: None known

Qualities: Dry, neutral

Typical dosage: 15–30 ml per week

Inula helenium

Common names: Elecampane

Family: Asteraceae

Part used: Root

Description: The genus Inula has diverse biological activities including anticancer, antibacterial, hepaprotective, cytotoxic, and anti-inflammatory properties. Various species are distributed in Asia, Europe and Africa. In Greek mythology, Helen of Troy was said to have been the most beautiful woman

69

in the world, and to have carried this flower in her hair as she was abducted from her homeland. The Eclectics recommended it for coughs and colds, pulmonary irritation and chronic bronchitis.

Constituents: Helonin (alant-camphor), alantolactones, essential oil, inulin, isoalantolactones, sesquiterpene lactones, sesquiterpenes, sterols, thymol derivative, triterpenes.

Primary actions: Antiseptic (respiratory tract), Antispasmodic (respiratory tract), Expectorant (stimulating).

All actions: Anthelmintic, Antiasthmatic, Antimicrobial, Antipyretic, Antiseptic (respiratory tract), Antispasmodic (respiratory tract), Antitussive, Diaphoretic, Expectorant (stimulating).

Indications:

* Asthma, Bronchitis, Cough, Emphysema, Infection; respiratory tract, Pertussis, Pleurisy.
* **BHP:** Bronchial or tracheal catarrh, cough of pulmonary tuberculosis, and irritating cough in children. Specific indications: irritating cough of bronchitis, phthisis.

Cautions: Do not use during pregnancy without professional advice. Allergic contact dermatitis has been reported as an adverse effect.

Contraindications: Strongly discouraged during lactation. Contraindicated in those with known sensitivity to plants in Asteraceae (Compositae) family and other plants containing sesquiterpene lactones.

Qualities: Dry, warm

Typical dosage: 20–40 ml per week

Inula racemosa

Common names: Inula

Family: Asteraceae

Part used: Root

Description: Traditionally used for cough, dysponoea and precordial chest pain and for ischaemic heart disease. Antianginal activity demonstrated in an open trial. A combination of *Inula racemosa* and *Commiphora mukul* was shown to be superior to nitroglycerin in reducing the chest pain and dyspnea associated with angina. Specifically indicated for chronic bronchitis with cardiac complications. Pharmacological research suggests a potential for use of isoalantolactone and *Inula racemosa* in the management of diabetes (combine with gymnema). Root extract found to have antimutagenic and antiapoptotic effects.

Constituents: Sesquiterpene lactones (alantolactones)

Primary actions: Antiangina, Antispasmodic (respiratory tract), Cardioprotective.

All actions: Antiangina, Antispasmodic (respiratory tract), Antispasmodic (uterus), Bronchodilator, Cardioprotective, Nrf2-pathway activator, Selective

oestrogen receptor modulator (SERM).

Indications:

* Angina pectoris, Arteriosclerosis, Asthma, Atherosclerosis, Bronchitis, Cardiac debility, Congestive heart failure, Myocardial ischaemia.

Contraindications: None known

Qualities: Dry, hot

Typical dosage: 30–60 ml per week

Iris versicolor

Common names: Blue flag

Family: Iridaceae

Part used: Root

Description: Chiefly used for its alterative (blood purifying) properties. Considered a stimulant to the liver and intestines and is used in constipation and biliousness.

Constituents: Essential oil, iriversical, oleoresin, plant acids (acidic mucilage), tannin, triterpenoids.

Primary actions: Cholagogue, Depurative/Alterative, Laxative.

All actions: Cholagogue, Diuretic, Laxative, Lymphatic.

Indications:

* Constipation, Eczema, Lymphadenopathy, Psoriasis, Weight loss; to assist.
* **BHP:** Skin diseases, biliousness with constipation and liver function. Specific indication: cutaneous eruptions.

Cautions: Care needs to be taken to reduce the prospect of exacerbating chronic skin conditions. Large doses may cause nausea, vomiting and intestinal colic.

Contraindications: None known

Qualities: Cold, dry

Typical dosage: 20–40 ml per week

Isatis tinctoria

Common names: Isatis, ban lan gen, woad, Chinese indigo

Family: Brassicaceae

Part used: Root

Description: *Isatis tinctoria* is an important herbal medicine in both Eastern and Western herbal traditions. It is used to remove heat and toxins, cool the blood and clear the throat. The term 'Isatis' derives from the latin word 'Isazein' and the greek word 'Isadso' and refers to its ancient use in the treatment of wounds. The term 'tinctoria' refers to its use as a dye. Clinically, it is recommended for the prevention and treatment of colds and malignant infectious diseases, especially SARS and H1N1.

Constituents: Alkaloids, including isatin, indican, isatan A and B, tryptanthrin, indirubin, and indolinone, phenolic compounds, polysaccharides, glucosinolates, carotenoids, volatile constituents, and fatty acids.

Primary actions: Anti-inflammatory, Antimicrobial, Antiviral (systemically).

All actions: Analgesic, Anti-inflammatory, Anticancer, Antimicrobial, Antiviral (systemically).

Indications:

- Cancer; including prevention/supportive treatment, Conjunctivitis (locally as eye lotion), Eczema, Fever, Gastroenteritis, Haemorrhoids, Infection; respiratory tract, Infection; viral, Influenza, Laryngitis, Mumps, Pharyngitis, Psoriasis, Shingles, Tonsillitis, Ulcer (topically), Viral pneumonia, Wounds.

Cautions: Patients with sulfonylurea (antidiabetic) or sulfonamide (antibiotic) allergies may also experience allergic reactions to this herb.

Typical dosage: 25–70 ml per week

Isodon rubescens

Synonym or related species: Rabdosia rubescens

Common names: Dong ling cao, Chinese sage bush, rabdosia

Family: Lamiaceae

Part used: Leaf

Description: Isodon, comprised of about 150 species worldwide, is mainly distributed throughout the tropical and subtropical Asia and south-western China. I. rubescens is a perennial herb widely used in China to treat inflammation, bacterial infections, respiratory and gastrointestinal diseases and cancer. Used in TCM to clear heat and remove toxicity, activate blood and stop bleeding.

Constituents: Alkaloids, flavonoids, diterpenoids, diterpene glucosides including oridonin, ponicidin, pedalitin, phenolics and glucosidic iridoids.

Primary actions: Anti-inflammatory, Antibacterial, Anticancer.

All actions: Anti-inflammatory, Antibacterial, Anticancer, Anticatarrhal, Chemoprotective.

Indications:

- Cancer; including prevention/supportive treatment, Catarrh; naso-pharyngeal congestion, Cerebral ischaemia, Cough, Dementia, Gingivitis, Headache, Hepatitis, Infection; bacterial, Rheumatoid arthritis, Tonsillitis, Tracheitis.

Qualities: Sweet, bitter, cooling

Typical dosage: 30–70 ml per week

Juglans cinerea

Common names: Butternut bark, white walnut, lemon walnut

Family: Juglandaceae

Part used: Bark

Description: Mainly used as a laxative for constipation, hepatobiliary dysfunction, and exudative skin eruptions.

Constituents: Anthraquinone glycosides

Primary actions: Cholagogue, Depurative/Alterative, Laxative.

All actions: Anthelmintic, Cholagogue, Depurative/Alterative, Laxative.

Indications:

- Constipation, Gallbladder disorders, Liver insufficiency.

- **BHP:** Constipation, hepatic dysfunction, exudative skin eruptions. Specific indication: chronic constipation associated with dyspepsia.

Contraindications: None known

Qualities: Cold, pungent

Typical dosage: 25–50 ml per week

Juglans nigra

Common names: Black walnut

Family: Juglandaceae

Part used: Green hull, leaf

Description: The black walnut preparation is produced from the green hull of the edible walnut (J. nigra). It is not to be confused with another medicine based on an extract of the English walnut (J. regia). Walnut leaf has alterative, laxative, anthelmintic and astringent properties for the treatment of worms, constipation and inflammatory skin disorders. Another similar medicine is butternut, an extract of J. cinerea mainly used for constipation.

Constituents: The main active ingredients in the walnut hulls are tannins such as galloyglucose and ellagitannins, and juglone (5-hydroxy-alphanapthaquinone). L. nigra leaf oils is dominated by sesquiterpenes, (E)-caryophyllene (17.3–20.4%), germacrene D (7.1–22.5%), δ-cadinene (3.8–8.7%), α-humulene (1.1–4.2%), and α-muurolene (2.4–2.8%), and the monoterpene α-pinene (6.3–11.4%). There were also notable quantities of juglone (1.0%–8.8%) and α-hydrojuglone (1.0–9.5%). The activity of J. regia leaf oil can be attributed to the major aromatic components methyl salicylate and eugenol. J. regia has been found to contain 0.015% essential oil comprising of eugenol (27%), methyl salicylate (16%), germacrene (21%), and faresene (11%). Little research has been done on J. nigra. It is conjecture as to whether the information known about J. regia is applicable to J. nigra. J. nigra leaf oil is largely inactive against bacteria, fungi, and tumour cells, and this may explain the apparent absence of use of J. nigra leaves in Native American traditional medicine.

Primary actions: Anthelmintic, Antibacterial, Astringent.

All actions: Anthelmintic, Anti-inflammatory, Antibacterial, Antifungal, Antiviral (systemically), Astringent, Depurative/Alterative.

Indications:

- Diarrhoea, Eczema, Intestinal worms, Parasites.

Typical dosage: 10–40 ml per week

Juniperus communis

Common names: Juniper

Family: Cupressaceae

Part used: Fruit

Description: In traditional medicine, preparations made from juniper berries were used to relieve flatulence and indigestion and to stimulate the appetite. The cone berries should contain not less than 10 ml/kg of essential oil. Juniper essential oil distilled from the dried ripe fruit is used for abdominal cramps, flatulence and a feeling of fullness. Added to baths to stimulate blood circulation of the skin. Used as a diuretic. The dried herbal substance is used in a dose of 2 g with a maximum of 10 g per day which corresponds to 20 and 100 mg essential oil, respectively. The oil is used in dosages of 2–4 drips per day. In Germany soft capsules containing 100 mg essential oil is used for dyspeptic complains. In Denmark, juniper is combined with essential oils of peppermint, anise, eucalyptus and fennel.

Constituents: Monoterpenes (about 58% of the essential oil); the essential oil contains mainly α-pinene (20%), limonene (8.7%), myrcene (8.5%) and β-pinene, myrcene, sabinene, 1,4-cineol, camphene, Δ³-carene, terpinen-4-ol, terpinolene, 4-terpineol, β-elemene-7-ol; Sesquiterpenes: delta-cadinene, α-cadinene, β-cadinene; Diterpenic acids: isocommunic acid; labdane diterpenes; C12 terpenoid: geijerone; Tannins: proanthocyanidines (condensed), gallocatechin and epigallocatechin; Flavonoids: amentoflavone, quercitin, isoquercitrin, apigenin and various glucosides; Invert sugar (30%); glucose + fructose (about 30%) and pectin; Organic acids: malic acid, ascorbic acid, glucuronic acid; lignan: pesoxypodophyllotoxin; resins.

Primary actions: Antirheumatic, Antiseptic, Diuretic.

All actions: Antirheumatic, Antiseptic (GIT), Carminative, Diuretic, Stomachic.

Indications:

- Cystitis, Flatulence, Rheumatism.
- **BHP:** Acute or chronic cystitis, flatulent colic, rheumatism. Topically for rheumatic pain in joints or muscles. Specific indication: cystitis in the absence of renal inflammation.
- **Commission E:** Dyspepsia.
- **ESCOP:** Widely documented as a remedy to enhance the renal elimination of water and for dyspeptic complaints, but published scientific evidence does not yet adequately support these therapeutic indications.

Cautions: It may influence glucose levels in diabetics. According to many herbal texts, juniper is to be used with caution in renal disease, and is not suitable for long-term use due to the irritant effect

of the essential oil from the juniper berries on the kidneys. This assumption, however, is most likely misleading due to poor manufacturing methods used in earlier times, and poor research methods leading to faulty conclusions. However, caution is still recommended in treatment of acute renal inflammation, and with the use of juniper oil.

Contraindications: Acute and chronic inflammation of the kidney. During pregnancy and lactation

Qualities: Dry 1st degree, hot 3rd degree

Typical dosage: 10–20 ml per week

Justicia adhatoda

Synonym or related species: Adhatoda vasica

Common names: Basak, vasaka, Malabar nut

Family: Acanthaceae

Part used: Leaves

Description: Adhatoday, known as *basak* in Bangladesh, contains the alkaloid vasicine, from which the mucolytic drug bromhexine was developed.

Constituents: Approx 0.08% essential oil, 1% alkaloids. Of the alkaloids, vasicine makes up 75–90% and is considered the major active constituent. Other alkaloids are vasicinone and vasicinol.

Primary actions: Antiasthmatic, Antispasmodic (respiratory tract), Mucolytic.

All actions: Antiasthmatic, Antispasmodic (respiratory tract), Bronchodilator, Expectorant (relaxing), Mucolytic, Oxytocic.

Indications:

- Asthma, Bronchitis, Gingivitis, Haemorrhage; post-partum, Respiratory catarrh, Uterine contractions.

Contraindications: During pregnancy except at delivery.

Qualities: Drying

Typical dosage: 10–25 ml per week

Lamium album

Common names: White dead nettle

Family: Lamiaceae

Part used: Aerial parts

Description: The 'dead' in the common name refers to white dead nettle having no sting. It is used as an expectorant and to resolve mucus in catarrhal conditions. Also used in gynaecological conditions and for gastrointestinal complaints including irritation of the gastric mucosa, bloating, and flatulence. Externally used as a poultice for swelling of the skin, boils, varicose veins and gouty nodules.

Constituents: 6-desoxylamalbide, albosides A and B, caryoptin, catechins, choline, histamine (biogenic amine), iridoids, isoquercetin (flavonoid), kaempferol, lamalbide, methylamine (biogenic amine), mucilage, oligosaccharides, tyramine (biogenic amine).

Primary actions: Antihaemorrhagic (uterine), Astringent, Wound healing/Vulnerary.

All actions: Antihaemorrhagic (uterine), Astringent, Depurative/Alterative, Wound healing/Vulnerary.

Indications:

- Dysmenorrhoea, Flatulence, Gastritis, Gastrointestinal catarrh, Leucorrhoea, Leucorrhoea and vaginitis (douche), Menstrual irregularity, Uterine bleeding; dysfunctional, Wounds (topically).

Contraindications: None known

Qualities: Cold, moist, secondary drying effect

Typical dosage: 20–40 ml per week

Lavandula angustifolia

Synonym or related species: Lavandula officinalis, Lavandula vera

Common names: Lavender

Family: Lamiaceae

Part used: Flowers

Description: Inhalation therapy for symptomatic treatment of anxiety, restlessness and to induce relaxation. Externally in balneotherapy (the treatment of disease by bathing in mineral springs) for the treatment of circulation disorders. Symptomatic treatment of insomnia, and as a carminative for the treatment of gastrointestinal disorders of nervous origin.

Constituents: Essential oil including linalyl acetate, linalool, borneol, camphor and geraniol; coumarins including herniarine, umbelliferone and santonine. Also tannins, triterpenes, flavonoids and sesquiterpenes (caryophyllene).

Primary actions: Antidepressant, Antispasmodic (muscles), Sedative.

All actions: Antidepressant, Antirheumatic, Antispasmodic (muscles), Carminative, Sedative.

Indications:

- Anxiety, Colic, Depression, Depression; post natal, Digestive complaints, Digestive weakness, Dyspepsia; flatulent, Headache, Menopausal symptoms, Menopause; depression.

- **BHP:** Flatulent dyspepsia, colic, depressive headache. Topically as oil for rheumatic pain. Specific indication: depressive states associated with digestive dysfunction.

- **Commission E:** Restlessness or insomnia and nervous stomach irritation, Roehmheld's syndrome (roseola, a rose-colored skin rash that sometimes appears with diseases including measles, syphilis or scarlet fever), meteorism and nervous intestinal discomfort, and for the treatment of functional circulatory disorders (balneotherapy).

- **WHO:** Inhalation therapy for symptomatic treatment of anxiety, restlessness and to induce relaxation. Externally in balneotherapy for the treatment of circulation disorders. Symptomatic treatment of insomnia, and as a carminative for the treatment of gastrointestinal disorders of nervous origin.

Cautions: Allergic contact dermatitis has been reported in some patients. Essential oils should be used with caution in children and during lactation.

Contraindications: Contraindicated in cases of known allergy to the plant material (Labiatae family). Essential oil should not be used internally during pregnancy due to emmenagogue properties.

Drug interactions: Lavender may increase or potentiate the CNS depressant effects of sedative-hypnotics; observe patient. May have additive effects when used with antidepressants; use with caution.

Qualities: Dry 3rd degree, hot 3rd degree

Typical dosage: 15–30 ml per week

Leonurus cardiaca

Synonym or related species: Leonurus artemisia

Common names: Motherwort

Family: Lamiaceae

Part used: Aerial parts

Description: Traditional use for cardiac debility, simple tachycardia, and in gynaecology including amenorrhoea. The BHP lists the specific indication as cardiac symptoms including palpitations associated with neurosis.

Constituents: Bitter glycoside, caffeic acid, flavonoids, leonuride (iridoid glucoside), leonurin (alkaloids), stachydrine (alkaloid), tannin, urosol (triterpene).

Primary actions: Antispasmodic (uterus), Cardiotonic, Sedative.

All actions: Anti-inflammatory, Antiarrhythmic, Antiplatelet, Antiproliferative, Antispasmodic (uterus), Cardiotonic, Sedative.

Indications:

- Amenorrhoea, Arrhythmia, Cardiac debility, Graves' disease, Hyperthyroidism, Nervous tachycardia, Neurasthenia, Tachycardia.

- **BHP:** Cardiac debility, simple tachycardia, amenorrhoea. Specific Indication: cardiac symptoms associated with neurosis.

- **Commission E:** Nervous cardiac disorders and as an adjuvant for thyroid hyperfunction.

Cautions: Do not use in pregnancy without professional advice.

Contraindications: None known

Qualities: Cool, dry

Typical dosage: 20–40 ml per week

Leptospermum scoparium

Common names: Manuka, tea tree

Family: Myrtacease

Part used: Leaf

Description: Leaves used as a substitute for tea. Manuka is from the same family as Australian tea tree (*Melacleuca alternifolia*) and share some medicinal properties. Manuka honey is a dark monofloral honey rich in phenolic content with antimicrobial activity. The antibacterial potency of Manuka honey is related to the Unique Manuka Factor (UMF) rating, which is correlated with the methylglyoxal and total phenols content. In addition to bacterial growth inhibition, glyoxal and methylglyoxal from Manuka honey can enhance wound healing and tissue regeneration by their immunomodulatory properties. Galenical extracts are likely to share such medicinal properties. Manuka decoction was traditionally used for urinary complaints, as a febrifuge and for rubbing in to sore muscles and joints. The steam from leaves boiled in water was inhaled for head colds.

Constituents: Essential oil, triketones approximately 20%, sesquiterpenes 60–70%, and monoterpene about 5%, especially α-pinene and β-pinene monoterpenes.

Lipophilic flavones which have been shown to interact with benzodiazepine receptors, and a significant amount of tannis.

The activity of manuka honey is largely due to the presence of methylglyoxal (MGO), which is produced non-enzymatically from dihydroxyacetone (DHA) present in manuka nectar.

Primary actions: Anti-inflammatory, Antibacterial, Febrifuge.

All actions: Anti-inflammatory, Antibacterial, Antifungal, Antimicrobial, Antispasmodic (muscles), Anxiolytic, Astringent, Diuretic, Febrifuge, Gastroprotective, Sedative.

Indications:

- Anxiety, Common cold, Enuresis, Gingivitis, Incontinence, Infection; skin, Influenza, Insomnia, Wounds (topically).

Cautions: Take away from meals as tannins may interfere with nutrient absorption.

Typical dosage: 20–60 ml per week

Ligustrum lucidum

Common names: Glossy privet, nu zhen zi, joteishi

Family: Oleaceae

Part used: Fruit

Description: Used in TCM to nourish and tonify the liver and kidneys and in the treatment of yin deficiency of the same organs. The Chinese name *nu zhen zi* translates as 'the fruit of a chaste woman', apparently referring to the virtues of women as the tree is an evergreen, even in the harshness of winter.

Constituents: Volatile components, triterpenes, flavonoids, polysaccharides, secoiridoid glucosides salidroside, ligustroside, nuezhenoside, and nuezhenoside, oleanolic and ursolic acids, and phenolic compounds.

Primary actions: Anti-inflammatory, Immunomodulator, Tonic.

All actions: Anti-inflammatory, Antiageing, Anticancer, Antidiabetic, Antihyperlipidemic, Antiosteoporotic, Diuretic, Hepatoprotective, Hypoglycaemic, Immunomodulator, Renal protective, Tonic.

Indications:

- Age-related macular degeneration, Cancer; including prevention/supportive treatment, Debility, Diabetes, Fatigue, Hepatic steatosis, Menopausal symptoms, Metabolic syndrome, Osteoporosis prevention, Rheumatism.

Qualities: Bitter, sweet, neutral

Typical dosage: 30–80 per week

Lobelia inflata

Common names: Indian tobacco, Indian pukeweed

Family: Campanulaceae

Description: Lobelia has a long history as a respiratory herb by native Americans. It was recommended for asthma by Culter. In the vitalist system of Samuel Thomson (1769–1843) lobelia was the key herb to restore the natural heat of the body. It is indigenous to Eastern USA and Canada. Lobelia is relaxing at lower dosages but emetic at higher dosages. 'If lobelia be chewed, it gives rise to an acrid, prickling, and persistently pungent sensation in the throat and fauces, accompanied by slight nausea and a feeling of warmth and distension along the esophageal tract and in the stomach. The sensation is not very unlike that produced by tobacco. The salivary and buccal glands are impressed, pouring out saliva and mucus in abundance. A sense of epigastric depression succeeds, followed by profound nausea, and if the amount chewed be large enough, severe and thorough emesis results.' *King's American Dispensary*, 1898.

Part used: Above ground parts.

Constituents: The principal constituent is lobeline, an alkaloid with similar, but less potent, properties to nicotine. Piperidine-type alkaloids (0.2–0.4% including lobeline, lobelanine, lobelanidine, norlobelanine, lelobanidine, norlelobanidine, norlobelanidine and lobinine; bitter glycodise (lobelacrin), chelidonic acids, fats, gum, resin and volatile oil. Lobeline causes initial CNS stimulation followed by respiratory depression.

Primary actions: Antiasthmatic, Expectorant, Emetic.

All actions: Antiasthmatic, Antispasmodic, Antidepressant, Anticonvulsant, Antimicrobial, Diaphoretic, Expectorant, Emetic, Respiratory

Stimulant, Sialogogue, Sedative

Indications:
- Asthma, Bronchial asthma, Bronchitis, Emphysema, Fever, Whooping cough.

- **Other Uses:** Low, sub-emetic doses used traditionally to enhance the effects of other herbs in a formula. Priest & Priest states that lobelia equalises the çirculation and relieves vascular tension. They also recommend lobelia to relax tension and spams due to trauma, for pertussis and pleurisy, hepatitis, jaundice and hepatic congestion; hypertension and neurasthenia. Lobelia is also used as an antismoking agent although a clinical trial found that a sublingual formulation of lobeline sulfate did not appear to be an effective smoking cessation aid. The emetic property was traditionally used during the height of an asthma attack, a practice that is no longer recommended. Lobelia may also help appetite and indigestion with flatulence. Also used for tension headaches.

- **BHP:** Bronchitic asthma, chronic bronchitis. Topically for myositis and rheumatic nodules. Specific indication: Spasmodic asthma with secondary bronchitis. Combines well with capsicum, grindelia, drosera, Symplocarpus foetidus, euphorbia and ephedra in asthma.

Cautions: Overdose may cause side effects similar to nicotine toxicity including nausea, vomiting, diarrhoea, coughing, tremors, dizziness and hypotension, which can be fatal although there have not been any serious adverse events or confirmed death from lobelia.

Pregnancy/Lactation: Not recommended in pregnancy or lactation.

Contraindications: Lobelia is contraindicated in all cardiac diseases and pneumonia. Avoid with CNS depressants.

Qualities: Bitter, neutral

Dosages: Fluid extract 4–12 ml per week

Tincture 0.2–0.6 ml three times daily

Lomatium dissectum

Common names: Fern-leaf biscuit root, tohza, desert parsley

Family: Apiaceae

Part used: Root

Description: Known as *tohza* by the Shoshone native American tribe, lomatum was a prized food, medicine and ceremonial plant. It is traditionally used for arthritis, burns, respiratory tract infections, stomach and musculoskeletal disorders.

Constituents: Furanocoumarins, flavonoids, ichthyotoxic tetronic acids, Z-ligustilide, terpenes, sesquiterpenes, volatile oil.

Primary actions: Antimicrobial, Antiviral (systemically), Expectorant (stimulating).

All actions: Antibacterial, Antimicrobial, Antiviral (systemically), Expectorant (stimulating), Immunomodulator.

Indications:
- Asthma, Candidiasis, Common cold, Fever, Gingivitis, Infection; respiratory tract, Infection; urinary tract, Infection; viral, Influenza, Periodontitis, Rheumatism, Shingles, Viral pneumonia, Warts (topically), Wounds (topically).

Cautions: In susceptible individuals, lomatium can cause an allergic skin reaction.

Contraindications: Safety in pregnancy and lactation has not been established.

Typical dosage: 15–40 ml per week

Lycopus spp.

Synonym or related species: Lycopus europaeus, L. virginicus

Common names: Bugleweed, gypsy wort

Family: Lamiaceae

Part used: Aerial parts

Description: Traditionally used in mild forms of hyperthyroidism. High doses have been shown to cause a reduction of TSH or thyroid hormone levels in animal experiments, whereas in hyperthyroid patients treated with low doses of Lycopus, an improvement of cardiac symptoms has been reported without major changes in TSH or thyroid hormone concentrations. One study found that the raised body temperature was reduced very effectively even by the low dose of the plant extract, whereas the reduced gain of body weight and the increased food intake remained unaffected by any treatment. No significant changes of thyroid hormone concentrations or TSH levels were observed. Lycopus extract and atenolol reduced the increased heart rate and blood pressure. The cardiac hypertrophy was alleviated significantly by both treatment regimens. Beta-adrenoceptor density in heart tissue was significantly reduced by the Lycopus extract or the beta-blocking agent showing an almost equal efficacy. Although the mode of action remains unclear, these organo-specific anti-T4-effects seem to be of practical interest, for example in patients with latent hyperthyroidism. Shown in a pilot study to increase urinary excretion of T4 which was associated with a reduction in hyperthyroid symptoms such as increased heart rate in the morning.

Constituents: Phenolic acids and flavonoids, with a predominance of rosmarinic acid and luteolin-7-O-glucuronide; other phenolic acid derivatives including caffeic, chlorogenic, and ellagic acids; volatile oil; tannins; and isopimarane diterpenes including euroabienol.

Primary actions: Antibacterial, Antimicrobial, Antithyroid.

All actions: Antibacterial, Antimicrobial, Antithyroid.

Indications:

- Cough, Graves' disease, Hyperthyroidism, Nervous tachycardia, Tachycardia, Thyrotoxicosis with dyspnoea.

- **BHP:** Nervous tachycardia, Graves' disease with cardiac involvement, irritating cough with copious sputum, haemoptysis. Specific indication: thyrotoxicosis with dyspnoea, tachycardia and tremor

Cautions: Caution in women trying to conceive. Taper dose when ceasing treatment. Adverse effects include enlarged thyroid, increase in hyperthyroid symptoms, and headache.

Contraindications: Contraindicated during pregnancy and lactation, and in patients with hypothyroidism.

Drug interactions: Avoid concurrent use with preparations containing thyroid hormone.

May interfere with diagnostic procedures using radioactive isotopes (case report).

Qualities: Cool, dry

Typical dosage: 20–40 ml per week

Macropiper excelsum

Synonym or related species: Piper excelsum

Common names: Kawakawa, New Zealand peppertree

Family: Piperaceae

Part used: Leaf

Description: Tonic herb in traditional Maori medicine. Botanically related to kava (*Piper methsticum*). The fruit, bark and leaves of the kawakawa all have medicinal properties. Analgesic property is a key indication.

Constituents: Amides, lignans-demethoxyexcelsin, diagyangambin, epielxelsin, excelsin, piperin and volatile oils including myristicin (anti-inflammatory, antifungal larvicidal, analgesic activities) and elemicin (antifungal and potential anticholinergic activities).

Primary actions: Analgesic, Depurative/Alterative, Diuretic.

All actions: Analgesic, Anthelmintic, Anti-inflammatory, Antimicrobial, Antispasmodic (muscles), Carminative, Circulatory stimulant, Depurative/Alterative, Diaphoretic, Diuretic, Laxative.

Indications:

- Boils, Bruises (topically), Cystitis, Eczema, Gastritis, Inflammation; skin (topically), Migraine, Rheumatism, Visceral pain.

- **Other uses:** Generally used for gastrointestinal disorders, pain and infections but also for dysmenorrehoea. Suitable for paediatric use: colic, diarrhoea, poor appetite, intestinal parasites/helminths, skin disorders including eczema and boils, common cold, influenza and cough. Externally used to heal cuts, boils, bruises, rheumatism, and nettle stings. For

acute headache or migraine, take 10 ml of 1:2 hydroalcoholic leaf extract and repeat some time later if required.

Cautions: Laxative and mildly sedative effects.

Qualities: Warming

Typical dosage: 20–60 ml per week

Magnolia officinalis

Common names: Magnolia, Hou po

Family: Magnoliaceae

Part used: Bark

Description: The thick bark is a medicine from the Chinese and Japanese herbal traditions. It is a constituent of prominent combinations Saiboku-to (bronchial asthma, antiallergic) and Hange-koboku-to (prokinetic, used for nausea, vomiting and abdominal distention). It is considered a vital energy tonic. Magnolia is now popular in the treatment of anxiety and depression. The main body systems affected are gastrointestinal, immune, nervous, endocrine and cardiovascular. The constituent, honokiol, has neuroprotective, anti-inflammatory, anti-angiogenic and anticancer properties.

Constituents: Honokiol, magnolol, 4-O-methylhonokiol and obovatol. Alkaloids, flavonoids, coumarins and terpenoids.

Primary actions: Antidepressant, Anxiolytic, Tonic.

All actions: Anti-inflammatory, Antiatherosclerotic, Anticancer, Antidepressant, Antiobesity, Antispasmodic/Spasmolytic, Anxiolytic, Cardioprotective, Neuroprotective, Nrf2-pathway activator, PPARgamma agonist.

Indications:

- Anxiety, Asthma, Atherosclerosis, Cancer; including prevention/supportive treatment, Cardiovascular disease prevention, Constipation, Dementia, Depression, Dyspepsia, Insomnia, Irritable bowel syndrome, Memory and concentration; poor, Metabolic syndrome, Nausea, Obesity, Rheumatism.

Typical dosage: 30–70 ml per week

Marrubium vulgare

Common names: White horehound

Family: Lamiaceae

Part used: Aerial parts

Description: Traditional herb for cough, acute bronchitis, and catarrh of the respiratory tract. Expectorant with secretolytic activity. Dyspeptic complaints such as fullness and flatulence. Laxative in large doses. Loss of appetite. Expressed juice from fresh horehound herb can be taken as 10–20 ml three times daily.

Constituents: Traces of essential oil (0.05–0.06%) with monoterpenes such as camphene, p-cymol, fenchene, lomonene, α-pinene, sabinene, and α-terpinolene; diterpenes of labdane-type with marrubiin (0.12–1%) and its precursor pre-marrubiin (0.13%), marrubenol, a labdane-hemiacetale, marrubiol, peregrinol and vulgarol; tannins (up to 7%) and hydroxylcynamic acid-derivates, e.g., acteoside, chorogenic acid, caffeic acid, 1-caffeoylquinic acid and cryptochlorogenic acid, but no rosmarinic acid. Acteoside is used as qualitative marker. Flavonoids: flavone and flavonol glycosides and their respective aglycones (e.g., apigenin, luteolin, quercetin).

Primary actions: Bitter tonic, Digestive tonic, Expectorant (relaxing).

All actions: Anti-inflammatory, Antispasmodic (respiratory tract), Bitter tonic, Digestive tonic, Expectorant (relaxing), Gastroprotective.

Indications:

- Anorexia, Bronchitis, Cough, Dyspepsia, Pertussis.

- **BHP:** Acute or chronic bronchitis, pertussis. Specific indications: bronchitis with non-productive cough.

- **Commission E:** Loss of appetite and dyspepsia with bloating and flatulence.

Cautions: Do not use during pregnancy without professional advice.

Qualities: Dry 3rd degree, hot 2nd degree

Typical dosage: 15–40 ml per week

Matricaria chamomilla

Synonym or related species: Matricaria recutita, Chamomilla recutita

Common names: Chamomile, German chamomile

Family: Asteraceae

Part used: Flowers

Description: Used in the treatment of mild gastrointestinal disorders including colic and bloating, irritation of the oropharyngeal mucosa and of the upper respiratory tract. Inflammations in the oral cavity and pharynx, periodontal disease, acute gingivitis, after tooth extraction and during teething, gum irritation caused by dentures; catarrh of larynx, inflammation of vocal cords, sore throat.Topical use as emollient, antiseptic and antipruritic treatment of dermatological conditions. For treatment of weeping or pruritic eczema, to support wound healing, eczema in anal area.

Constituents: Essential oil (0.3–1.9%): proazulenes like matricin and matricarin, which are at least partially converted during steam distillation into azulenes like chamazulene; flavonoids (up to 6%) such as apigenin-7-glucoside (0.5%), apigenin and luteolin; sesquiterpene lactones such as matricin (0.03–0.2%); coumarins (0.01%–0.08%) such as herniarin and umbelliferone; spiroethers (cis- and trans en-in-dicycloethers); phenolic acid and polysaccharides. Major constituents of the essential oil: sesquiterpenes: azulenes (2–18%), especially chamazulene (-)-alpha-bisabolol (up to 50%),

bisabolol oxides A and B; trans-β-farnesene (up to 45%); spiroethers (20–30%).

Primary actions: Anti-inflammatory (GIT), Antispasmodic/Spasmolytic, Wound healing/Vulnerary.

All actions: Anti-inflammatory, Anti-inflammatory (GIT), Antiallergic, Antidiarrhoeal, Antimicrobial, Antiseptic, Antispasmodic/Spasmolytic, Anxiolytic, Bitter tonic, Carminative, Cholagogue, Digestive tonic, Galactagogue, Gastroprotective, Sedative, Wound healing/Vulnerary.

Indications:

- Allergies/Sensitivities, Anorexia, Anxiety, Asthma, Boils, Colic; childhood, Colic; intestinal, Colitis, Diarrhoea, Dyspepsia, Dyspepsia; flatulent, Dyspepsia; nervous, Eczema (topically), Flatulence, Gastritis, Gastrointestinal catarrh, Gastrointestinal tract dysbiosis, Gingivitis, Gout, Haemorrhoids (topically), Hayfever, Herpes simplex, Indigestion, Inflammation; gastrointestinal tract, Inflammation; oral cavity, Inflammatory bowel disease, Insomnia, Irritability, Irritable bowel syndrome, Nausea, Pruritus ani (topically), Restlessness, Ulcer; gastrointestinal, Wounds (topically).

- **BHP:** Flatulent nervous dyspepsia, travel sickness, nasal catarrh, nervous diarrhoea, restlessness. Topically for haemorrhoids, mastitis, leg ulcers. Specific indication: gastrointestinal disturbance with associated nervous irritability in children.

- **Commission E:** Gastrointestinal spasms and inflammatory diseases. Topically for inflammation and infections of the skin and mucous membranes.

- **ESCOP:** Internal use: Symptomatic treatment of gastrointestinal complaints such as minor spasms, epigastric distention, flatulence and belching. External use: Minor inflammation and irritations of skin and mucosa, including the oral cavity and the gums, the respiratory tract and the anal and genital area.

- **WHO:** Internal: symptomatic treatment of digestive ailments such as dyspepsia, epigastric bloating, impaired digestion, and flatulence. Infusion for treatment of restlessness and in mild cases of insomnia due to nervous disorders. External: inflammation and irritations of the skin and mucosa (skin cracks, bruises, frostbite, and insect bites), mouth, gums and haemorrhoids. Inhalation: relief of irritations of the respiratory tract due to the common cold.

Cautions: Allergic reactions are mostly due to contamination with *Athemis cotula* (cotains anthecotulide, a contact allergen). Pollens are not likely to be present or active in aqueous alcohol extracts of chamomile.

Contraindications: Known sensitivity or allergy to members of the Compositae (Asteraceae) family

Qualities: Dry 1st degree, hot 1st degree
Typical dosage: 20–40 ml per week

Melissa officinalis

Synonym or related species: Calamintha officinalis, *Melissa graveolens*

Common names: Lemon balm, Melissa

Family: Lamiaceae

Part used: Leaves

Description: Human studies have found moderate evidence for the use of *Melissa officinals* in dementia, heart palpitation, glycaemic control in type 2 diabetes, improved lipid profiles, agitation, anxiety, depression, insomnia, memory and mood. Also used for IBS and for colic in infants. Topically Melissa exhibits antiviral properties.

Constituents: Caffeic acid, caryophyllene oxide, chlorogenic acid, citral, citronellal, citronellol, essential oil, eugenol acetate, ferulic acid, flavonoids, geraniol, linalool, polyphenolics, rosmarinic acid, terpenes, triterpenoids.

Primary actions: Antiviral (topically), Carminative, Diaphoretic.

All actions: Antimicrobial, Antipyretic, Antispasmodic (muscles), Antiviral (topically), Carminative, Diaphoretic, Emmenagogue, Gastroprotective, Sedative, Stomachic.

Indications:

- Anxiety, Colic; flatulent, Common cold, Depression, Dyspepsia; flatulent, Dyspepsia; nervous, Fever, Fever; childhood, Flatulence, Herpes (topically), Herpes simplex, Inflammatory bowel disease, Influenza, Insomnia, Irritable bowel syndrome, Migraine, Neuralgia, Neurasthenia, Restlessness.

- **BHP:** Flatulent dyspepsia, neurasthenia, and depressive illness. Specific indications: dyspepsia associated with anxiety or depressive states.

- **Commission E:** Insomnia, anxiety and restlessness, and functional gastrointestinal complaints.

- **ESCOP:** Internal use: Tenseness, restlessness and irritability, symptomatic treatment of digestive disorders such as minor spasms. External use: Cold sores.

- **WHO:** Externally, for symptomatic treatment of herpes labialis. Orally as a carminative for gastrointestinal disorders, and as a sedative for treatment of nervous disturbances of sleep.

Contraindications: None known

Drug interactions: Observe patients taking lemon balm extract with pentobarbital due to increased sedative effect.

Qualities: Cool, pungent

Typical dosage: 20–40 ml per week

Mentha pulegium

Common names: Pennyroyal

Family: Lamiaceae

Part used: Aerial parts

Description: Traditionally used for flatulent dyspepsia, intestinal colic, common cold and topically for cutaneous eruptions. The BHP includes the indication 'delayed menstruation' – could also be a euphimism for pennyroyal being an abortifacient. Abortifacients pose toxicity risks to the mother, including kidney and liver damage. Abortifacients are contraindicated during pregnancy and herbal abortion is not a recommended method of terminating a pregnancy.

Constituents: Flavonoid glycosides (diosmin, hesperidin)

Primary actions: Antipyretic, Carminative, Diaphoretic.

All actions: Antipyretic, Carminative, Diaphoretic, Emmenagogue.

Indications:

- Colic; flatulent, Colic; intestinal, Dyspepsia, Flatulence, Menstrual irregularity.

- **BHP:** Flatulent dyspepsia, intestinal colic, common cold, delayed menstruation. Topically: cutaneous eruptions, formication, gout. Specific indication: delayed menstruation due to chill or nervous shock.

Cautions: Administration to children is not advised. Do not use excessive doses. When taken by mouth, pennyroyal oil is highly toxic and has been linked to several instances of toxic liver injury and death.

Contraindications: Contraindicated during pregnancy and lactation due to toxicity of pulegone.

Qualities: Cooling followed by a warming potential

Typical dosage: 20–40 ml per week

Mentha x piperita

Common names: Peppermint, Bo He

Family: Lamiaceae

Part used: Leaves

Description: Peppermint oil has been reported to increase alertness. Essential oils of ginger, spearmint, peppermint, and cardamom have been shown to be beneficial for postoperative nausea. Peppermint gel, lanolin ointment, and placebo gel can be used to prevent nipple crack in breastfeeding women. Prophylactic peppermint gel in breastfeeding lactating women is associated with fewer nipple cracks and is more effective than lanolin and placebo. Peppermint gel has a positive effect in the prevention of pressure injuries in patients with head trauma admitted to ICUs. Sage, thyme and peppermint hydrosol oral rinse has promising results in alleviating oral mucositis induced by chemotherapy.

Constituents: Menthol, menthone, menthyl acetate as major ingredients. Minor ingredients include 1,8-cineole, pulegone, bitter substances, caffeic acid, flavonoids, and tannins.

Primary actions: Antiemetic, Carminative, Diaphoretic.

All actions: Antibacterial, Antiemetic, Antispasmodic (muscles), Aromatic, Carminative, Diaphoretic.

Indications:

- Colic; childhood, Colic; intestinal, Common cold, Crohn's disease, Dysmenorrhoea, Dyspepsia; flatulent, Fever, Fever; childhood, Flatulence, Flavouring, Gastric reflux, Halitosis, Indigestion, Inflammatory bowel disease, Irritable bowel syndrome, Menstrual irregularity, Morning sickness, Nausea, Ulcerative colitis.

- **BHP:** Dyspepsia, flatulence, intestinal colic, biliary disorders.

- **Commission E:** As a leaf preparation for spastic complaints of the gastrointestinal tract, gallbladder and bile ducts.

- **ESCOP:** Internal use: Symptomatic treatment of digestive disorders such as flatulence, irritable bowel syndrome and for the symptomatic relief of coughs and colds. External use: Relief of coughs and colds, symptomatic relief of rheumatic complaints, tension-type headache, pruritis, urticaria and pain in irritable skin conditions.

- **WHO:** Internally for symptomatic treatment of irritable bowel syndrome, and digestive disorders such as flatulence and gastritis. Externally for treatment of myalgia and headache. Internally and externally for the symptomatic treatment of catarrh and coughs.

- **Other uses:** Spearmint (*Mentha spicata*) has been shown to have antiandrogenic activity.

Cautions: Do not administer during pregnancy or lactation without medical supervision. Avoid if gallstones are present. Patients with achlorhydria (due to medication with histamine H2 receptor antagonists) should only use enteric-coated preparations.

Contraindications: Peppermint oil is contra-indicated for bile duct obstruction, gallbladder inflammation, gastro-oesophageal reflux, constipation, iron-deficiency anaemia and severe liver damage, and for use on or near the nose (including face) of infants or small children (potential risk of spasms of tongue or respiratory arrest). Do not use if there is contact sensitivity to peppermint oil or menthol.

Qualities: Dry, secondary cooling effect, warm

Typical dosage: 10–30 ml per week

Mitchella repens

Common names: Partridgeberry

Family: Rubiaceae

Part used: Whole plant

Description: Ellingwood considered it the partus preparatory par excellence: 'If a good preparation of mitchella be administered once or twice daily for the sixth and seventh months of pregnancy, three times daily for the eighth month, and in larger doses as confinement approaches, the influence upon the entire system will be most marked. Erratic pains and unsatisfied longings are removed, the nervous system assumes a tranquil condition, reflex symptoms abate, the urinary function is performed normally, the bowels become regular, imperfect digestion is improved, and the appetite becomes natural. Labor approaches, devoid of the irritating, aggravating complications, the preparatory stage is simple, the dilatation is completed quickly, the expulsive contractions are strong, unirritating, and effectual, and are much less painful than without the remedy; involution is rapid and perfect, there are no subsequent complicating conditions to contend with, the patient's strength is not abated, and the function of lactation is in its best condition.' *American Materia Medica*, 1919.

Constituents: No recent or reliable research, but the following have been reported: alkaloids, bitter glycoside, dextrin, emodin, mucilage, resin, saponins, tannin, wax.

Primary actions: Partus praeparator, Postpartum tonic, Uterine tonic.

All actions: Antihaemorrhagic (uterine), Antispasmodic (uterus), Astringent, Diuretic, Emmenagogue, Galactagogue, Partus praeparator, Postpartum tonic, Uterine tonic, Wound healing/ Vulnerary.

Indications:

- Amenorrhoea, Childbirth recovery, Colitis, Dysmenorrhoea, Gastrointestinal catarrh, Haemorrhage; postpartum, Menstrual irregularity, Pregnancy; to prepare uterus for labour, Uterine bleeding; dysfunctional, Uterine contractions.

- **BHP:** Dysmenorrhoea, pregnancy, catarrhal colitis. Specific indication: facilitation of parturition.

Contraindications: Contraindicated in first trimester of pregnancy.

Qualities: Cool, pungent

Typical dosage: 20–40 ml per week

Momordica charantia

Common names: Bitter melon, bitter gourd, African or wild cucumber

Family: Cucurbitaceae

Part used: Fruit, whole plant

Description: Traditionally used for diabetes. Type 1 diabetes: supportive treatment, reduction in long-term complications. Type 2 diabetes: blood sugar control and reduction of long-term complications, metabolic syndrome (insulin resistance, obesity and cardiovascular symptoms), obesity; to reduce risk of diabetic development, and digestive complaints including ulceration, hyperlipidaema. Traditionally also used to treat intestinal colic, peptic ulcers, worms, malaria, constipation, dysmenorrhea, eczema, gout, jaundice, kidney stone, leprosy, leucorrhoea, piles, pneumonia, psoriasis, rheumatism, chickenpox, measles and scabies.

Constituents: Glycosides, saponins, alkaloids, fixed oils, triterpenes, proteins and steroids. The hypoglycemic constituents are a mixture of steroidal saponins (charantins), insulin-like peptides and alkaloids, and are concentrated in the fruits. Momorcharins, momordenol, momordicins, cucurbitins, cucurbitacins, HIV inhibitory proteins code named MRK29, trypsin, elastase and gyanylate cyclase inhibitors and lectins have also been isolated; momordicins are important for the nemiticidal activity.

Primary actions: Antihyperlipidemic, Hypoglycaemic.

All actions: Anthelmintic, Antihyperlipidemic, Antimicrobial, Antiobesity, Antiviral (systemically), Bitter tonic, Digestive tonic, Gastroprotective, Hypoglycaemic, Immunomodulator.

Indications:

- Colic; intestinal, Dyslipidaemia, Dyspepsia, Ulcer; gastrointestinal.

Contraindications: Due to possible anti-fertility, teratogenic and abortifacient effects of certain constituents, and due to a lack of detailed information, the use of bitter melon extract is not recommended during pregnancy or women wishing to conceive.

Drug interactions: May have additive effects when consumed concomitantly with other hypoglycemic agents. Use with caution.

Qualities: Cooling

Typical dosage: 10–30 ml per week

Myrica cerifera

Common names: Bayberry, candleberry, wax myrtle

Family: Myricaceae

Part used: Root bark

Description: The use of bayberry in herbal medicine has declined since its peak in popularity in the 19th century. Today the plant is mainly used in the treatment of fever and diarrhoea.

Constituents: Flavonoid myricitrin, together with tannins and triterpenoids (myricadiol, taraxerol, taraxerone), acrid resins, astringent resins.

Primary actions: Antidiarrhoeal, Astringent, Diaphoretic.

All actions: Antidiarrhoeal, Astringent, Diaphoretic, Emetic.

Indications:

- Colitis, Common cold, Diarrhoea, Fever, Leucorrhoea and vaginitis (douche), Sore throat (gargle).

- **BHP:** Diarrhoea, colds, sort throat (gargle), leucorrhoea (douche), indolent ulcers (topically). Specific indication: mucous colitis.

Contraindications: None known.

Drug interactions: May interfere with steroid treatment and blood pressure medication.

Qualities: Cooling potential, warm

Typical dosage: 15–40 ml per week

Nepeta cataria

Common names: Catnip, catmint, Jing Jie

Family: Lamiaceae

Part used: Leaves and flowering tops

Description: Mostly used as a diaphoretic during fevers. Nervous dyspepsia, colic in children, colds, headache, insomnia. Topically as ointment in haemorrhoids.

Constituents: Essential oil rich in nepatalactone, nepatalic acid, epinepetalacone, caryophyllene, citral, citronellol, linonen, geraniol and camphor.

Primary actions: Antipyretic, Carminative, Diaphoretic.

All actions: Antipyretic, Astringent, Carminative, Diaphoretic, Sedative.

Indications:

- Colic, Common cold, Dyspepsia; nervous, Headache, Inflammatory bowel disease, Insomnia.

- **BHP:** Nervous dyspepsia, colic in children, colds, headache, insomnia. Topically as ointment in haemorrhoids. Specific indications: flatulent colic in children, common cold.

Contraindications: None known.

Qualities: Cool, dry

Typical dosage: 25–50 ml per week

Nigella sativa

Common names: Black cumin

Family: Ranunculaceae

Part used: Seed

Description: Nigella seeds have long been used in folk medicine in the Arabian Gulf region, Far East Asia, and Europe. According to common Islamic and Arabic belief, black cumin (habbatul barakah) is a remedy for all ailments (universal healer). Black Seed is also mentioned as the curative 'black cumin' in the Bible and is described as Melanthion by Hippocrates and Dioscorides and as Gith by Pliny.

Constituents: Volatile oil containing thymoquinone (major compound), carvone, thymol, nigellone, nigellicine, nigellimine, nigellimine – N oxide, melanthin and melanthingenin. It also contains approximately 0.5–1.5% of volatile oil mainly comprised of *p*-cymene, ethyl linoleate, α-pinene, ethyl hexadecanoate, ethyl oleate, and β-pinene. Other constituents identified include fixed oil, resins, proteins, reducing sugars, tannins, bitter principles, glycosidal saponins, various glycerides, various glucosides, and amino acids such as crystine, lysine, aspartic acid, glutamic acid, alanine and tryptophan.

Primary actions: Anticancer, Antidiabetic, Hepatoprotective.

All actions: Anodyne, Anthelmintic, Anti-inflammatory, Antiasthmatic, Antibacterial, Anticancer, Anticonvulsant, Antidiabetic, Antimicrobial, Bronchodilator, Cardioprotective, Carminative, Digestive stimulant, Diuretic, Emmenagogue, Expectorant (general), Galactagogue, Hepatoprotective, Immunomodulator, Sedative, Uterine tonic.

Indications:

- Allergies/Sensitivities, Amenorrhoea, Anorexia, Autoimmune disease, Cancer; including prevention/supportive treatment, Cough, Diabetes, Dysentery, Dyslipidaemia, Dysmenorrhoea, Dyspepsia, Fever, Haemorrhoids, Headache, Hepatitis, Hypertension, Infection; urinary tract, Intestinal worms, Jaundice, Metabolic syndrome, Obesity, Polycystic ovarian syndrome.

Contraindications: Contrary to other sources, nigella seed preparation appears not to be contraindcated in pregnancy nor a particular concern in patients with anaemia.

Drug interactions: Nigella seed oil found to protect against methotrexate-induced hepatotoxicity in children with acute lymphoblastic leukemia.

Results of pharmacodynamics and pharmacokinetics studies suggested that simultaneous administration of fenugreek or *N. sativa* with amlodipine improves the pharmacological response of amlodipine in hypertensive rats, though there was no remarkable change in pharmacokinetic parameters.

Qualities: Spicy, bitter, warming

Typical dosage: 30–80 ml per week

Ocimum tenuiflorum

Common names: Tulsi, Holy basil

Family: Lamiaceae

Part used: Whole plant (predominantly leaf and seed)

Description: Traditionally, whole herb, leaf, seed and its essential oil are employed in the treatment of diabetic and respiratory conditions. According to the Indian Ayurvedic system of medicines they have been used to balance vata and kapha.

Constituents: Major compounds identified and isolated from the essential oil of the plant include eugenol, carvacrol, nerol, eugenolmethylether, menthol, menthone, isomenthone, 1,8-cineole, α-pinene, β-pinene, limonene, neomenthol, and menthofuran. In addition, leaves have been reported to contain ursolic acid, apigenin, luteolin, apigenin-7-O-glucuronide, luteolin-7-O-glucuronide, orientin and molludistin.

Primary actions: Antidiabetic, Antimicrobial, Antispasmodic (respiratory tract).

All actions: Analgesic, Antidiabetic, Antimicrobial, Antispasmodic (respiratory tract).

Indications:

- Asthma, Asthma; bronchial, Bronchitis, Common cold, Cough, Diabetes, Fever, Influenza, Rhinitis, Sinusitis.

- **WHO:** In the treatment of arthritis, asthma, bronchitis, common cold, diabetes, fever, influenza, peptic ulcer, rheumatism, earache, epilepsy, heart disease, malaria, sinusitis, snake bites, stomach ache, vomiting, anthelminthic, to stimulate lactation, to prevent hair loss, and as a tonic.

Qualities: Pungent, bitter, lightness, dryness, hot potency.

Typical dosage: 20–50 ml per week

Olea europaea

Common names: Olive tree

Family: Oleaceae

Part used: Leaves

Description: Fresh olives need to be processed due to their bitter and acrid taste. Olive oil helps maintain healthy blood lipid levels. Olive leaf has also been used to treat diabetes, hypertension, inflammation, diarrhoea, respiratory and urinary tract infections, stomach and intestinal diseases, asthma, hemorrhoids, rheumatism, and as a laxative, a mouth cleanser, and vasodilator.

Constituents: Leaf: secoiridoids (oleuropein, hydroxytyrosol, ligustroside, oleacein), triterpenoids (oleanolic acid, uvaol), sterols, flavonoids (hesperidin, rutin, apigenin, chrysoeriol, luteolin glycoside, kaempferol), phenolic acids. Olive oil represents about 30% of the ripe fruit, and is rich in triglycerides (oleic acid, linoleic acid).

Primary actions: Antihyperlipidemic, Cardioprotective, Vasodilator.

All actions: Antihyperlipidemic, Antioxidant, Cardioprotective, Cardiotonic, Diuretic, Vasodilator.

Indications:

- Dyslipidaemia, Gout, Hypertension, Infection; gastrointestinal system.

Qualities: Bitter, cool, dry

Typical dosage: 20–50 ml per week. Ideally standardised to oleuropein.

Paeonia lactiflora

Synonym or related species: Paeonia albiflora

Common names: Peony, white peony, bai shao

Family: Ranunculaceae

Part used: Root

Description: Key indications are PMS and PCOS.

The central activity seems to be that paeonia is an ovulation normaliser. Also used with *Angelica polymorpha* for menopausal hot flushes. Also used for postmenopausal symptoms associated with androgen excess such as androgenic alopecia (long term treatment).

Constituents: 8-debenzoylpaeoniflorin, albiflorin, benzoic acid, monoterpenoid glycosides, oxypaeoniflorin, paeoniflorin, palbinone, pentagalloyl glucose, peonan SA and SB, phenols, phytosterol, polysaccharides, sitosterol, terpenoids, triterpenoids.

Primary actions: Antihyperprolactinaemic, Hypothalamic-pituitary-ovarian (HPO) regulator, Menstrual cycle regulator.

All actions: Analgesic, Anti-inflammatory, Antiallergic, Antiandrogenic, Anticonvulsant, Antiepileptic, Antihyperprolactinaemic, Antispasmodic (muscles), Antispasmodic (uterus), Astringent, Hypothalamic-pituitary-ovarian (HPO) regulator, Immunomodulator, Menstrual cycle regulator, Nootropic, Sedative, Selective oestrogen receptor modulator (SERM).

Indications:

*   Acne, Acne (topically), Adenomyosis, Amenorrhoea, Androgen excess, Angina pectoris, Arteriosclerosis, Benign breast disease, Cramps; muscular spasm; muscular tension, Dysmenorrhoea, Dysmenorrhoea; spasmodic, Endometriosis, Epilepsy, Fibroids, Infertility, Irritable bowel syndrome, Leucorrhoea, Leucorrhoea and vaginitis (douche), Luteal phase complaints, Mastalgia, Memory and concentration; poor, Menopausal symptoms, Menstrual irregularity, Metrorrhagia, Migraine, Miscarriage; threatened, Myalgia, Ovarian cyst, Ovulation; eratic, Polycystic ovarian syndrome, Uterine bleeding; dysfunctional.

*   **WHO:** As an analgesic, anti-inflammatory and antispasmodic drug in the treatment of amenorrhoea, dysmenorrhoea, and pain in the chest and abdomen. Also used to treat dementia, headache, vertigo, spasm of the calf muscles, liver disease, and allergies, and as an anticoagulant.

Contraindications: None known.

Qualities: Sour, bitter, slightly cold

Typical dosage: 30–60 ml per week

Panax ginseng

Synonym or related species: Korean ginseng

Common names: Ginseng, Ren Shen

Family: Araliaceae

Part used: Fresh or mostly dried root

Description: Revered general tonic for both men and women. Adaptogens are indicated for fatigue and overwork. Other key indications include weakness, loss of physical stamina, diminished concentration, poor memory and menopausal hot flushes.

Depression commonly accompanies menopausal flushing, particularly when sleep is disturbed. Some of the most reliable herbs are *Hypericum perforatum*, *Lavandula officinalis*, combined with *Withania somnifera* and the ginsengs.

Constituents: Triterpenoid saponins (ginsenosides), also polyacetylenes (ginsenoynes A-K) and small amounts of essential oil.

Primary actions: Adaptogen, Cytoprotective, Immunomodulator.

All actions: Adaptogen, Anti-inflammatory, Antiarrhythmic, Antiasthmatic, Anticancer, Cardioprotective, Cardiotonic, Chemoprotective, Cytoprotective, Hepatoprotective, Hepatotonic, Hypoglycaemic, Immunomodulator, Male tonic, Selective oestrogen receptor modulator (SERM), Tonic.

Indications:

*   Angina pectoris, Arrhythmia, Asthma, Cancer; including prevention/supportive treatment, Cardiovascular disease prevention, Chemotherapy; to minimise the side effects of, Chronic fatigue syndrome, Congestive heart failure, Convalescence, Debility, Depression, Emphysema, Erectile dysfunction, Exhaustion, Immune deficiency, Impotence, Infection; to improve resistance to, Libido; low, Longevity, Memory and concentration; poor, Menopausal symptoms, Mental exhaustion, Radiation; side effects of, Sperm count; low, Stress.

*   **Commission E:** Tonic for invigoration and fortification in times of fatigue and debility or declining capacity for work and concentration; also during convalescence.

*   **ESCOP:** Decreased mental and physical capacities such as weakness, exhaustion, tiredness and loss of concentration, as well as during convalescence.

*   **WHO:** Prophylactic and restorative agent for enhancement of mental and physical capacities, in cases of weakness, exhaustion, tiredness, and loss of concentration, and during convalescence.

Cautions: May aggravate insomnia. Caution when administering during pregnancy or to diabetics.

Contraindications: Contraindicated in hypertension, acute asthma, acute infections with fever, signs of heat, excessive menstruation, nose bleeds and in persons who are very hot, overstimulated and tense. BHC contraindicates use concurrent with stimulants including excessive caffeine.

Drug interactions: Ginseng extracts may have an antioestrogenic effect in premenopausal women and a mild oestrogenic effect in postmenopausal women. There are no indications that ginseng interferes with the effect of oral contraceptives. Ginseng may reduce the adverse effects of postmenopausal hormone therapy. Coadministration of ginsenosides has been shown to prevent bone loss in ovariectomised animals. May interact with warfarin (positive animal studies, one case report and negative effect in clinical trials). May potentiate adverse effect of imatinib (case report) and HIV integrase inhibitors (case report). May potentiate the effects on hypoglycaemic medication. May increase side effects of MAO inhibitors (case reports). May decrease midazolam blood levels. May potentiate sildenafil.

Ginseng for one week significantly increased the plasma concentration of metformin, with increased half-life and urinary excretion of metformin following oral administration of metformin (50 mg/kg), which could be attributed to the increased absorption of metformin in vivo. Combination therapy may improve the efficacy of metformin.

Qualities: Sweet, slightly bitter, warm

Typical dosage: 7–14 ml per week (standardised extract)

Panax notoginseng

Synonym or related species: Panax pseudoginseng

Common names: Tienchi ginseng (san qi, tian qi – Mandarin) Yunnan bayou

Family: Araliaceae

Part used: Root

Description: Yunnan Bai Yao, a patent medicine to stop bleeding from traumatic injury and haemorrhage. Can also be used externally as a poultice for bleeding. Also used for cardiovascular disorders including angina pectoris, hypertension, dyslipidaemia and ischaemia. Used in gynaecology for menorrhagia due to fibroids and dysfunctional bleeding and for heavy bleeding following childbirth.

Constituents: Ginsenosides (many common to *P. ginseng* but in differing ratios)

Primary actions: Antihaemorrhagic (uterine), Antihyperlipidemic, Cardioprotective.

All actions: Anti-inflammatory, Antiarrhythmic, Antihaemorrhagic (uterine), Antihyperlipidemic, Antiobesity, Cardioprotective, Cardiotonic.

Indications:

• Angina pectoris, Arrhythmia, Arteriosclerosis, Atherosclerosis, Blood stasis, Congestive heart failure, Fibroids, Haematemesis, Haematuria, Haemorrhage; postpartum, Myocardial ischaemia, Uterine bleeding; dysfunctional, Weight loss; to assist.

Cautions: Acute remedy usually prescribed at time of bleeding.

Contraindications: Traditionally contraindicated during pregnancy (TCM).

Drug interactions: Ginseng extracts may have an antioestrogenic effect in premenopausal women and a mild oestrogenic effect in postmenopausal women. Coadministration of ginsenosides has been shown to prevent bone loss in ovariectomised animals.

Qualities: Sweet, slightly bitter, warm

Typical dosage: 30–60 ml per week

Panax quinquefolium

Common names: American ginseng

Family: Araliaceae

Part used: Root

Description: Ginseng is generally viewed as an adaptogen, a substance which can help reduce the impact of environmental stress. There are different species of ginseng, the two most common being Asian (*Panax ginseng*) and American (*Panax quinquefolius*), both from the genus Panax of the Araliaceae family. Both Asian and American ginseng have a common mixture of active ingredients, the most important being ginsenosides, in varying amounts, strengths, and ratios and both ginseng preparations are thought to have broad and similar activity.

Constituents: Complex mixture of triperpenoid dammarane saponins known as ginsenosides or quinquenosides. *P. quionguefolium* also contains 24-R-pseudoginsenoside not found in *P. ginseng*. Other constituents are polysaccharides, polyacetylenes, resins and a volatile oil.

Primary actions: Adaptogen, Nootropic, Tonic.

All actions: Adaptogen, Antiageing, Anticancer, Anxiolytic, Aphrodisiac, Cardioprotective, Hepatoprotective, Immunomodulator, Neuroprotective, Nootropic, Radiosensitiser, Tonic.

Indications:

• Anxiety, Cancer; including prevention/supportive treatment, Cardiovascular disease prevention, Dementia, Dyspepsia, Exhaustion, Fatigue, Memory and concentration; poor, Menopausal symptoms, Mental exhaustion.

Cautions: Doses up to 3,000 mg have been studied with no significant toxicity being reported.

Contraindications: Traditionally not used during signs of heat, acute infection, hypertension, and menorrhagia. Avoid with stimulants such as excessive caffeine.

Drug interactions: Reduction of testicular toxicity during doxorubicin therapy, sensitisation of tumour cells to cytotoxic drugs and radiation.

Typical dosage: 7–40 ml per week

Passiflora incarnata

Synonym or related species: Passiflora kerii

Common names: Passion flower

Family: Passifloraceae

Part used: Aerial parts, particularly leaves

Description: Traditional herb for stress, anxiety and insomnia. Anxiolytic activity is mediated via the GABAergic system.

Constituents: Flavonoids (C-glycosides of vitexin, isovitexin, apigenin, luteolin), traces of volatile oil, cyanogenic glycoside

Primary actions: Anxiolytic, Hypnotic, Sedative.

All actions: Anodyne, Anxiolytic, Hypnotic, Sedative.

Indications:

- Anxiety, Insomnia, Nervous tachycardia, Neuralgia, Premenstrual syndrome, Restlessness.
- **BHP:** Neuralgia, generalised seizures, hysteria, nervous tachycardia, restlessness, nervous stress and spasmodic asthma. Specific indications: insomnia.
- **Commission E:** Nervous restlessness.
- **ESCOP:** Tenseness, restlessness, and irritability with difficulty in falling asleep.
- **WHO:** Internally as a mild sedative for nervous restlessness, insomnia and anxiety. Treatment of gastrointestinal disorders of nervous origin.
- **Other uses:** May be useful in supportive treatment for withdrawal from opiates, cannabis, and alcohol.

Contraindications: Contraindicated during pregnancy due to possibility of uterine contractions.

Qualities: Cool, dry

Typical dosage: 20–40 ml per week

Pelargonium sidoides

Common names: African geranium, umckaloabo

Family: Geraniaceae

Part used: Root

Description: Umckaloabo means severe cough in Zulu. A 2008 Cochrane review suggests that *P. sidoides* may be effective in alleviating symptoms of acute rhinosinusitis and the common cold in adults. It may be effective in relieving symptoms in acute bronchitis in adults and children, and sinusitis in adults. The overall quality of the evidence was, however, considered low for main outcomes in acute bronchitis in children and adults, and very low for acute sinusitis and the common cold. A 2015 review found strong evidence for *A. paniculata* and ivy/primrose/thyme-based preparations and moderate evidence for *P. sidoides* being significantly superior to placebo in alleviating the frequency and severity of patients' cough symptoms. Another review supports the efficacy of extract EPs 7630 in adults with the common cold. This extract is also efficacious in children.

Constituents: Oligomeric and polymeric proanthocyanidins (polyphenols), cinnamic acids, tannins, flavonoids, and coumarins.

Primary actions: Antiviral, Immunomodulator, Mycolytic.

All actions: Antibacterial, Antimicrobial, Antiviral (systemically), Immunomodulator, Mycolytic.

Indications:

- Bronchitis, Common cold, Influenza, Pharyngitis, Sinusitis, Tonsillitis.
- **Other uses:** Traditionally used to treat dysentery,

diarrhoea, hepatic complaints, wounds, colds, fatigue, fevers, generalised weakness, and infections of the respiratory tract, including tuberculosis.

Cautions: Minor gastrointestinal complaints (e.g. gastric pain, heartburn, nausea, diarrhoea) reported in clinical studies.

Contraindications: None known.

Typical dosage: 20–40 ml per week.

Perilla frutescens

Common names: Perilla, su zi, shisu

Part used: Leaf, stem, seed

Description: Perilla is an annual plant native to Eastern Asia, and one of the most popular species in these communities. Used as an ingredient for flavour and as a spice in cooking, soups, salads and sushi, and as a garnish and food colourant. It is also used to wrap and eat cooked food in Japan, India, and Korea. The seed is mainly used for its high oil content. The salty Japanese umeboshi plum is coloured by the addition of special red perilla leaves. In China, perilla has been used to reduce the risk of food poisoning by cooking seafood with the leaf. In TCM, perilla seed is used for cough and wheezing with copious mucus. In recent times certain compounds (monoterpines) isolated from the oil are being trialed as an anticancer treatment while the defatted seed extract is used in the treatment of allergies.

Constituents: The **leaf** contains henolic compounds including caffeic acid, faffeic acid-3-O-glucoside, coumaroyl tartaric acid, ferulic acid, rosmarinic acid. Flavonoids including catechin, apigenin, catechin, luteolin and several varieties, scutellarein. Anthocyanins including chrysontenin, cyanin, malonylshisonin, shisonin. Triterpenes and a volatile oil containing terpenoids, and aromatic and aliphatic compounds.

The **seed** is rich in polycosanols, tocopherols, phytosterols and fatty acids. Defatted perilla seed extract is a concentrated ethanolic extract rich in phenolics including 30-dehydroxyl-rosmarinic acid-3-O-Glucoside, caffeic acid, ferulic acid, rosmarinic acid and its metyl ester and glucoside, vanillic acid. Flavonoids including catechin, apigenin, catechin, cimidahurinine, luteolin. Normally flavonoids exist as glycosides in plants, however, in perilla seed extract they occur as their aglycones (free flavonoids) that have more potent activity. The defatted extract is free of perilla ketone, perilla aldehyde and perillyl alcohol.

Primary actions: Anti-inflammatory, Antiallergic.

All actions: Anti-inflammatory, Antiallergic, Antibacterial, Anticancer, Antidiabetic, Antioxidant, Hepatoprotective.

Indications:

- Allergies/Sensitivities, Asthma, Diabetes, Diabetic neuropathy, Hayfever, Periodontitis, Rhinitis.

Contraindications: Insufficient information is

available to determine the safety of perilla during pregnancy.

Typical dosage: 30–70 ml per week

Petroselinum crispum

Common names: Parsley root

Family: Apiaceae

Part used: Root

Description: Parsley is believed to be cultivated in the Mediterranean regions since the third century BC. It was brought to England and apparently first cultivated in Britain in 1548.

Constituents: Phenolic compounds, flavonoids (particularly apigenin, apiin and 6-acetylapiin) and essential oils – mainly myristicin and apiol.

Primary actions: Antilithic, Carminative, Diuretic.

All actions: Anticancer, Antilithic, Antirheumatic, Antispasmodic/Spasmolytic, Carminative, Diuretic, Emmenagogue, Expectorant (general).

Indications:

* Colic; flatulent, Cystitis, Dyspepsia; flatulent, Menstrual irregularity, Urinary gravel.
* **BHP:** Flatulent dyspepsia, tormina, cystitis, dysuriea, bronchitic cough in the elderly. Dysmennorhoea, functional amenorrhoea. Myalgia – internal and topical use. Specific indications: Flatulent dyspepsia with intestinal colic.
* **Other uses:** In Persian medicine, the seeds are used as anti-infectives, antispasmodics, sedatives, antidotes, carminatives, digestives, astringents, gastrotonics, and in the management of gastrointestinal disorders, inflammation, halitosis, kidney stones, and amenorrhoea. Root extracts have been shown to have cytotoxic and antiproliferative action in cancer cell lines.

Cautions: Photosensitising furocoumarines bergapten and isoimperatorin in the root may increase the photosensitivity of the skin.

Typical dosage: 40–80 ml per week

Peumus boldus

Common names: Boldo

Family: Monimiaceae

Part used: Leaves

Description: A chilean tree whose leaves have been traditionally employed in folk medicine, especially for gall stones. A review of pharmacological actions found cytoprotective, antitumour promoting, anti-inflammatory, antidiabetic, antiatherogenic actions, vasorelaxant, antitrypanocidal, immuno- and neuromodulator, cholagogic and/or choleretic actions. Based on the pharmacological and toxicological data now available, further research needs and recommendations are suggested to define the clinical potential of boldo.

Constituents: Aprophine alkaloids (bolding),

essential oil (p-cymene, ascaridole, 1,8-cineole, linalool, minor monoterpenoids), flavonols and their glycosides (boldoglucin, isorhamnetin).

Primary actions: Cholagogue, Hepatotonic, Laxative.

All actions: Anthelmintic, Cholagogue, Diuretic, Hepatotonic, Sedative.

Indications:

* Cholecystitis, Cystitis, Dyspepsia, Gall stones (cholelithiasis), Gallbladder disorders, Rheumatism.
* **BHP:** Gall stones, pain in liver or gallbladder, cystitis, rheumatism. Specific indications: cholelithiasis.
* **Commission E:** For mild dyspepsia and spastic gastrointestinal complaints.
* **ESCOP:** Minor hepatobiliary dysfunction and symptomatic treatment of mild digestive disturbances.
* **Other uses:** Dry boldo extract prolongs orocaecal transit time.

Cautions: Pure oil not suitable for internal use (toxic). Continuous long-term use not recommended. Use with caution in unconjugated hyperbilirubinaemia, acute or severe hepatocellular disease, septic cholecystitis, intestinal spasm, or ileus or liver cancer.

Contraindications: Contraindicated during pregnancy and lactation, and in patients with biliary obstruction.

Drug interactions: Possible interaction with warfarin leading to increased anticoagulant activity of the drug; monitor prothrombin times and INR values.

Qualities: Bitter, cold

Typical dosage: 5–15 ml per week

Phyllanthus spp.

Synonym or related species: Phyllanthus amarus, Phyllanthus urinaria, Phyllanthus niruri, Phyllanthus fraternus

Common names: Phyllanthus

Family: Euphorbiaceae

Part used: Aerial parts

Description: Traditionally used on the Indian subcontinent for disorders of the stomach, genitourinary system, liver, kidney and spleen, and to treat chronic fever.

Constituents: Tannin (geraniin), lignan (hypo-phyllanthin), lignan (phyllanthin)

Primary actions: Antiviral (systemically), Hepatoprotective, Hepatotonic.

All actions: Antiviral (systemically), Blood sugar regulator, Chemoprotective, Cytoprotective, Hepatoprotective, Hepatotonic, Hypoglycaemic.

Indications:

* Diabetes, Fever, Gastroenteritis, Hepatitis, Infection; viral, Splenic enlargement.

85

Contraindications: None known.

Qualities: Cool

Typical dosage: 15–40 ml per week

Phytolacca americana

Synonym or related species: Phytolacca decandra

Common names: Poke root, pokeweed

Family: Phytolaccaceae

Part used: Root

Description: Native Americans and early settlers used pokeweed as an emetic and purgative, and a salve composed of a mixture of the root and lard was used to treat rheumatism. Poisoning can occur from ingestion of any part of the plant or from skin contact with the plant. Severe emesis and diarrhoea, accompanied by tachycardia, have been observed after ingestion of raw leaves and after drinking tea prepared from the powdered root.

Constituents: Alkaloids (betacyanins, betanidine, betanine, phytolaccine), triterpenoid saponins, lectin (pokeweed mitogen), antiviral protein (pokeweed antiviral protein), neolignans (isoamericanin A and others).

Primary actions: Antirheumatic, Immunomodulator, Lymphatic.

All actions: Anti-inflammatory (topically), Antirheumatic, Immunomodulator, Lymphatic.

Indications:

* Acne, Acne (topically), Glands; swollen, Inflammation; respiratory tract, Laryngitis, Lymphadenitis, Lymphadenopathy, Mammary abscess (poultice), Mastitis, Mumps, Rheumatism, Tinea (topically), Tonsillitis, Tracheitis.

* **BHP:** Chronic rheumatism, chronic respiratory catarrh, tonsillitis, laryngitis, adenitis, mastitis, mumps. Externally as ointment in scabies, tinea, sycosis, acne. Poultice in mammary abscess, mastitis. Specific indications: inflammatory conditions of the upper respiratory tract, lymphatic adenitis.

Cautions: Very low dosage; toxic in medium to large doses (nausea, abdominal pain, diarrhoea, haematemesis, hypotension and tachycardia have been reported). Do not use for longer than 6 months. Avoid contact with the eyes. Use with caution in patients with pre-existing cholestasis, coeliac disease, fat malabsorption, and vitamins A, D, E and K deficiency.

Contraindications: Contraindicated during pregnancy and lactation, and in patients with lymphocytic leukaemia and gastrointestinal irritation. Do not apply to broken or ulcerated skin.

Drug interactions: Avoid concurrent use with immunosuppressive drugs.

Qualities: Cool, pungent

Typical dosage: 1–5 ml per week

86

Picrorhiza kurroa

Common names: Kutki

Family: Scrophulariaceae

Part used: Root

Description: Traditional Ayurvedic herb for liver and bronchial disorders. Kutkin, a mixture of iridoid glycosides picroside I and kutkoside has hepatoprotective properties. Androsin, a phenolic glycoside, has antiasthmatic, antiplatelet and antiallergic properties. Picroliv (Sabinsa Corporation) a standardised extract (4% catkin) has been shown to have anti-inflammatory, apoptotic, hepatoprotective, immunomodulating, antiparasitic, anticarcinogenic properties and protect against repercussion injury, promote epithelialisation and angiogenesis in wounds, prevent of cadmium toxicity and reduce inflammation in colitis.

Constituents: Iridoid glycosides (kutkin), cucurbitacin glycosides (highly oxygenated triterpenes) including cucurbitacin B, apocynin, androsin.

Primary actions: Antiallergic, Hepatoprotective, Immunomodulator.

All actions: Anti-inflammatory, Antiallergic, Antiasthmatic, Anticancer, Antiseptic (GIT), Antiseptic (respiratory tract), Bitter tonic, Choleretic, Hepatoprotective, Hepatotonic.

Indications:

* Allergies/Sensitivities, Asthma, Autoimmune disease, Cancer; including prevention/supportive treatment, Hepatitis, Immune deficiency, Infection; systemic, Non-alcoholic fatty liver disease (NAFLD), Rheumatoid arthritis.

Cautions: May cause severe abdominal cramping. Start with 10 ml per week, and do not exceed recommended dose. Combine with antispasmodic or carminative herbs.

Contraindications: None known

Qualities: Bitter, cold

Typical dosage: 10–20 ml per week

Pimpinella anisum

Synonym or related species: Anisum officinarum

Common names: Aniseed

Family: Apiaceae

Part used: Ripe dried fruits

Description: The seed contains anethole with phyto-oestrogenic properties used to promote breast milk production and alleviate hot flushes during menopause. Foeniculum vulgare, Anethum graveolens, Pimpinella anisum, Nigella sativa, and Vitex agnus-castus are among the most effective galactogogues. Anise oil is beneficial in IBS (enteric coated capsules) and to treat hair lice. The carminative action combines well with laxative herbs.

Constituents: 5% essential oil (trans-anethole, estragole, anise ketone, anisaldehye, anisic acid), flavonoids (rutin, quercetin, agigenin), coumarins (bergapten), fatty oil, choline, Vit B, potassium, calcium, iron, magnesium.

Primary actions: Carminative, Galactagogue, Selective oestrogen receptor modulator (SERM).

All actions: Antiparasitic, Carminative, Expectorant (general), Galactagogue, Laxative, Selective oestrogen receptor modulator (SERM).

Indications:

- Bronchitis, Colic; flatulent, Cough, Flatulence, Inflammatory bowel disease, Pertussis, Respiratory catarrh, Tracheitis.

- **BHP:** Bronchial catarrh, pertussis, spasmodic cough, flatulent colic. Topically for pediculosis, scabies. Specific indications: bronchitis, tracheitis with persistent cough.

- **ESCOP:** Dyspeptic complaints such as mild spasmodic gastrointestinal complaints, bloating and flatulence. Catarrh of the upper respiratory tract.

- **WHO:** Treatment of dyspepsia and mild inflammation of the respiratory tract.

- **Other uses:** The internal dosage of aniseed essential oil is 3–5 drops on a lump of sugar or honey several times daily.

Contraindications: Persons with known sensitivity to anethole and aniseed should avoid aniseed. Preparations containing the essential oil or alcohol extracts should not be used during pregnancy or lactation. Due to reports of anethole toxicity in infants, use in children under the age of 12 years is contraindicated.

Qualities: Dry, warm

Typical dosage: 20–40 ml per week

Pinus pinaster

Common names: Maritime bark

Family: Pinaceae

Part used: Bark

Description: Maritime pine bark extract was developed by Masquelier who named the active extract pycnogenol; a term no longer used in the scientific community today except as a trademark for oligomeric proanthocyanidins (OPCs) derived from French maritime pine bark. Pycnogenol® contains oligomeric proanthocyanidins (OPCs) as well as several other bioflavonoids: catechin, epicatechin, phenolic fruit acids (such as ferulic acid and caffeic acid), and taxifolin.

Constituents: Maritime pine bark contains polyphenolic compounds classified as monomeric and oligomeric flavan-3-ols. Condensed flavanols (oligomers and polymers) are also known as proanthocyanidins or oligomers of proanthocyanidines (OPCs). The name stems from the Greek works anthos meaning flower and kyanos meang blue, referring to the water-soluble pigments responsible for the blue, violet or red colours of many flowers and fruits. Proanthocyanidins are an integral part of the human diet, found in high concentrations in fruits such as apple, pear, and grapes, and in chocolate, wine, and tea. Grape seed extract is also a rich source of OPCs/flavan-3-ols.

Primary actions: Antioedematous, Antioxidant, Vasoprotective.

All actions: Antioedematous, Anti-inflammatory, Anticancer, Antioxidant, Antiviral (systemically, Vasoprotective.

Indications:

- Asthma, Diabetes, Diabetic retinopathy, Dyslipidaemia, Fluid retention, Gingivitis, Hypertension, Venous insufficiency, Venous leg ulcers.

Cautions: Due to its very astringent taste and occasional minor stomach discomfort, it may be best to take maritime pine bark extract with or after meals. The ability of OPCs to form complex protein is referred to as astringency and is responsible for the 'puckery' sensation when tea, red wine or an OPC-rich extract comes in contact with saliva and buccal tissue.

Drug interactions: An in vitro study has showed that an OPC extract may improve the efficacy of acetylsalicylic acid in the inhibition of platelet function. Whether this has any clinical relevance needs to be demonstrated. OPCs may reduce adverse effects of common chemotherapy drugs cyclophosphamide and doxorubicin. An animal study found that OPCs inhibit thymus DNA synthesis induced by cyclophosphamide. An in vitro study found that an OPCs may have a protective effect on the cardio-toxicity of doxorubicin. In a clinical trial with an OPC-rich extract, it was shown to reduce the need for the Calcium channel blocker nifedipine in mildly hypertensive patients. A case report of a 10 year-old with attention deficit hyperactivity disorder (ADHD) suggests that the OPC-rich extract in addition with dexedrine (dextroamphetamine) may decrease hyperactive and impulsive behaviour.

Typical dosage: Extracts containing 100–200 mg OPCs daily.

Piper methysticum

Common names: Kava

Family: Piperaceae

Part used: Rhizome, root

Description: Kava is traditionally used in the South Pacific island nations (mainly Vanuatu, Fiji, Tonga, Samoa and New Caledonia) for the preparation of a recreational drink with relaxing effect. The safety and the anxiolytic effects of kava have been examined in observational and controlled clinical trials. The observed hepatotoxicity is probably related to the use of the inferior kava cultivar known as 'two-day kava' and the use of acetone as a solvent by some European companies. 'Two-day kava' is known locally to produce a two day hangover effect and is generally avoided by the islanders.

Constituents: Fat-soluble kava lactones (kavapyrones), mainly methysticin, dihydromethysticin, kavain, dihydrokavain, desmethoxyangonin, flavonoids (flavokavains).

Primary actions: Anaesthetising (mucous membranes), Anxiolytic, Sedative.

All actions: Anaesthetising (mucous membranes), Analgesic, Anodyne, Antiepileptic, Antihypertensive, Antimicrobial, Antispasmodic (muscles), Antispasmodic/Spasmolytic, Anxiolytic, Hypnotic, Sedative.

Indications:

- Anxiety, Cramps; muscular spasm; muscular tension, Depression; postnatal, Headache, Hypertension, Insomnia, Menopausal symptoms, Menopause; depression, Muscular tension, Nervous tension, Night cramps, Premenstrual syndrome, Stress.
- **BHP:** Cystitis, urethritis, rheumatism. Topically for joint pains. Specific indications: genito-urinary tract infection.
- **ESCOP:** Anxiety, tension and restlessness arising from various causes of non-psychotic origin.
- **WHO:** Short-term symptomatic treatment of mild states of anxiety or insomnia, due to nervousness, stress or tension.

Cautions: No adverse effects are to be expected on vital signs and physical findings when exposed to the recommended doses of kava extract, and even with overdoses. The only known finding is the kava dermopathy syndrome producing scaly skin, possibly due to concomitant alcohol abuse, which is reversible upon cessation.

Contraindications: Kava has no hallucinogenic effects and does not cause addiction. There is therefore no typical abuse phenomenon as observed with illicit drugs. Tolerance effects have never been observed with kava use, be it traditional kava drinking of the application of kava extracts. There is no known requirement for dose increases over time or a reduction of efficacy with continued application. Withdrawal effects have never been observed with kava use, neither with traditional kava drinking for with the application of kava extracts in herbal medicinal products. The clinical data do not point towards a requirement for tapering off the intake.

The effect on cognition and the ability to drive have been examined in dedicated studies with kava extract, showing no negative effect in the relevant dose range.

No information is available on the safety of kava during pregnancy and lactation. As lipophilic substances, kavalactones might theoretically pass into breast milk, but there are no data confirming this suspicion. Kava not recommended for the use by pregnant or breastfeeding women. There is insufficient experience with respect to the use in children.

Drug interactions: Avoid with benzodiazepines (e.g. Alprazolam, Xanax), as co-prescription may increase sedation. Kava may decrease the effectiveness of levodopa (Madopa, Sinemet) because of dopamine antagonism. May reduce the effectiveness of levodopa in the treatment of symptoms of Parkinson's disease.

Kava does not significantly modify Pgp and would probably not have any drug–botanical interactions with drugs such as digoxin. Kava extract is a potent inhibitor of CyP 1A2, CyP 2C9, and CyP 2C19 and a weak inhibitor of CyP 2D6 and 3A4, based on studies conducted using crude extracts from the rhizomes of kava in human liver microsomes. A subsequent study similarly demonstrated that kava causes concentration-dependent decrease in CyP 3A4 activity in primary human hepatocytes. However, kava did not affect CyP 1A2, 3A4, or 2D6 activities in human studies.

Qualities: Dry, neutral

Typical dosage: 20–60 ml per week (standard extract)

Piscidia piscipula

Synonym or related species: Piscidia erythrina

Common names: Jamaican dogwood

Family: Fabaceae

Part used: Root bark

Description: Traditionally used to control pain and relieve general distress: 'If given during the course of inflammatory fever of any character, and in inflammatory rheumatism, it is a useful and grateful remedy. It does not oppose other indicated agents, and induces the often needed sleep. In violent spasmodic cough it produces relief, and in the irritating persistent cough of bronchitis it is of service as an auxiliary to cough syrups. In phthisis it controls the night cough and induces restful sleep.' – Ellingwood, *American Materia Medica*, 1919.

Constituents: Isoflavonoids (erythbigenin, piscidone, ichthynone, jamaicin, lisetin, rotenone), organic acids (piscidic, fukiic, methylfukiic), tannins, beta-sitosterol

Primary actions: Anodyne, Hypnotic, Sedative.

All actions: Anodyne, Anti-inflammatory, Antispasmodic/Spasmolytic, Antitussive, Hypnotic, Sedative.

Indications:

- Cough, Dysmenorrhoea, Insomnia, Migraine, Nervous tension, Neuralgia, Rheumatism, Stress.
- **BHP:** Neuralgia, migraine, insomnia, dysmenorrhoea. Specific indications: insomnia due to neuralgia or nervous tension.

Cautions: Strongly discouraged in breastfeeding;

do not use without medical supervision. May cause nausea and headache in susceptible patients. Caution when using in patients with depression and insomnia marked by increasing restlessness during the early hours of the morning; monitor closely. Prescribe with caution for pain in children, neurological disease, liver and kidney disease, or a history of allergic or anaphylactic reactions. Caution is advised in women wishing to conceive. Prescription should be limited in duration.

Contraindications: Contraindicated in pregnancy, bradycardia and cardiac insufficiency.

Qualities: Cool, pungent

Typical dosage: 20–40 ml per week

Plantago lanceolata

Common names: Ribwort, narrow-leaved plantain

Family: Plantaginaceae

Part used: Leaves

Description: A mucilagenous herb for the treatment of wounds and dry cough caused by pharyngitis. Due to its positive benefit–risk ratio *Plantago lanceolata* is suitable for the treatment of moderate chronic irritative cough in children. A variety of pharmacological effects have been reported for plantago lanceolata extracts and other preparations and for iridoid glycoside and aucubin. Most of the investigations are quite old, while more recent investigations have mainly been performed with isolated compounds of the plant, making it difficult to assess the clinical relevance.

Constituents: Iridoid glycosides: mainly aucubin and catalpol; mucilage polysaccharides; flavonoids: mainly apigenin and luteolin; phenylethanoids: acteoside, plantamajoside; phenol carboxylic acids and tannins.

Primary actions: Anticatarrhal, Demulcent, Expectorant (general).

All actions: Anti-inflammatory, Anti-inflammatory (urinary), Antibacterial, Anticatarrhal, Antiseptic, Antispasmodic (respiratory tract), Astringent, Demulcent, Expectorant (general), Immunomodulator, Wound healing/Vulnerary.

Indications:

• Allergies/Sensitivities, Bronchitis, Catarrh; naso-pharyngeal congestion, Cough, Eczema, Haemorrhoids, Laryngitis, Rhinitis, Sinusitis, Ulcer (topically), Ulcer; mouth, Wounds.

• **ESCOP:** Catarrhs of the respiratory tract. Temporary, mild inflammations of the oral and pharyngeal mucosa.

Cautions: The oral administration has been investigated in a post-marketing study in 598 patients which confirms the safe use in elderly, adults, adolescents and children between 3 and 12 years of age. As there is only limited data on the use of *Plantago lanceolata* in children under 3 years and due to their special medical conditions, oral use is not recommended for this age group.

Contraindications: None known.

Qualities: Cold, dry

Typical dosage: 20–40 ml per week

Plantago major

Common names: Plantain, broad-leaved plantain, Che Qian Zi

Family: Plantaginaceae

Part used: Leaves harvested just prior to flowering

Description: Traditionally used for cystitis with haematuria, and externally for bleeding haemorrhoids. *Plantago major* has been shown to have equivalence to chlorhexidine and sodium bicarbonate solutions in the treatment of oral mucositis in cancer patients. An aloe vera and *P. major* gel has shown some promise in the treatment of diabetic foot ulcer in a pilot study. Contrary to traditional properties, *P. major* is not diuretic as defined by increased urinary output.

Constituents: Iridoids (aucubin), flavonoids (apigenin, luteolin, baicalein), tannins, organic acids, mucilage, vitamins C and K, calcium, potassium, sulphur, trace minerals.

All actions: Anti-inflammatory, Antiseptic, Astringent, Demulcent.

Indications:

• Cystitis, Cystitis with haematuria, Haematuria, Haemorrhoids, Mucositis, Ulcer; mouth, Wounds (topically).

• **BHP:** Cystitis with haematuria, haemorrhoids. Specific indications: haemorrhoids with bleeding and irritation.

• **Other uses:** Chemotherapy-induced mucositis.

Contraindications: None known.

Qualities: Cold 2nd degree, dry 2nd degree

Typical dosage: 15–30 ml per week

Plectranthus barbatus

Synonym or related species: Coleus forskohlii

Common names: Coleus, makandi

Family: Lamiaceae

Part used: Root

Description: Traditional medicinal of Ayurvedic medicine, as well as in the folk medicine of Brazil, tropical Africa and China. Used for intestinal disturbance and liver fatigue, respiratory disorders, heart diseases and certain nervous system disorders.

Constituents: Labdane diterpene (aka forskohlin or coleonol), essential oils. Forskolin is an adenylyl cyclase activator that underlies the wide range of pharmacological properties.

Primary actions: Antiangina, Antiasthmatic, Cardiotonic.

All actions: Anti-inflammatory, Antiallergic,

Antiangina, Antiasthmatic, Anticancer, Antihypertensive, Antiobesity, Antiplatelet, Antipsoriatic, Antispasmodic (muscles), Antispasmodic (respiratory tract), Bronchodilator, Cardiotonic, Digestive tonic, Lipolytic, Sialogogue, Thyroid stimulant, Vasodilator.

Indications:

- Angina pectoris, Anorexia, Asthma, Bronchitis, Cardiovascular disease prevention, Cerebrovascular disease, Digestive complaints, Digestive weakness, Hayfever, Hypertension, Myocardial ischaemia, Psoriasis, Thyroid gland; impaired, Weight loss; to assist.
- **Other uses:** Congestive cardiac failure, thrombosis, chronic obstructive pulmonary disease, glaucoma.

Cautions: Large doses of forskolin were found to cause a depressant action on the central nervous system in mice.

Contraindications: Hypotension and gastric ulcer.

Drug interactions: Antiplatelet activity of forskolin may theoretically interact with antiplatelet and anticoagulant drugs. Shown to reduce the anticoagulant activity of warfarin in vivo. May potentiate the effects of antihypertensive medication.

Qualities: Neutral

Typical dosage: 40–90 ml per week

Poria cocos

Common names: Hoelen, China root, sclerotium of tuckahoe, fu ling (Mandarin) and bukuryo (Japanese)

Family: Polyporaceae

Part used: Sclerotium

Description: Combined in cinnamon and hoelen combination for dysmenorrhoea, menorrhagia and adenomyosis (*Paeonia lactiflora* and *P. suffruticosa, Poria cocos, Cinnamomum cassia* and *Prunus persica*). Needs to be prescribed over long periods, usually until menopause, as symptoms often return if the formula is stopped.

Constituents: Pachyman polysaccharides, triterpene acids (pachymic acid, tumulosic acid, eburicoic acid, pnicolic acid, poricodic acid A and B, hydroxylanostatriendioic acid, trienoic acid, hydroxytrametenoic acid, dehydropahcymic acid, epidehydrotumulosic acid, dehydroeburiconic acid, polyporenic acid C, poricoric acid D and AM), ergosterol, choline, histidine, adenine, lecithin and potassium

Primary actions: Anti-inflammatory, Immunomodulator, LH-RH antagonist.

All actions: Anti-inflammatory, Antidiarrhoeal, Antiemetic, Antioxidant, Antiviral (systemically), Digestive tonic, Diuretic, Immunomodulator, LH-RH antagonist.

Indications:

- Anxiety, Benign breast disease, Cancer; including

prevention/supportive treatment, Congestive heart failure, Diarrhoea, Dysmenorrhoea, Fibroids, Fluid retention, Gastritis, Infertility, Inflammation, Insomnia, Leucorrhoea, Longevity, Memory and concentration; poor, Nausea, Nephritis, Nervous exhaustion, Nervous tension.

- **Other uses:** Traditionally used for disorders of the female reproductive tract including hypermenorrhea, dysmenorrhoea, fibroids, leucorrhoea and infertility. Hoelen increases progesterone secretion from the corpus luteum. Cinnamon and hoelen combination (Cinnamomum cassia, Paeonia lactiflora, Paeonia suffruticosa, Prunus persica) is used in the treatment of gynaecological disorders such as hypermenorrhea, dysmenorrhoea and infertility, decreases in LH, FSH and oestradiol. Non-specific fluid retention, renal and cardiac oedema, nephritis, difficult urination and neurasthenia. Gastrointestinal bleeding, burn injury, premature ageing, inflammatory conditions, cancer prevention, cardiac disease.

Contraindications: Contraindicated in patients with frequent, copious urine from deficiency cold (TCM diagnosis).

Qualities: Cooling

Typical dosage: Liquid extract: 40–80 ml per week

Propolis

Common names: Propolis

Part used: Resin

Description: Resin produced from flower nectar collected and processed by bees.

Constituents: Flavonoids (acacetin, galangin, pinocembrin), quercetin glucosides

Primary actions: Antimicrobial, Antiseptic (topically), Gastroprotective.

All actions: Antimicrobial, Antiseptic (GIT), Antiseptic (topically), Antiviral (systemically), Gastroprotective, Immunomodulator, Wound healing/Vulnerary.

Indications:

- Gastrointestinal tract dysbiosis, Gingivitis, Infection; fungal, Infection; gastrointestinal system, Infection; protozoal, Infection; respiratory tract, Infection; viral, Inflammation; oral cavity, Stomatitis, Ulcer (topically), Ulcer; gastrointestinal, Ulcer; mouth, Ulcerative colitis, Wounds (topically).

Cautions: Low incidence of contact dermatitis in beekeepers (about 1 in 2000). Caution should be exercised with patients who have a history of allergies, especially skin rashes.

Contraindications: None known.

Qualities: Neutral, pungent

Typical dosage: 15–30 ml per week

Prunus serotina

Synonym or related species: Cerasus serotina

Common names: Wild cherry, black cherry

Family: Rosaceae

Part used: Bark

Description: Native American herb for cough, especially a dry cough, as prunasin inhibits the cough reflex. Also considered a digestive tonic and also used for diarrhoea.

Constituents: Tannins, flavonoids, cyanogenic glycosides (prunasin), scopoletin

Primary actions: Antispasmodic (respiratory tract), Antitussive, Expectorant (general).

All actions: Antispasmodic (respiratory tract), Antitussive, Astringent, Expectorant (general), Sedative.

Indications:

• Bronchitis, Cough, Dyspepsia; nervous, Pertussis.

• **BHP:** Persistent cough, pertussis, and nervous dyspepsia. Specific indications: irritable and persistent cough of bronchitis, cough due to increased irritability of respiratory mucosa, pertussis.

Cautions: Do not use during pregnancy without professional advice. Use only as needed and limit use as soon as possible.

Contraindications: None known.

Qualities: Cool, dry

Typical dosage: 15–30 ml per week

Pseudowintera colorata

Common names: Horopito

Family: Winteraceae

Part used: Leaf

Description: Horopito is commonly known as New Zealand pepperwood due to the hot, peppery flavour of its leaves. Traditionally, the indigenous Maori population used the leaves and berries as a flavouring agent for food and medicinally for a variety of diseases including sexually transmitted infections, ringworm, chafed skin and skin diseases. Skin complaints were historically treated using bruised leaves or inner bark, which had been steeped in water or chewed before application. The inhibition of bacterial triggers for autoimmune disease, suggests a possible use for the prevention of autoimmune diseases including rheumatoid arthritis, ankylosing spondylitis, multiple sclerosis and rheumatic fever.

Constituents: Volatile oils containing eugenol and sesquiterpene dialdehydes polygodial and 9-deoxymuzigadial responsible for its hot, peppery flavour, anthocyanins, flavonols, dihydroflavonols, hydroxycinnamic acids and tannins.

Primary actions: Anti-inflammatory (GIT), Antifungal, Circulatory stimulant.

All actions: Anti-inflammatory, Anti-inflammatory (GIT), Antiallergic, Antibacterial, Antifungal, Antifungal (topically), Astringent, Circulatory stimulant, Gastroprotective, Rubefacient.

Indications:

• Asthma, Candidiasis, Chilblains; unbroken (topically), Circulation; peripheral, Common cold, Cough, Infection; bacterial, Infection; fungal, Inflammation, Inflammation; skin (topically), Intermittent claudication, Raynaud's syndrome.

• **Other uses:** More recently, modern herbalists have used Horopito for the management of digestive and skin conditions. It is also the featured ingredient in products marketed for the treatment of fungal infections, as it has been shown clinically to be particularly effective against *Candida albicans.*

Cautions: Case report of contact vulvitis in a 16-yearold patient following vaginal application of a Horopito-containing cream.

Contraindications: Acute gastritis, peptic ulcers.

Drug interactions: None known.

Qualities: Warming

Typical dosage: 10-30 ml per week

Pueraria lobata

Common names: Kudzu

Family: Leguminosae

Part used: Root

Description: Kudzu has been traditionally used in TCM to treat alcoholism, diabetes, gastroenteritis, cardiovascular diseases, diarrhoea, dysentery, fever, and deafness. Limited evidence suggests that kudzu may improve signs and symptoms of unstable angina, improve insulin resistance, and have a positive effect on cognitive function in postmenopausal women.

Some, but not all, animal and human studies have found kudzu decreased alcohol intake. Subjects in the human study reported feeling intoxicated earlier and apparently slowed their consumption accordingly. Additionally, no side effects were noted.

Constituents: Isoflavonies including daidzin, daidzein, puerarin (daidzein-8-C-glucoside), genistin, genistein, tectorigenin, glycitin, tectoridin, 6-O-xylosyltectoridin, 6-O-xyloglycitin, biochanin A, isoflavonoids, triterpenoids, and spinasterol. Puearin is considered the main active compound which is also used in its pure form intravenously at 200–500 mg per day.

Primary actions: Antiaddictive, Cardioprotective, Hepatoprotective.

All actions: Anti-inflammatory, Antiaddictive, Antiarrhythmic, Anticancer, Antidiabetic, Antihyperlipidemic, Antihypertensive, Antihyperuricaemic, Antinociceptive, Antiosteoporotic, Cardioprotective, Hepatoprotective,

Neuroprotective, Selective oestrogen receptor Modulator (SERM), Vasodilator, Vasoprotective.

Indications:

- Alcoholism, Angina pectoris, Cardiovascular disease prevention, Diabetes, Diabetic neuropathy, Diabetic retinopathy, Dyslipidaemia, Hypertension, Osteoporosis.

- **Other uses:** The data from the reviewed studies demonstrated that 200–500 mg IV puerarin decreased the urinary albumin excretion rate in diabetic neuropathy patients with few adverse events, suggesting that puerarin may be a beneficial therapy for treating diabetic neuropathy.

Cautions: High dosages may cause gastrointestinal distress, such as nausea, dyspepsia, vomiting and bloating.

Contraindications: There is a lack of data on the use of kudzu during pregnancy or lactation.

Qualities: Pungent, cooling.

Typical dosage: 25–90 ml per week

Punica granatum

Common names: Pomegranate

Family: Punicaceae

Description: All parts of the pomegranate have a long history of use in traditional medicines in the Middle East and across Asia. The seed oil has SERM activity, the fruit is rich in phenolic compounds with strong antioxidant activity. The fruit and bark of pomegranate are used against intestinal parasites, dysentery, and diarrhoea. The juice and seeds are considered a tonic for throat and heart. Externally used to stop nose and gum bleeds and treat haemorrhoids.

Constituents: 50% of the total fruit weight corresponds to the peel, which is an important source of bioactive compounds. Ellagitannins (hydrolysable tannins) as esters of hexahydroxydiphenic acid and apolyol, usually glucose or quinic acid and glycosides including punicalagin, punicalin, pedunculagin and their hydrolysis products e.g. ellagic acid. Ellagitannins are not absorbed but reach the colon and release ellagic that is metabolised by the human microflora. Flavonoids including luteolin, quercetin, and kaempferol, proanthocyanidins including cyanidin, pelargonidin, and delphinidin as well as polysaccharides and fatty acids.

Primary actions: Antimicrobial, Antiparasitic, Astringent.

All actions: Anti-inflammatory, Anticancer, Antidiabetic, Antidiarrhoeal, Antihyperlipidemic, Antimicrobial, Antioxidant, Antiparasitic, Antiviral (systemically), Astringent.

Indications:

- Cancer; including prevention/supportive treatment, Diabetes, Diarrhoea, Dyslipidaemia, Haemorrhoids (topically), Hepatitis, Infection; viral,

Parasites, Periodontitis, Sore throat (gargle).

Cautions: No observed-adverse-effect level (NOAEL) for this standardised pomegranate fruit extract was determined as 600 mg/kg body weight/day, the highest dose tested.

Typical dosage: 40–125 ml per week

Quercus robur

Common names: Oak bark

Family: Fagaceae

Part used: Bark

Description: The European oak tree is traditionally used in tanning and as medicine. Both the bark and leaves of the oak tree have been used medicinally. Its astringent effects were used to treat diarrhoea, vomiting, mouth ulcers, sore throats and leucorrhoea. The tree was sacred to the Druids and much folklore exists about its magical uses, including the acorns being used for fertility. The acorns were also soaked, dried and ground into a flour, and used by the peasants and for fodder. Oak barrels releasing ellagitannins are used to store and flavour wine.

Constituents: Tannins including roburins (A–E) including grandinin and ellagitannins including gallic acid, ellagic acid, vescalagin, and castalagin. Oak also includes flavonoid glycosides (including rutin), and proanthocyanidins. Robuvit® contains tannins e.g., gallic acid, ellagic acid, vescalagin, and castalagin. The extract is standardised according to its HPLC profile and its polyphenol content (> 40%).

Primary actions: Antimicrobial, Astringent, Lithotryptic.

All actions: Anti-inflammatory, Antimicrobial, Antioxidant, Astringent, Diuretic, Lithotryptic.

Indications:

- Calculi; kidney and bladder, Diarrhoea, Eczema, Eczema (topically), Fatigue, Haemorrhoids, Haemorrhoids (topically), Lymphoma treatment; as an adjunct to, Pharyngitis, Psoriasis, Sore throat (gargle), Tonsillitis.

- **BHP:** Diarrhoea, pharyngitis, tonsillitis, haemorrhoids. Topical: haemorrhoids (enema), leucorrhoea (douche).

- **Commission E:** Non-specific, acute diarrhoea, inflammatory skin disorders, Topical: mild inflammation of the oral cavity and pharyngeal region, and genital and anal area, eczema.

- **Other uses:** Robuvit®, 300 mg standardised extract of Q. robur, shown to be beneficial in the treatment of lymphoedema, and to improve fatigue in healthy volunteers and in patients recovering from influenza. Robuvit® has been shown to rejuvenate mitochondrial function which may account for its beneficial effects on energy levels. Also found to stimulate mitophagy.

- Urocalun®, extract of Q. salicina, has been clinically used for the treatment of urolithiasis in

Japan since 1969. Two tablets (containing 225 mg extract) three times daily.

Non-standardised liquid extracts may not provide the same benefits as Urocalun® and Robuvit®.

Cautions: Not be used in high doses for long periods. Tannin-containing herbs may reduce absorption of nutrients and medical drugs. Administer away from food and other medications.

Contraindications: Avoid tannins in constipation and iron-deficient anaemia.

Typical dosage: 20-40 ml per week

Rehmannia glutinosa

Synonym or related species: Rehmannia chinensis

Common names: Rehmannia, sheng di huang (uncured), shu di huang (cured), Chinese foxglove

Family: Scrophulariaceae

Part used: Root

Description: Common ingredient in multiherb TCM formulations for inflammation and autoimmune disorders including nephritis, nephropathy, diabetes, benign prostatic hyperplasia, obesity, stress, diabetic foot ulcers, menopausal symptoms, PCOS, metabolic syndrome, dementia, periodontal disease, SLE, osteoporosis, ankylosing spondylitis, aplastic anaemia, radiation toxicity. Combined with *Angelica polymorpha* in chronic obstructive pulmonary disease.

Constituents: Iridoid compounds (jioglutosides, rehmaglutins, jioglutins), other glycosides

Primary actions: Adaptogen, Anti-inflammatory, Immunomodulator.

All actions: Adaptogen, Anti-inflammatory, Antihaemorrhagic (uterine), Antipyretic, Immunomodulator.

Indications:

- Allergies/Sensitivities, Amenorrhoea, Anaemia, Autoimmune disease, Chronic fatigue syndrome, Convalescence, Exhaustion, Haematuria, Menstrual irregularity, Metrorrhagia.

- **WHO:** Internally for the symptomatic treatment of fevers, diabetes, hypertension, rheumatoid arthritis, skin eruptions and maculation, sore throat, hypermenorrhoea and polymenorrhoea. As a tonic to stimulate the immune system.

Cautions: Transient diarrhoea, abdominal pain, oedema, fatigue, vertigo and heart palpitations have been reported. Do not administer during pregnancy or lactation or to children without medical supervision.

Contraindications: Contraindicated in chronic liver or gastrointestinal diseases, and diarrhoea. In TCM, uncured Rehmannia is contraindicated in pregnant women with deficient blood, deficient spleen, or deficient stomach.

Qualities: Uncured: bitter, cold, sweet. Cured: sweet, slightly warm

Typical dosage: 30-60 ml per week

Reynoutria multiflora

Synonym or related species: Fallopia multiflora, Polygonum multiflorum

Common names: He Shou Wu, Fo-Ti

Family: Polygonaceae

Part used: Root

Description: He Shou Wu is a traditional Chinese medicine with a long history for promoting hair growth and prevention of greying. The crude herb seems better in this regard compared to the processed root commonly used as the preferred medicine. A clinical study found He Shou Wu extract to improve Ability of Daily Living Scale scores in patients with Alzheimer's disease.

TGA warning: Health professionals should be aware that, in rare circumstances, some complementary medicines may cause liver damage in some individuals. When treating patients presenting with symptoms of liver damage, health professionals should consider whether a complementary medicine could be involved.

Constituents: Anthraquinones, tannins, phospholipids (lecithin), trace elements, tetrahydrostilbene glycoside.

Primary actions: Antihyperlipidemic, Bitter tonic, Nervine tonic.

All actions: Antihyperlipidemic, Antioxidant, Bitter tonic, Nervine tonic.

Indications:

- Connective tissue disorders, Epilepsy, Insomnia, Longevity, Neurasthenia, Neuritis, Tinnitus, Visual fatigue.

- **Other uses:** Neurasthenia especially with insomnia, hypercholesterolaemia, ageing (tonic for elderly), connective tissue weakness, tinnitus, dizziness, blurred vision, possibly in nervous system disorders such as epilepsy, neuritis and schizophrenia.

Cautions: Unprocessed root can cause loose stools or diarrhoea.

Qualities: Bitter, sweet, astringent, warm

Typical dosage: 50-90 ml per week

Rhamnus frangula

Common names: Alder buckthorn

Family: Rhamnaceae

Part used: Bark

Description: Documented use since the 16th century as a laxative. Due to its purgative properties, also used for other conditions such as diseases of the liver, gallbladder and spleen, and for dropsy (oedema) and scabies. The administration of an aqueous suspension of 0.6 g pulverised bark (12 mg anthranoids (glucofrangulin and frangulin) had a laxative effect in humans after 6 to 24 hours.

Long-term use of stimulant laxatives should be avoided, as use for more than a brief period of treatment may lead to impaired function of the intestine and dependence on laxatives.

Constituents: Emodin-di-and mono-glycosides: the diglycosides glucofrangulin A and glucofrangulin B and the monoglycosides frangulins A, B, C and emodin-8-0-β-D-glucoside. Also contains small quantities of other anthraquinone glycosides, dianthrones and the aglycones emodin and emodin-9-anthrone.

Primary actions: Laxative.

All actions: Anti-inflammatory, Antifungal, Antiviral (systemically), Laxative.

Indications:

- Constipation.
- **Commission E:** Short-term use in occasional constipation.
- **ESCOP:** Short-term use in occasional constipation.
- **WHO:** Short-term use in occasional constipation.

Cautions: As for all anthranoid-containing laxative, major symptoms of overdose/abuse are griping pain and severe diarrhoea with consequent losses of fluids and electrolytes, which should be replaced. Diarrhoea may cause potassium depletion, in particular. Potassium depletion may lead to cardiac disorders and muscular asthenia, particularly where cardiac glycosides, diuretics or adrenocorticosteroids are being taken at the same time.

Treatment should be supported with generous amounts of fluid. Electrolytes, especially potassium, should be monitored. This is especially important in the elderly.

Furthermore, chronic ingestion of overdoses of anthranoid-containing medicinal products may lead to toxic hepatitis.

Contraindications: The use in children is contraindicated.

Drug interactions: Chronic use or abuse of frangula bark may lead to hypokalaemia similar to the abuse of all anthranoid-containing laxatives. This hypokalaemia and the increased loss of potassium may increase the activity of cardiac glycosides and interfere with the action of antiarrythmic agents (interaction with antiarrhythmic medicinal products, which induce reversion to sinus rhythm, e.g. quinidine) and medicinal products inducing QT-prolongation. Concomitant use with medicinal products inducing hypokalaemia (e.g. diuretics, adrenocorticosteroids and liquorice root) may aggravate electrolyte imbalance. The hypokalaemia can be aggravated by thiazide diuretics and by loop diuretics, in particular, but not by potassium-sparing diuretics such as amiloride.

Typical dosage: 20–40 ml per week

94

Rhamnus purshiana

Synonym or related species: Frangula purshiana

Common names: Cascara sagrada (sacred bark), Californian buckthorn

Family: Rhamnaceae

Part used: Dried trunk and aged stem bark

Description: Very astringent herbal medicine with laxative properties.

Constituents: Hydroxyanthraquinone glycosides (cascarosides A, B, C and D; also aloin A, B)

Primary actions: Antiparasitic, Laxative, Purgative.

All actions: Antiparasitic, Astringent, Laxative, Purgative.

Indications:

- Constipation.
- **BHP:** Occasional constipation, conditions in which soft stool is desirable (anal fissure, haemorrhoids).
- **Commission E:** Constipation.
- **ESCOP:** For short term use in cases of occasional constipation.
- **WHO:** For short term treatment of occasional constipation.

Cautions: For short-term use only (1–2 weeks); use only if no effect can be obtained through a change of diet or by the use of bulk-forming laxatives. Do not administer during lactation without professional advice. Single doses may result in cramp-like discomfort of the gastrointestinal tract. May cause griping colic, diarrhoea, potassium and fluid loss, and possible hepatic reactions.

Contraindications: Intestinal obstruction and stenosis, atony, inflammatory diseases of the colon (ulcerative colitis, irritable bowel syndrome, Crohns disease), appendicitis, abdominal pain of unknown origin, severe dehydration states with water and electrolyte depletion, or chronic constipation. Contraindicated in patients with cramps, colic, haemorrhoids and nephritis. Do not administer during pregnancy or to children less than 10 years.

Drug interactions: Do not administer concurrently with digoxin or thiazide diuretics as they may be exacerbated by, or cause, potassium loss.

Qualities: Cool, pungent

Typical dosage: 20–40 ml per week

Rheum palmatum

Common names: Da Huang, Chinese rhubarb

Family: Polygonaceae

Part used: Root and rhizome

Description: Rhubarb belongs to the stimulating laxatives containing hydroxyanthracene derivatives (senna, aloe, frangulae cortex and cascara) used for short-term use in constipation. Due to the content of tannins, rhubarb preparations are also used for diarrhoea, for gastritis and enteritis, and as a styptic. In vivo studies have found benefits in renal failure and emodin has anticancer properties.

Constituents: Anthraquinone glycosides, emodin.

Primary actions: Astringent, Laxative, Styptic.

All actions: Anti-inflammatory, Anti-inflammatory (GIT), Anti-inflammatory (urinary), Antiseptic (GIT), Astringent, Laxative, Purgative, Stomachic.

Indications:

- Cholecystitis, Constipation, Diarrhoea, Dyspepsia, Liver congestion, Renal insufficiency.
- **ESCOP:** For short-term use in cases of occasional constipation.
- **WHO:** Short term treatment of occasional constipation.

Cautions: Short term use only (1–2 weeks). Should be used only if no effect can be obtained through a change of diet or use of bulk-forming laxatives. Single doses may cause cramp-like discomfort of the gastrointestinal tract. Do not administer during pregnancy or lactation without medical advice.

Drug interactions: Chronic use or abuse of rhubarb preparations may lead to hypokalaemia as in the abuse of all anthranoid-containing laxatives. This hypokalaemia and the increased loss of potassium may increase the activity of cardiac glycosides and interfere with the action of antiarrythmic agents (interaction with antiarrhythmic medicinal products, which induce reversion to sinus rhythm, e.g. quinidine) and medicinal products inducing QT-prolongation. Concomitant use with medicinal products inducing hypokalaemia (e.g. diuretics, corticosteroids and liquorice root) may aggravate electrolyte imbalance.

Qualities: Bitter, cold

Typical dosage: 10–30 ml per week

Rhodiola rosea

Common names: Golden root, rose root, arctic root

Part used: Root

Description: Clinical studies have found moderate benefit in anaerobic exercise performance, anxiety, chronic obstructive pulmonary disease (mixed results), depression, stress-related fatigue, poor sleep, and metabolic syndrome. Reduction in oral mucositis induced by chemotherapy. ADAPT-232 (a standardised fixed combination of *Rhodiola rosea, Schisandra chinensis,* and *Eleutherococcus senticosus*) has been shown to improve cognitive functions in healthy volunteers.

Constituents: Phenylpropanoids (rosarin, rosavin, tyrosol and rosin), salidroside (a hydroxyphenethyl glucoside) and rosiridin. Extracts are often standardised to rosavin and salidroside.

Primary actions: Adaptogen, Anti-inflammatory, Immunomodulator.

All actions: Adaptogen, Anti-inflammatory, Anticancer, Antidepressant, Antihypertensive, Antioxidant, Cardioprotective, Hepatoprotective, Immunomodulator, Nootropic.

Indications:

- Amenorrhoea, Anxiety, Cancer; including prevention/supportive treatment, Depression, Exhaustion, Memory and concentration; poor, Mucositis, Myalgia, Nervous exhaustion, Post-viral syndromes, Stress.
- **Other uses:** To increase physical endurance, work productivity, longevity, resistance to altitude sickness, and to treat fatigue, depression, anaemia, impotence, gastrointestinal complaints, infections and nervous system disorders. For chronic immune deficiency; fatigue; physical stress; to enhance mental performance, and to improve physical fitness, muscle strength, speed, and reaction time, to aid mental performance, concentration and memory, especially when under stress; chronic fatigue, fibromyalgia, post-viral syndromes, erectile dysfunction, anxiety and depression. Mild thyroid insufficiency.

Cautions: The ethanol extract is quite astringent and should not be taken on an empty stomach, as it is likely to cause upset stomach and nausea.

Contraindications: None known

Typical dosage: Liquid extract standardised to contain 3.0 mg/ml rosavins and 1.0 mg/ml salidroside: 20–40 ml per week

Rosa canina

Common names: Rosehip, dog rose

Family: Rosaceae

Part used: Dried ripe fruit with or without seeds

Description: Rosehip powder from the seeds and pods is used for osteoarthritis and rheumatoid arthritis, kidney stones, urinary tract infections, gastrointestinal ailments, hypertension and respiratory problems such as bronchitis, cough and cold. Some of the ethnomedical indications of rose hip, such as nephroprotective and gastroproetctive actions, have been confirmed by pre-clinical pharmacological studies.

Lipophilic constituents are involved in the anti-inflammatory actions and much of the research is based on the products Litozin and Hypervital. Litozin has shown moderate effect in osteoarthritis, rheumatoid arthritis and low back pain.

There is also a rationale behind the use of Litozin in weight loss as part of a hypocaloric diet based on the prebiotic, stool-regulating and smooth muscle-relaxing actions of rose hip powder supported by the lipid-lowering, anti-obesity and gastroprotective effects.

HybenVital may ameliorate aging-induced skin conditions and reduce pain and improve general wellbeing in patients with osteoarthritis. The extent of how much hydro-ethanol extracts may share some of these properties is not known.

Constituents: Ascorbic acid, pectins, carotenoids (rubixanthin, lycopene, beta-carotene), flavonoids, tannins, organic acids (malic and citric), sugars, y-linolenic acid and linoleic acid.

Primary actions: Anti-inflammatory (musculoskeletal), Astringent.

All actions: Anti-inflammatory (musculoskeletal), Antidiarrhoeal, Astringent, Gastroprotective, Stomachic.

Indications:

- Arthritis, Common cold, Diarrhoea, Gastritis, Osteoarthritis.
- **BHP:** Polydipsia, avitaminosis C.
- Specific indications: dietary supplement as natural source of vitamin C, together with small amounts of A and B vitamins.
- **Other uses:** Source of vitamin C

Contraindications: None known

Qualities: Sour, warm

Typical dosage: 20–40 ml per week

Rubus idaeus

Common names: Raspberry leaf

Family: Rosaceae

Part used: Leaf

Description: Considered a uterine tonic and partus praeparator. Also drunk as a tea for dysmenorrhoea and menorrhagia, and during pregnancy to prevent or reduce nausea, to ease labour and to assist with lactation. A review of 12 original publications with focus on safety or efficacy during pregnancy, pharmacology and in vitro tests explaining mode of action or constituents in *Rubus idaeus* concluded that limited documentation exists and part of it is 50 years old or older. Only the latest animal study indicates an increased risk for the unborn child; however, all the studies are small and cannot rule out negative effects on pregnancy outcome. The efficacy of raspberry leaf is not convincingly documented by published evidence.

Constituents: Tannins (gallotannins, dimeric ellagitannins), flavonoids (rutin, quercetin), volatile oils, organic acids (gallic acid), vitamin C

Primary actions: Galactagogue, Partus praeparator, Uterine tonic.

All actions: Antidiarrhoeal, Antispasmodic/Spasmolytic, Astringent, Galactagogue, Partus praeparator, Uterine tonic.

Indications:

- Diarrhoea, Inflammation; oral cavity, Menorrhagia, Pregnancy; to prepare uterus for labour.
- **BHP:** Diarrhoea, pregnancy, stomatitis, tonsillitis (mouthwash), conjunctivitis (eye lotion). Specific indication: to facilitate parturition.
- **Other uses:** Tonsillitis, conjunctivitis (locally as eye lotion), stomatitis.

Cautions: Use under professional supervision in the first trimester of pregnancy, due to uterine stimulant

properties. May decrease absorption of iron, calcium and magnesium as well as of some drugs; separate administration by at least 2 hours. Use cautiously in highly inflamed or ulcerated conditions of the gastrointestinal tract.

Contraindications: Avoid in constipation, iron deficiency anaemia and malnutrition due to high tannin content.

Qualities: Cool, dry

Typical dosage: 30–80 ml per week

Rumex crispus

Common names: Yellow dock, curled dock

Family: Polygonaceae

Part used: Root

Description: Traditional alterative herbal medicine used in chronic skin disease, obstructive jaundice, psoriasis and constipation. Interestingly, a water extract of yellow dock has been found to significantly suppress RANKL-induced trabecular bone loss by preventing microstructural deterioration. In vitro, the extract increased osteoblast mineralisation by enhancing the transcription of runt-related transcription factor 2 and its transcriptional coactivators, and by stimulating extracellular signal-regulated kinase phosphorylation. Furthermore, the extract significantly inhibited osteoclast differentiation by suppressing the activation of the RANKL signalings (via MAPK and NF-κB). This study suggests that yellow dock extract could possibly protect against osteoporosis although there is not yet any clinical evidence to support this use.

Constituents: Anthraquinone glycosides, chrysophanol, emodin, essential oil, rhein, tannins, resin.

Primary actions: Astringent, Depurative/Alterative, Laxative.

All actions: Anti-inflammatory, Antimicrobial, Astringent, Cholagogue, Depurative/Alterative, Laxative, Purgative, Tonic.

Indications:

- Arthritis, Constipation, Eczema, Gout, Indigestion, Jaundice, Liver congestion, Liver insufficiency, Liver toxicity, Psoriasis.
- **BHP:** Chronic skin disease, obstructive jaundice, and constipation. Specific indications: skin disease especially psoriasis with constipation.

Cautions: As with all laxatives, do not use continuously or in high doses for prolonged periods, as habituation to any laxative other than bulking agents can cause potassium loss (reversible after cessation). Start at a low dose and increase to the point of producing a normal motion. Griping may be caused due to free anthraquinones. Correct any griping with the addition of carminative herbs. Do not use during pregnancy or lactation, or in young children without professional advice.

Contraindications: Contraindicated in persons with

intestinal obstruction or inflammatory diseases of the gastrointestinal tract.

Drug interactions: Excessive use may add to potassium depletion caused by agents such as thiazide diuretics or licorice.

Qualities: Cold, dry

Typical dosage: 15–30 ml per week

Ruscus aculeatus

Common names: Butcher's broom, box holly

Family: Ruscaceae or Asparagaceae

Part used: Rhizome and root

Description: Key herb for chronic venous insufficiency such as pain and heaviness, leg cramping, itching and swelling and also for haemorrhoids with itching and burning. Also indicated for orthostatic hypotension and osteopenia. A meta-analysis of clinical trials of Cyclo 3 Fort, a combination of root extract of *Ruscus aculeatus* (150 mg per capsule), hesperidin methyl chalcone (150 mg) and ascorbic acid (100 mg), in patients with chronic venous insufficiency found that the medicine significantly reduced the severity of pain, cramps, heaviness, oedema and paraesthesia compared to placebo.

Constituents: Steroidal saponins (ruscin, ruscoside) and corresponding aglycones (ruscogenin and neoruscogenin), fatty acids, flavonoids, sterols (sitosterol, campesterol, stigmasterol), benzofuranes. Ruscogenin has been shown to inhibit TNF-alpha-induced over expression of TNF-alpha-induced intercellular adhesion molecule-1 both at the mRNA and protein levels and suppressed NF-kappaB activation considerably by decreasing NF-kappaB p65 translocation and DNA binding activity.

Primary actions: Anti-inflammatory, Antioedematous, Venotonic.

All actions: Anti-inflammatory, Antioedematous, Diaphoretic, Diuretic, Venotonic.

Indications:

- Haemorrhoids, Varicose veins, Venous insufficiency, Weight loss; to assist.
- **Commission E:** For chronic venous insufficiency such as pain and heaviness, leg cramping, itching and swelling and also for symptoms of haemorrhoids such as itching and burning.
- **ESCOP:** Supportive therapy for symptoms of chronic venous insufficiency such as painful, tired and heavy legs, tingling and swelling. Supportive therapy for symptoms of haemorrhoids such as itching and burning.
- **Other uses:** Oedema, urinary lithiasis.

Cautions: Do not administer during pregnancy or lactation without professional advice. Use with caution in coeliac disease, fat malabsorption, and vitamins A, D, E and K deficiency, and some upper digestive system irritations. Caution in patients with pre-existing cholestasis.

Contraindications: Do not apply to broken or ulcerated skin.

Qualities: Cool, dry

Typical dosage: 30–50 ml per week

Ruta graveolens

Common names: Rue

Family: Rutaceae

Part used: Leaf

Description: Rue is a traditional medicine having been described by Dioscorides and Galen as an abortifacient and emmenagogue. It was also recommended as a specific remedy against pulmonary diseases. Leaves and also roots and seeds, were administered for internal use by Hippocratic physicians after having been soaked in wine or mixed with honey or its derivatives.

Constituents: Rue contains coumarins (coumarin, herniarin, gravelliferon, rutaretin), furanocoumarins (bergapten, psoralen, rutamarin), furanoquinoline alkaloids (dictamnine, skimmianine, rutacridone) and the flavonoids rutin and quercetin. Methyl nonyl ketone is a major component of the volatile oil and is used in perfumery and flavourings.

Primary actions: Antispasmodic (uterus), Antitussive, Emmenagogue.

All actions: Anticancer, Antihypertensive, Antimicrobial, Antispasmodic/Spasmolytic, Antitussive, Emmenagogue, Uterine tonic.

Indications:

- Colic; intestinal, Cough, Fibroids, Hypertension, Intestinal worms, Rheumatism.
- **BHP:** Atonic amenorrhoea.
- **Other uses:** Rue is traditionally used for a very wide range of ailments including menstrual disorders, spasm, loss of appetite, dyspeptic complaints, circulatory disorders, fever, high blood pressure, heart palpitations, inflamed mucosa, toothache, hysteria, arthritis, sprains, injuries and skin diseases.

Cautions: Rue furocoumarins have photosensitising effects. Topical as well as oral exposure may lead to photodermatitis. Acute phyto-photodermatitis with systemic upset in a two-year-old child after contact with rue growing in a garden has been reported.

Contraindications: Rue has been used as an abortifacient, but may potentially cause multiple organ system failure and death. Do not use for this purpose.

Drug interactions: Rue extract has been shown to inhibit aldehyde oxidase activity (89–96%) at 100 µg/ml in vitro, which was comparable with 10 µM of menadione, a specific potent inhibitor of aldehyde oxidase. Rutin and especially quercertin showed strong inhibition. Aldehyde oxidase is a drug-metabolising enzyme and this suggest rue has the potential to interact with medical drugs.

Typical dosage: 10–20 ml per week

Salix spp.

Synonym or related species: S. purpurea, S. fragilis, S. alba

Common names: Willow bark, white willow

Family: Salicaceae

Part used: Bark

Description: A Cochrane Review found that *Harpagophytum procumbens, Salix alba,* and *Capsicum frutescens* seems to reduce pain more than placebo. For treating mild or fairly severe cases of gonarthrosis (knee arthritis) and coxarthrosis, the effect of willow bark extract is comparable to that of standard therapies, without the corresponding side effects. Coxarthrosis is a disorder of the physiological balance between the strength of the articular cartilage and articular bone, and between the pressures exerted on the joint. It is a disease with a slow progressive and long course. However, two other studies found willow bark extract showed no relevant efficacy in patients with OA or RA.

Salix extracts can be used as a basic treatment in the long-term therapy of painful musculoskeletal disorders and can be combined with NSAIDs and other antiarthritic medications if necessary.

Constituents: Phenolic glycosides (salicylates, salicortin, salicin, tremulacin; syringin, triandrin), phenolic acids (chlorogenic acid), oligomeric proanthocyanidins, tannins, flavonoids

Primary actions: Analgesic, Anti-inflammatory (musculoskeletal), Antirheumatic.

All actions: Analgesic, Anodyne, Anti-inflammatory, Anti-inflammatory (musculoskeletal), Antihydrotic, Antiplatelet, Antipyretic, Antirheumatic, Astringent.

Indications:

- Arthritis, Gout, Influenza, Osteoarthritis, Rheumatoid arthritis.
- **BHP:** Muscular and arthroidal rheumatism with inflammation and pain, influenza and respiratory catarrh, gouty arthritis, ankylosing spondylitis. Specific indications: rheumatoid arthritis and other systemic connective tissue disorders characterised by inflammatory changes.
- **Commission E:** Diseases accompanied by fever, rheumatic ailments, headaches.
- **ESCOP:** Relief of low back pain, symptomatic relief of mild osteoarthritic and rheumatic complaints.
- **Other uses:** Respiratory catarrh

Cautions: No serious adverse effects were reported from trials of willow bark extracts delivering 120–240 mg salicin (the purported active constituent) daily for up to eight weeks (no adverse events are expected with even longer term use). Use cautiously in patients with a history of allergic or anaphylactic reactions.

Contraindications: Contraindicated in those with salicylate sensitivity and glucose-6-phosphate dehydrogenase deficient patients.

Drug interactions: May potentiate the effects of warfarin due to antiplatelet activity.

Qualities: Cold 2nd degree, dry 2nd degree

Typical dosage: 25–50 ml per week

Salvia miltiorrhiza

Common names: Dan shen (Mandarin), red root sage

Family: Lamiaceae

Part used: Root

Description: In vivo and in vitro studies showed that the tanshinone IIA and salvianolate have a wide range of cardiovascular effects including antioxidative, anti-inflammatory, endothelial protective, myocardial protective, anticoagulation, vasodilation, and anti-atherosclerosis, as well as significantly help to reduce proliferation and migration of vascular smooth muscle cells.

In addition, some of the clinical studies reported that the *S. miltiorrhiza* preparations in combination with Western medicine were more effective for treatment of various cardiovascular diseases including angina pectoris, myocardial infarction, hypertension, hyperlipidemia, and pulmonary heart diseases.

Constituents: Diterpene diketones (tanshinones, cryptotanshinone, isotanshinones)

Primary actions: Antiarrhythmic, Cardioprotective, Hepatoprotective.

All actions: Antiarrhythmic, Antibacterial, Anticancer, Antifibrotic, Antimicrobial, Antiplatelet, Cardioprotective, Fibrinolytic, Hepatoprotective, Hepatotonic, Neuroprotective, Renal tonic, Vasodilator, Wound healing/Vulnerary.

Indications:

- Acne, Angina pectoris, Autoimmune disease, Buerger's disease, Cardiac debility, Cerebrovascular disease, Circulation; peripheral; impaired, Congestive heart failure, Diabetes, Diabetic neuropathy, Endometriosis, Hypertension, Intermittent claudication, Lymphoma treatment; as an adjunct to, Myocardial ischaemia, Nephritis, Nerve damage, Palpitations, Pulmonary fibrosis, Scleroderma.

Contraindications: Contraindicated in patients with a bleeding tendency and during pregnancy.

Drug interactions: May decrease midazolam levels (clinical trial). May potentiate warfarin (case report). Coadministration of a dan shen formulation improved the anti-dyslipidaemic effects of atorvastatin (synergistic effect) in vivo.

Qualities: Bitter, cold 1/2 degree

Typical dosage: 25–50 ml per week

Salvia officinalis

Common names: Sage

Family: Lamiaceae

Part used: Aerial parts

Description: Clinical trials have been small, single studies, probably with bias and other methodological problems. However, the body of evidence is growing for the use of *S. officinalis* in PMS, vulvovaginal candidiasis (in the form of vaginal tablet, alone and when combined with Clotrimazole), Alzheimer's disease (*S. officinalis* extract produced a significantly better outcome on cognitive functions than placebo), mood and cognitive performance in healthy and aged populations, menopausal hot flushes, acute pharyngitis (as a spray), and hyperlipidaemia. Sage tea-thyme-peppermint hydrosol oral rinse has promising results in alleviating oral mucositis induced by chemotherapy. A combined topical sage-rhubarb preparation has been shown to be as effective as topical aciclovir cream in lip herpes infections and an echinacea-sage preparation was as efficacious and well tolerated as a chlorhexidine/lidocaine spray in the treatment of acute sore throats.

Constituents: Essential oil (salviol, thujone rich, cineole, camphor), phenolic acids (rosmarinic), flavonoids, diterpenoids, triterpenes, steroids, flavones, flavonoid glycosides, tannins including salviatannin.

Primary actions: Antigalactagogue, Antihydrotic, Antiseptic (respiratory tract).

All actions: Antifungal (topically), Antigalactagogue, Antihydrotic, Antihyperlipidemic, Antiseptic (respiratory tract), Antiviral (topically), Carminative, Nootropic.

Indications:

- Dementia, Dyspepsia; flatulent, Galactorrhoea, Hyperhydrosis including sweating with menopause, Inflammation; oral cavity, Menopausal symptoms, Night sweats, Sore throat (gargle), Sweating; excessive, Tonsillitis, Tracheitis.

- **BHP:** Flatulent dyspepsia, pharyngitis, uvulitis, stomatitis, gingivitis, glossitis (internally or as gargle/mouthwash), hyperhydrosis, galactorrhoea. Specific indications: inflammation of the mouth, tongue or throat, as gargle/mouthwash.

- **Commission E:** For dyspeptic symptoms and excessive perspiration (internally), and externally for inflammations of mucous membranes of nose and throat.

- **ESCOP:** Inflammations and infections of the mouth and throat such as stomatitis, gingivitis and pharyngitis. Used to treat hyperhidrosis.

Cautions: Caution is required with the use of alcoholic preparations because of the presence of thujone. Thujone is a monoterpene ketone found in varying quantity in a several plants, including *Salvia officinalis*, *Salvia sclarea*, *Tanacetum vulgare*, *Artemisia artemisia*, and *Thuja occidentalis*. Allergic reactions are also possible.

Contraindications: Contraindicated during pregnancy or lactation (except to stop milk flow) due to potential toxicity.

Qualities: Dry 2nd degree, hot 2nd degree

Typical dosage: 15–30 ml per week

Salvia rosmarinus

Synonym or related species: *Rosmarinus officinalis*

Common names: Rosemary

Family: Lamiaceae

Part used: Leaves

Description: Reviews of rosemary and its constituents, especially caffeic acid derivatives such as rosmarinic and carnosic acids, have a therapeutic potential in treatment or prevention of bronchial asthma, spasmogenic disorders, peptic ulcers, inflammatory diseases, hepatotoxicity, cataract, cancer, poor sperm motility, arthritis, gout, muscular pain, neuralgia, and wound healing. Rosemary oil can also be rubbed into hair for stimulating hair growth. Rosemary is also undervalued in the prevention and management of dyslipidaemia and other cardio-metabolic diseases. Rosemary is of course also known to improve memory!

Constituents: Essential oil (cineole, pinene, camphor and smaller amounts of beta-pinene, borneol, limonene, terpineol and verbinol), phenolic acids (rosmarinic and carnosic acids), bitter diterpenes (carnosol, rosmanol), triterpenes (oleanic betulinic and ursolic acids), triterpene alcohols, flavonoids and their glycosides (diosmetin, luteolin, genkwanin).

Primary actions: Antimicrobial, Carminative, Sedative.

All actions: Analgesic, Anti-inflammatory, Antiatherosclerotic, Anticancer, Antidiabetic, Antihyperlipidemic, Antihypertensive, Antimicrobial, Antioxidant, Cardioprotective, Carminative, Hepatoprotective, Hypoglycaemic, Sedative.

Indications:

- Alopecia neurotica, Anxiety, Asthma; bronchial, Cancer; including prevention/supportive treatment, Cardiovascular disease prevention, Debility, Depression, Dyslipidaemia, Dyspepsia; flatulent, Headache, Hepatitis, Memory and concentration; poor, Myalgia, Neuralgia, Neuralgia (topically), Ulcer; gastrointestinal.

- **BHP:** Flatulent dyspepsia associated with psychogenic tension, headaches (migrainous or hypertensive). Topically for myalgia, sciatica, intercostal neuralgia. Specific indications: depressive states with general debility and indications of cardiovascular weakness.

- **Commission E:** For dyspeptic complaints (internally) and rheumatic diseases and circulatory problems (externally).

- **ESCOP:** Internal use: Improvement of hepatic and biliary function and in dyspeptic complaints. External use: Adjuvant therapy in rheumatic conditions, peripheral circulatory disorders, promotion of wound healing and as a mild antiseptic.

- **Other uses:** NRF2 activator (carnosic acid) Dimethyl fumarate (DMF) is an electrophilic compound previously called BG-12 and marketed under the name Tecfidera®. It was approved in 2013 by the US Food and Drug Administration and the European Medicines Agency for the treatment of relapsing multiple sclerosis. One mechanism of action of DMF is stimulation of the nuclear factor erythroid 2-related factor 2 (NRF2) transcriptional pathway that induces anti-oxidant and anti-inflammatory phase II enzymes to prevent chronic neurodegeneration. However, electrophiles such as DMF also produce severe systemic side effects, in part due to non-specific S-alkylation of cysteine thiols and resulting depletion of glutathione. NRF2 activators such as carnosic acid may avoid these side effects.

Contraindications: Hypersensitivity to rosemary leaf and its preparations, especially those containing carnosol.

Qualities: Dry 2nd degree, hot 2nd degree

Typical dosage: 15–30 ml per week

Sambucus nigra

Synonym or related species: Sambucus arborescens

Common names: Elder, elderflower, elderberry, sambuco

Family: Caprifoliaceae

Part used: Flowers or berries

Description: Elderberry juice and syrup have been used traditionally, and in some observational and clinical studies, as supportive agents against the common cold and influenza. Pharmacological studies suggest the antiviral effects are associated with production of inflammatory cytokines (IL-1 beta, TNF-alpha, IL-6, IL-8). A review has found that elderberry substantially reduces symptoms of upper respiratory tract viral infections. The review was based on four studies (N=180). The majority of the studies were based on elderberry syrup (Sambucol) which is dosed at 20–60 ml daily in divided dosages. Hydroethanol extracts can be based on the flowers and leaves. Elderflowers are rich in rutin, a di-p-coumaroylquic acid and chlorogenic acid.

Constituents: **Elderberries** predominantly contain anthocyanins (primarily cyanidin 3-glucoside and cyanidin 3-sambubioside), flavonols including rutin, isoquercetin and caffeoylquinic acid. Sambucol is standardised to three flavonoids. Analysis of the patent suggests that Sambucol contains triterpenes (0.9% mass weight), flavonoid glycosides 2–3%, rutin 0.2%, quercetin 0.02%, caffeic acid

derivatives 1–3%, anthocyanidins 0.2–1%. **Flowers** predominantly contain rutin, di-p-coumaroylquic acid and chlorogenic acid; with lesser amounts of Quercetin 3-O-glucoside (isoquercitrin) and isorhamneton 3-O-rutinoside (narcissin). **Leaves** also contain sambunigrin (cyanogenic glycoside).

Primary actions: Anticatarrhal, Antipyretic, Antiviral (systemically).

All actions: Anticatarrhal, Antimicrobial, Antipyretic, Diaphoretic, Diuretic.

Indications:

- Catarrh; naso-pharyngeal congestion, Catarrhal deafness, Common cold, Cough, Fever, Influenza, Sinusitis.

- **BHP:** Influenzal colds, chronic nasal catarrh with deafness, sinusitis. Specific indication: common cold.

- **Commission E:** Common cold.

- **WHO:** As a diaphoretic for treatment of fever and chills, and as an expectorant for treatment of mild inflammation of the upper respiratory tract. Also for symptomatic treatment of the common cold.

Cautions: Administer with caution during pregnancy or lactation.

Contraindications: None known.

Qualities: Dry, neutral, secondary cooling effect

Typical dosage: 20–40 ml per week

Schisandra chinensis

Common names: Bei-Wuweizi, Schisandra, Chinese magnolia vine, Wu Wei Zi

Family: Schisandraceae

Part used: Seeds and fruit

Description: A major adaptogen and liver tonic, Schisandra also exerts a protective effect against skin photoaging, osteoarthritis, sarcopenia, senescence, and mitochondrial dysfunction, and improves physical endurance and cognitive/behavioural functions, which can be linked with its general anti-aging potency. Also used for menopausal symptoms, especially for hot flushes, sweating, and heart palpitations. Combines with *Rhodiola rosea* and *Eleutherococcus senticosus* for pneumonia.

Pharmacological research has demonstrated that most of the biological actions and pharmacological effects of wuweizi can be attributed to its lignan constituents, particularly the dibenzocyclooctadiene-type lignans, which can lower the serum glutamate-pyruvate transaminase level, inhibit platelet aggregation, and show antioxidative, calcium antagonism, antitumor-promoting, and anti-HIV effects. The dried ripe fruits of both *Schisandra chinensis* and *Schisandra sphenanthera* have long been used as wuweizi, although their chemical constituents and contents of the bioactive components are quite different. Since 2000, they have been accepted as two different crude drugs, bei-wuweizi and nan-wuweizi, respectively, by the Chinese Pharmacopoeia. *S. sphenanthera* markedly increased the concentration of tacrolimus in the blood of liver transplant patients, improved liver function and reduced the incidence of tacrolimus-associated side effects.

Constituents: Dibenzocyclo-octane lignans (schizandrins, schizabdrols, schisantherins, gomisins), malic, tartaric, nigranoic and citric acids, resins, pectin, vitamins A, C and E, niacin, beta-carotene, sterols, tannins, several minerals.

Primary actions: Adaptogen, Hepatotonic, Neuroprotective.

All actions: Adaptogen, Anticancer, Antidiabetic, Antihyperlipidemic, Antioxidant, Antitussive, Cardioprotective, Hepatoprotective, Hepatotonic, Nervine tonic, Neuroprotective, Nootropic, Renal tonic, Tonic, Uterine tonic.

Indications:

• Cancer; including prevention/supportive treatment, Cardiovascular disease prevention, Chronic fatigue syndrome, Convalescence, Dyslipidaemia, Hepatitis, Liver congestion, Liver insufficiency, Liver toxicity, Longevity, Memory and concentration; poor, Mental exhaustion, Nervous tension, Stress.

• **WHO:** For the treatment of psychosis, gastritis, hepatitis and fatigue associated with illness.

Cautions: Minor adverse effects such as heartburn, acid indigestion, stomach pain, anorexia, allergic skin reactions and urticaria have been reported. Not recommended during lactation or for paediatric use.

Contraindications: In pregnancy except to facilitate childbirth. Early stages of cough or rash.

Drug interactions: Schisandra may increase the metabolism of oestrogens. Coadministration may lower drug effect, although the clinical significance of this is unknown. Interaction inconclusive; schisandra has been shown to decrease serum oestradiol levels. Coadministration may affect the efficacy of OCP and HRT and cause lowered serum drug levels. May decrease blood levels of sirolimus (observations in liver transplant recipients and in a clinical trial with volunteers).

Qualities: Sour, warm

Typical dosage: 30–60 ml per week

Scrophularia nodosa

Common names: Figwort

Family: Scrophulariaceae

Part used: Open flowering aerial parts

Description: 'Figwort is alterative, diuretic, and anodyne; reputed highly beneficial in hepatic diseases, scrofula, secondary syphilis, cutaneous diseases, dropsy, and as a general deobstruent to the glandular system, when used in infusion or syrup. Externally, in the form of fomentation, or ointment,

it is valuable in bruises, mammary inflammation, ringworm, piles, painful swelling, itch, and cutaneous eruptions of a vesicular character.' – *King's American Dispensatory*, 1898. *Scrophularia nodosa* is similar in clinical effect to the related species *S. ningpoensis* (Xuan Shen), used in Traditional Chinese Medicine.

Constituents: Saponins, cardio-active glycosides, flavonoids (diosmin, hesperidin), iridoid glycosides (harpagoside, harpagide, procumbide, aucubin, catalpol), phenolic acids (vanillic, cholorogenic and caffeic)

Primary actions: Anti-inflammatory, Depurative/Alterative, Diuretic.

All actions: Anodyne, Anti-inflammatory, Depurative/Alterative, Diuretic, Lymphatic.

Indications:

• Eczema, Pruritus, Psoriasis.

• **BHP:** Chronic skin disease. Specific indications: eczema, psoriasis, pruritus.

Contraindications: Contraindicated in tachycardia and diabetes. Should not be used internally by pregnant or lactating women.

Qualities: Cool, dry

Typical dosage: 20–40 ml per week

Scutellaria baicalensis

Synonym or related species: Scutellaria grandiflora

Common names: Baikal skullcap, baical skullcap, Chinese skullcap, Huang qin (Mandarin), ogon (Japanese)

Family: Lamiaceae

Part used: Root

Description: Used in TCM for hepatitis, diarrhoea, vomiting and high blood pressure. Extracts of *S. baicalensis* and its major chemical constituents have been reported to possess antiviral, antitumor, antibacterial, antioxidant, anti-inflammatory, hepatoprotective, and neuroprotective activities. Baicalin and baicalein has been shown to be active against hyperglycemia, insulin resistance, type 2 diabetes, hyperlipidemia, obesity, and non-alcoholic fatty liver. Wogonin has long been used as an active anticancer drug in Chinese medicine practice. In recent past wogonin has been shown to possess notable anti-inflammatory, and antiallergic properties, antiviral, and also antithrombotic properties. Wogonin has shown to alleviate apoptosis, and *endoplasmic reticulum* stress in the cells and this property can also be used in the treatment of cardiovascular diseases. Notably, wogonin has been documented to have an extensive margin of safety, as well as displaying little or no organ toxicity following extended intravenous administration. Baicalin effectively prevents neurodegenerative diseases through various pharmacological mechanisms, including antioxidative stress, antiexcitotoxicity, antiapoptotic, anti-inflammatory, stimulating neurogenesis, promoting the expression of neuronal protective factors.

Constituents: Numerous flavonoids and their glycosides (baicalin, baicalein, wogonoside and wogonin; lower levels of others such as skullcap flavone I and II and chrysin), resin, tannins.

Primary actions: Antiallergic, Antimicrobial.

All actions: Aldose reductase inhibitor, Anti-inflammatory, Antiallergic, Antiasthmatic, Antiemetic, Antifibrotic, Antihyperlipidemic, Antimicrobial, Antioxidant, Antiplatelet, Antipyretic, Antiseptic (GIT), Anxiolytic, Cardioprotective, Chemoprotective, Diuretic, Gastroprotective, Hypoglycaemic, Neuroprotective, Sedative.

Indications:

- Acne, Allergies/Sensitivities, Asthma, Atherosclerosis, Autoimmune disease, Cancer; including prevention/supportive treatment, Cataract and diabetic complications, Eczema, Hayfever, Hepatitis, Hypertension, Infection; gastrointestinal system, Infection; respiratory tract, Nausea, Rhinitis, Sinusitis, Urticaria.

- **WHO:** May stimulate the immune system and induce haematopoiesis. Treatment of fever, nausea and vomiting, acute dysentery, jaundice, coughs, carbuncles and sores, and threatened abortion.

- **Other uses:** Adjunctive therapy during treatment to reduce nausea and immune suppression, toxaemia of pregnancy, and restless foetus.

Cautions: Rare gastrointestinal discomfort and diarrhoea are associated with oral administration. Do not administer during pregnancy or lactation or to children under 12 years without professional advice.

Contraindications: Contraindicated in cold conditions in TCM, and during interferon therapy.

Drug interactions: May increase risk of bleeding if used concurrently with anticoagulants (warfarin): use with caution.

Qualities: Bitter, cold

Typical dosage: 30–60 ml per week

Scutellaria lateriflora

Common names: Blue skulcap

Family: Lamiaceae

Part used: Dried aerial parts

Description: Several Cherokee (Appalachian Mountain region) medicinal plants are still in use today as herbal medicines, including yarrow (*Achillea millefolium*), black cohosh (*Actaea racemosa*), American ginseng (*Panax quinquefolius*), and blue skullcap (*Scutellaria lateriflora*). Infusion of the S. *lateriflora* were used by the Cherokee for monthly periods and to treat diarrhea; root decoctions were used as an emetic to expel afterbirth and to remedy breast pains. The aerial parts, rather than the roots, are currently used as an herbal medicine as an anxiolytic, sedative and antispasmodic.

Constituents: Flavonoid glycosides (baicalin, 102

dihydrobaicalin, lateriflorin, ikonnikoside I, scutellarin, and oroxylin, flavonoid aglycones (baicalein, oroxylin A, wogonin, and lateriflorein), phenylpropanoids (caffeic acid, cinnamic acid, p -coumaric acid, and ferulic acid), and clerodane diterpenoids (scutelaterin A, scutelaterin B, scutelaterin C, ajugapitin, and scutecyprol A). The essential oil is composed largely of sesquiterpene hydrocarbons, delta-cadinene (27%), calamenene (15.2%), beta-elemene (9.2%), alpha-cubenene (4.2%), alpha-humulene (4.2%), and alpha-bergamotene (2.8%).

Primary actions: Anxiolytic, Nervine tonic, Sedative.

All actions: Analgesic, Anticonvulsant, Antispasmodic (muscles), Anxiolytic, Nervine tonic, Sedative.

Indications:

- Depression, Epilepsy, Insomnia, Menopause, Nervous tension, Neurasthenia, Premenstrual syndrome.

- **BHP:** Epilepsy, chorea, hysteria, nervous tension states. Specific indication: grand mal seizures.

Contraindications: None known.

Drug interactions: May increase drug levels of losartan and rosuvastatin.

Qualities: Cool, dry

Typical dosage: 15–30 ml per week

Serenoa repens

Synonym or related species: Sabal serrulata

Common names: Saw palmetto, cabbage palm, dwarf palmetto

Family: Arecaceae

Part used: Dried ripe fruit

Description: S. *repens* is a very well tolerated medical therapy alone or in combination with other symptom-relieving drugs for patients with male lower urinary tract symptoms/BPH. Fatty acids are the major constituents of saw palmetto extract. Lauric acid has been demonstrated to have a1-adrenergic receptor-binding activity as well as inhibitory effects on 5a-reductase, suggesting that the fatty acids reduce BPH symptoms via relaxation of muscle tone and inhibition of testosterone metabolism. Phytosterol (b-sitosterol) was found to effectively reduce prostatic inflammation.

In 2020, two meta-analyses examined the evidence for serenoa extract in the treatment of BPH. The first analysis found that serenoa extract did not show clinically meaningful improvement in male lower urinary tract symptoms (LUTS) secondary to benign prostatic enlargement, and peak flow. The analysis of 22 RCTs (n=8564) showed that the benefit over placebo was minimal and may not justify its clinical use before higher level of evidence will be available. However, the second analysis concluded that persistent prostatic inflammatory status plays a central role in both the development and progression of male LUTS/BPH. In men with

LUTS/BPH who have a high chance of harbouring persistent prostatic inflammatory status, serenoa extract will not only improve LUTS, but also reduce (underlying) inflammation. The authors of the second analysis suggest that the authors of the first analysis misundersood statistical analysis!

Constituents: Rich in short chain fatty acids (capric, caprylic, myristic and especially lauric acid) and their glycerides, phytosterols (sistosterol, beta-sitosterol, campesterol, cyclosartenol), essential oil, fixed oil, polysaccharides

Primary actions: Anti-inflammatory, Antiandrogenic, Antihyperprostatic.

All actions: Anti-inflammatory, Antiandrogenic, Antihyperprostatic, Antiseptic (urinary), Diuretic.

Indications:

- Benign prostatic hyperplasia, Cystitis, Prostatitis.

- **BHP:** Chronic or subacute cystitis, prostatic hypertrophy, genito-urinary catarrh, testicular atrophy, sex hormone disorders. Specific indications: prostatic enlargement.

- **ESCOP:** Symptomatic treatment of micturition disorders (dysuria, pollakisuria, nocturia, urine retention) in mild to moderate benign prostatic hyperplasia.

- **WHO:** Treatment of lower urinary tract symptoms (nocturia, polyuria, urinary retention) secondary to early BPH stages, in cases where diagnosis of prostate cancer is negative.

- **Other uses:** Genito-urinary catarrh, testicular atrophy

Cautions: Do not administer for difficulties with micturition without medical supervision. Consulation with a medical practitioner is required for all cases of acute retention of urine or blood in the urine. Symptom relief in people with enlarged prostate is generally experienced within 4–8 weeks: seek professional assessment if symptoms worsen. Minor gastrointestinal side effects have been reported.

Contraindications: During pregnancy, and in children under 12 years, due to hormonal effects.

Drug interactions: Caution for concurrent use with warfarin.

Qualities: Dry, warm

Typical dosage: 15–30 ml per week

Silybum marianum

Synonym or related species: Carduus marianus
Common names: St Mary's thistle, milk thistle, silymarin
Family: Asteraceae
Part used: Ripe seed
Description: Silybum marianum extract and silymarin have cytoprotective, anti-inflammatory and hepatoprotective properties. Bioavailability of silymarin is poor. Large doses of silymarin in solid dose form may be needed in serious disorders. S.

marianum extract or silymarin does not stimulate P450 liver enzymes or P-glycoprotein and it is unlikely to cause adverse drug interactions.

Constituents: The main active ingredient in milk thistle is a group of flavonolignans collectively called silymarin. Silymarin consists of silybin (silibinin) A B, silydianin, silychristin, dehydrosilybinin, isosilybinin A B and others. Silybin is the main biologically active flavonolignan in silymarin. *Silybum marianum* also contains a fixed oil containing linoleic, oleic and palmitic acids, tocopherol and sterols including campesterol, 5-stigmasterol, beta-sitosterol, 7-stigmasterol, avenasterol and spinasterol.

Primary actions: Antihyperlipidemic, Cytoprotective, Hepatoprotective.

All actions: Anti-inflammatory, Antiatherosclerotic, Antihyperlipidemic, Antihypertensive, Antiobesity, Antioxidant, Chemoprotective, Choleretic, Cytoprotective, Digestive tonic, Hepatoprotective, Hepatotonic, Neuroprotective.

Indications:

- Allergies/Sensitivities, Atherosclerosis, Digestive complaints, Dyslipidaemia, Gallbladder disorders, Hepatitis, Jaundice, Liver cirrhosis, Liver insufficiency, Liver toxicity, Metabolic syndrome, Obesity.

- **Commission E:** Dyspeptic complaints (crude preparations), supportive treatment in chronic inflammatory liver diseases and hepatic cirrhosis (standardised extracts).

- **WHO:** Supportive treatment of acute or chronic hepatitis and cirrhosis induced by alcohol, drugs or toxins. Treatment of dyspeptic complaints and gallstones.

- **Other uses:** Alcoholism, hypercholesterolaemia, nausea of pregnancy.

Cautions: Oral doses of silymarin up to 2.1 g per day were safe and well tolerated. The nonlinear pharmacokinetics of silybin A and silybin B suggests low bioavailability associated with customary doses of silymarin may be overcome with doses above 700 mg.

Contraindications: Contraindicated in people with known allergy to Compositae (Asteraceae) plant family.

Drug interactions: Milk thistle and black cohosh appear to have no clinically relevant effect on CYP3A activity in vivo (Gurley, Hubbard, et al. 2006). When compared with rifampin and clarithromycin, supplementation with these specific formulations of milk thistle or black cohosh did not appear to affect digoxin pharmacokinetics, suggesting that these supplements are not potent modulators of P-gp in vivo. May increase blood levels of domperidone (dose of 1000 mg silymarin in healthy volunteers). May improve insulin sensitivity. May decrease sirolimus clearance. May reduce losartan and metronidazole efficacy by increasing clearance. May delay absorption rate of nifedipine. May increase drug levels of talinolol and Ornidazole (clinical studies). Silymarin is not a potent CYP3A4 inhibitor in vivo. Silymarin has no apparent effect on indinavir plasma concentrations in healthy subjects. Exposure to milk thistle extract produced no significant influence on CYP1A2, CYP2C9, CYP2D6, or CYP3A4/5 activities.

Coadministration of silymarin with darunavir-ritonavir seems to be safe in HIV-infected patients; no dose adjustment for darunavir-ritonavir seems to be necessary.

Milk thistle in commonly administered dosages should not interfere with indinavir therapy in patients infected with the human immunodeficiency virus.

Qualities: Dry, warm

Typical dosage: 30–60 ml per week

Smilax ornata

Common names: Sarsaparilla

Family: Liliaceae

Part used: Root

Description: Main use is for inflammatory skin disorders but also gout and arthritis.

Constituents: Furostanol saponins and their sapogenins including sarsaparilloside B, sarsaparillosides, and parillin. Despite the long history of medicinal use of sarsaparilla and the extensive phytochemical characterisation of the above Smilax species, little is known about the chemical constituents of *S. ornata*. Erroneously claimed to contain testosterone and/or other anabolic steroids. While smilax is a rich source of steroidal saponins, it has never been proven to have any anabolic effects (nor has testosterone been found in any plant source).

Primary actions: Anti-inflammatory, Antirheumatic, Depurative/Alterative.

All actions: Analgesic, Anti-inflammatory, Antipruritic, Antirheumatic, Depurative/Alterative, Diaphoretic, Diuretic, Hepatoprotective, Tonic.

Indications:

- Arthritis, Eczema, Gout, Psoriasis, Rheumatism, Rheumatoid arthritis.

- **BHP:** Psoriasis and other cutaneous conditions, chronic rheumatism, rheumatoid arthritis, leprosy (adjunct to other treatment). Specific indications: psoriasis, especially with irritation and heavy desquamation.

Cautions: Ingestion of large dosages of saponins may cause gastrointestinal irritation.

Contraindications: None known.

Qualities: Moist, warm

Typical dosage: 20–40 ml per week

104

Solidago virgaurea

Common names: Goldenrod

Family: Asteraceae

Part used: Aerial parts

Description: In Europe its use centers around dysuria of different origin: hyperactive bladder with urine incontinence, urolithiasis, renal calculi, renal and bladder gravel, irritable bladder and infections of urinary tract. Also indicated for congestion of the upper respiratory tract.

Constituents: Flavonoids (1.5%) (quercetin, kaempferol and their glycosides, astragalin and rutoside) and antocyanidins, derivatives of cyanidin. Other constituents include triterpene saponins of the oleanane type (up to 2%), the bisdesmosidic phenol glycosides leiocarposide (0.08–0.48%) and virgaureoside A, diterpenoid lactones of the cis-clerodane type, phenolic acids (caffeic acid, chlorogenic acid (0.2–0.4%), ferulic acid, synapic and vanillin acids) and small amount of essential oil (cadinene, α and β pinene, myrcene, limonene, sabinene and germacren D).

Primary actions: Anti-inflammatory (urinary), Antibacterial, Diuretic.

All actions: Analgesic, Anti-inflammatory, Anti-inflammatory (musculoskeletal), Anti-inflammatory (urinary), Antibacterial, Anticatarrhal, Antifungal, Antiseptic (urinary), Antispasmodic/Spasmolytic, Diuretic.

Indications:

- Calculi; kidney and bladder, Catarrh; naso-pharyngeal congestion, Cystitis, Dysuria, Infection; throat, Influenza, Renal insufficiency, Rhinitis, Sinusitis.

- **ESCOP:** Irrigation of the urinary tract, especially in cases of inflammation and renal gravel, and as an adjuvant in the treatment of bacterial infections of the urinary tract.

- **Other uses:** Throat infection (gargle), flatulent dyspepsia.

Cautions: There is almost no information on the toxicity, genotoxicity, carcinogenicity and reproductive and developmental toxicology. Therefore the use in pregnancy and lactation is not recommended.

Contraindications: Contraindicated in those with known allergy to goldenrod or members of the Asteraceae (Compositae) family.

Qualities: Cool, dry

Typical dosage: 20–40 ml per week

Stachys officinalis

Synonym or related species: Stachys betonica, Betonica officinalis

Common names: Wood betony

Family: Lamiaceae

Part used: Aerial parts

Description: The plant was commonly grown in the gardens of apothecaries and monasteries for medicinal purposes. The British Medical Journal lists betony as an ingredient in pistoja powder for gout and arthritis. Betony has also been used in traditional Austrian medicine internally as tea, or externally as compresses or baths for treatment of disorders of the respiratory tract, gastrointestinal tract, nervous system, skin and gynaecological problems.

Constituents: Phenylethanoid glycosides, (betonyosides A-F) and acetoside, acetoside isomer, campneosides II, forsythoside B and leucosceptoside B.

Primary actions: Anxiolytic, Bitter tonic, Sedative.

All actions: Anti-inflammatory, Anxiolytic, Bitter tonic, Sedative.

Indications:

- Anxiety, Hypertension, Indigestion, Migraine, Neuralgia.
- **BHP:** Headache, vertigo, anxiety, neuralgia. Specific indication: Headache in neurasthenia.

Qualities: Bitter taste, cooling.

Typical dosage: 15–30 ml per week

Stellaria media

Common names: Chickweed, starweed

Family: Caryophyllaceae

Part used: Aerial parts

Description: Mostly used topically for wounds and inflammatory skin disorders.

Constituents: Triterpene saponins, coumarins, phytosterols, mucilage, flavonoids (apigenin C-glycosides, rutin) carotenoids, carboxylic acids as well as nitrate salts.

Primary actions: Anti-inflammatory, Antipruritic, Wound healing/Vulnerary.

All actions: Anti-inflammatory (GIT), Antipruritic, Antirheumatic, Antitussive, Demulcent, Emollient, Expectorant (general), Wound healing/Vulnerary.

Indications:

- Eczema, Eczema (topically), Infection; gastrointestinal system, Pruritus, Ulcer (topically), Ulcer; gastrointestinal, Urticaria.
- **BHP:** Rheumatism, topically as ointment for eczema, psoriasis, indolent ulcer, poultice for carbuncle or abscess. Specific indications: topical application as ointment in pruritic skin eruptions.

Cautions: Allergic skin reactions (dermatitis) can occur with topical use; test before applying widely.

Contraindications: Contraindicated in those with known allergy or sensitivity to chickweed.

Qualities: Cool, moist

Typical dosage: 20–40 ml per week as succus (expressed juice) or fresh plant tincture.

Stevia rebaudiana

Synonym or related species: Eupatorium rebaudianum

Common names: Stevia

Family: Asteraceae

Part used: Leaves

Description: Ingenous to Paraguay, widely used in South America and now worldwide as a natural sweetener. Stevia, a non-cariogenic sweetener, is almost 300 times sweeter than sucrose. Studies in diabetic type 1 and 2 subjects have shown that stevia did not alter systolic BP, diastolic BP, glucose and glycated hemoglobin (HbA1c) from baseline measurements, except for the placebo type 1 diabetics group where a significant difference was observed for systolic BP and glucose. Stevia extracts can be considered nonacidogenic and non-cariogenic. Antihypertensive properties demonstrated in some but not all clinical trials. Stevioside reduces postprandial blood glucose levels in type 2 diabetic patients but has little effect on other parameters.

Constituents: Several glycosides (including stevioside which is largely responsible for stevia's sweetness, rebaudioside A and B, steviol, steviolbioside).

Primary actions: Antidiabetic, Antihypertensive, Taste improver.

All actions: Antidiabetic, Antihypertensive, Hypoglycaemic, Taste improver, Vasodilator.

Indications:

- Diabetes, Hypertension.

Cautions: Higher doses may be necessary for therapeutic effect.

Contraindications: None known.

Typical dosage: 5–10 ml per week as a flavouring agent. Higher doses may be necessary for therapeutic effect.

Symphytum officinale

Common names: Comfrey, knitbone

Family: Boraginaceae

Description: Due to toxicity concerns, the use of comfrey is for external use only unless based on cultivars free of pyrrolizidine alkaloids. Multiple trials have demonstrated the efficacy of comfrey preparations for treatment of pain, inflammation, and swelling of muscles in degenerative arthritis, sprains, acute myalgia in the back, contusions, and strains after sport injuries.

Comfrey contains pyrrolizidine alkaloids (PAs). During hepatic biotransformation, toxic PA metabolites are produced, which can cause hepatic veno-occlusive disease. The lungs may also be affected leading to pulmonary arterial hypertension.

A systemic review of case reports of possible

pyrrolizidine alkaloid related harm from ingestion of comfrey, coltsfoot or borage identified 11 appropriate case reports, none of which involved borage. Nine reports were assessed for causality and indicated some degree of association between the material ingested and the adverse event. Some cases may have wrongly attributed the adverse event to comfrey or coltsfoot when other plants with established toxicity may have been the culprit.

References:

Avila, C., et al., *A systematic review and quality assessment of case reports of adverse events for borage (Borago officinalis), coltsfoot (Tussilago farfara) and comfrey (Symphytum officinale* Fitoterapia, 2020. 142: p. 104519.

Traumaplant Cream, produced by German company, Harras Pharma, is not only clinically tested, but also based on their own comfrey cultivar free of PAs.

Part used: Root, leaf

Constituents: Alkaloids: pyrrolizidine-type alkaloids (0.3%). Not all are toxic: two non-hepatotoxic pyrrolizidine alkaloids, sarracine and platyphylline, have been used for the treatment of gastrointestinal hypermobility and peptic ulcers; gums (arabinose, glucuronic acid, mannose, rhamnose, and xylose); mucilage; tannins; triterpenes; rosmarinic, chlorogenic and caffeic acids and allantoin (0.75–2.25%). Allantoin promotes tissue regeneration and wound healing.

Primary actions

Root: Cytoprotective, Demulcent, Vulnerary,

Leaf: Anti-inflammatory, Antirheumatic, Cytoprotective, Demulcent, Vulnerary

All actions:

Root: Vulnerary, cytoprotective, astringent, antihaemorrhagic, demulcent

Leaf: Vulnerary, demulcent, anti-inflammatory, styptic

Indications

- **Root:** Externally: injuries, bruises, myalgia, joint pain, inflammation, wounds, ulcers. Internally: Gastrointestinal ulcer, colitis
- **Leaf:** Externally: injuries, bruises, myalgia, joint pain, inflammation, wounds, ulcers, athlete's foot, mastitis.Internally: Gastrointestinal ulcer, colitis, rheumatic pain, arthritis.
- **Other Uses:** Considered a soothing demulcent to the gastrointestinal mucosa and by reflex action to the respiratory mucosa, hence also indicated for pruritis ani, irritated mucous membranes, coughs and colds. Traditionally also used for diarrhoea and leucorrhoea.

BHP Indications

- **Root:** Gastric and duodenal ulcer. Haematemesis. Colitis. Topically: ulcers, wounds, fractures, herniae by application of fresh root.
- **Leaf:** Gastric and duodenal ulcer. Rheumatic pain. Arthritis. Topically: as poultice or fomentation in bruises, sprains, athlete's foot, crural ulcers and mastitis.

- **Specific indications:** Gastric ulcer. Topical: Varicose ulcer. Combines well with *Filipendula ulmaria* and *Althaea officinalis* in gastric ulcer.

Cautions: In Australasia comfrey, coltsfoot and borage cannot be legally prescribed for internal use. In Germany and the Netherlands short-term use of a prescribed dose is recommended (up to six weeks use at dose levels of 1 µg/day), while the European Medicines Agency recommends two weeks as the maximum duration of use while insufficient safety data is established regarding a herbal medicine.

Pregnancy/Lactation: Not recommended in pregnancy or lactation.

Contraindications: PAs are poorly absorbed across intact skin. Use only PA-free products in the treatment of ulcers or for wounds healing.

Typical weekly dosage: Extract equivalent to not more than1 µg/day PAs daily for up to six weeks.

Syzygium aromaticum

Common names: Cloves

Family: Myrtaceae

Part used: Flower bud

Description: A traditional spice that has also been used for food preservation. Cloves are the dried, unopened flower bud. Native to Indonesia, now cultivated in coastal areas in tropical regions. The name clove derives from the French 'clou' (meaning 'nail'), as the buds vaguely resemble small irregular nails in shape. Important herb in many traditional medicine systems including TCM, Ayurveda and Unani. *S. cumini* (jambul) is listed in the BHP as an astringent and carminative for diarrhoea with griping.

Constituents: Sesquiterpenes, monoterpenes, hydrocarbon, and phenolic compounds. Eugenyl acetate, eugenol, and beta-caryophyllene are the most significant phytochemicals in clove oil, as well as hydroethanolic extracts, with significant activity against various pathogenic parasites, microorganisms and viruses. Hydroethanolic extracts of cloves may also contain flavonoids including quercetin and kaempferol.

Primary actions: Anthelmintic, Anti-inflammatory, Antiseptic.

All actions: Analgesic, Anthelmintic, Anti-inflammatory, Antibacterial, Antifungal, Antifungal (topically), Antinociceptive, Antioxidant, Antiparasitic, Antiseptic, Antiviral (systemically), Antiviral (topically), Astringent, Digestive tonic, Gastroprotective, Immunomodulator.

Indications

- Cough, Diabetes, Headache, Indigestion, Infection; bacterial, Infection; fungal, Intestinal worms, Irritable bowel syndrome, Laryngitis, Parasites, Periodontitis, Rheumatism.
- **Other uses:** Clove oil is used internally and externally for its antimicrobial activities. The internal dose is 20 mg per dose. As a cream in

chronic anal fissures. Clove oil is commonly used in dentistry due to its analgesic, anesthetic, and antiseptic effects.

Qualities: Acrid, pungent, sweet. Warming.

Typical dosage: 10–15 ml per week

Tanacetum parthenium

Synonym or related species: Pyrethrum parthenium, Chrysanthemum parthenium

Common names: Feverfew

Family: Asteraceae

Part used: Leaves

Description: Feverfew is mainly used for migraine prophylaxis. Greek medicinal literature mentions its anti-inflammatory properties and its use in relieving menstrual discomforts. The first documented use of feverfew for migraines was in 1972 when the wife of a Welsh physician ended her 50-year history of migraines following 10 months of therapy. Although the exact mechanism of feverfew's action is unknown, it is believed that a sesquiterpene lactone called parthenolide is the active ingredient and works by inhibition of several known mediators of migraine: cyclooxygenase-2, TNF-α, interleukin-1, and serotonin.

Constituents: Monoterpenes, sesquiterpenes, sesquiterpenes lactones (chrysanthemolids, chrysanthemonin, 10-epi-canin, magnonliolide, parthenolide), reynosin, santamarin, tanaparthins.

Primary actions: Anti-inflammatory, Antiallergic, Migraine prophylactic.

All actions: Analgesic, Anti-inflammatory, Antiallergic, Migraine prophylactic.

Indications:

- Allergies/Sensitivities, Arthritis, Migraine.
- **ESCOP:** Prophylaxis of migraine.
- **WHO:** Prevention of migraine.
- **Other uses:** Arthritis, endometriosis, menopausal symptoms.

Cautions: Do not administer during pregnancy or lactation without medical supervision. Do not administer to children without professional advice. May occasionally cause mouth ulceration, sore tongue, indigestion, gastric disturbance, urinary complications, swelling of lips, heart palpitations, heavy periods, weight gain, skin rashes/dermatitis, palpitations, dizziness and headache. Reduce dose gradually when ceasing treatment.

Contraindications: Hypersensitivity to feverfew or other members of the Compositae (Asteraceae) family.

Drug interactions: May increase bleeding in persons taking warfarin; monitor prothrombin times and INR values.

Qualities: Dry 2nd degree, hot 3rd degree

Typical dosage: 5–10 ml per week

Taraxacum officinale folia

Common names: Dandelion leaf, pu gong ying

Family: Asteraceae

Part used: Leaves

Description: Fresh leaf hydroethanolic extract has been shown to be a true diuretic. For the entire population (n=17) there was a significant (p < 0.05) increase in the frequency of urination in the five hour period after the first dose. There was also a significant (p < 0.001) increase in the excretion ratio in the five hour period after the second dose of extract. The third dose failed to change any of the measured parameters.

Constituents: Carotene, hydroxyphenolic acid, minerals, sesquiterpene lactones, taraxacin.

Primary actions: Antioedematous, Antirheumatic, Diuretic.

All actions: Antioedematous, Antirheumatic, Bitter tonic, Diuretic, Laxative.

Indications:

- Cholecystitis, Constipation, Digestive complaints, Dyspepsia, Fluid retention, Fluid retention; premenstrual, Gallbladder disorders, Oliguria, Weight loss; to assist.
- **Commission E:** Disturbances in bile flow, stimulation of diuresis, loss of appetite and dyspepsia (root with leaf).
- **ESCOP:** As an adjuvant to treatment where enhanced urinary output is desirable, for example, rheumatism and the prevention of renal gravel.
- **WHO:** To stimulate diuresis, increase bile flow and stimulate appetite, and for treatment of dyspepsia.

Cautions: Do not administer during pregnancy without professional advice. May cause stomach hyperacidity, as with all drugs containing amaroids.

Contraindications: Occlusion of the biliary or intestinal tract, acute gallbladder inflammation or gallbladder disease. Contraindicated in individuals with known allergy to members of the Asteraceae (Compositae) family.

Qualities: Bitter, cold

Typical dosage: 40–80 ml per week

Taraxacum officinale radix

Common names: Dandelion root

Family: Asteraceae

Part used: Root

Description: Time honoured traditional medicine to stimulate diuresis, stimulate appetite, increase bile flow and to restore hepatic and biliary function.

Constituents: Minerals, phenolic acids, sesquiterpene lactones, taraxacin, taraxacoside, triterpenes.

Primary actions: Bitter tonic, Cholagogue, Diuretic.

All actions: Antirheumatic, Bitter tonic, Digestive tonic, Diuretic, Hepatotonic, Laxative.

Indications:

- Anorexia, Cholecystitis, Constipation, Digestive complaints, Dyspepsia, Gallbladder disorders, Jaundice, Liver insufficiency, Liver toxicity, Rheumatism, Weight loss; to assist.
- **BHP:** Cholecystitis, gallstones, jaundice, atonic dyspepsia with constipation, muscular rheumatism, oliguria. Specific indications: cholecystitis and dyspepsia.
- **BHC:** hepato-biliary disorders, dyspepsia, lack of appetite, rheumatic conditions.approved by the Commission E (root with leaf) for disturbances in bile flow, stimulation of diuresis, loss of appetite and dyspepsia.
- **Commission E:** Root with leaf: for disturbances in bile flow, stimulation of diuresis, loss of appetite and dyspepsia.
- **ESCOP:** Restoration of hepatic and biliary function, dyspepsia, loss of appetite.
- **WHO:** To stimulate diuresis, increase bile flow and stimulate appetite, and for treatment of dyspepsia.

Cautions: May cause stomach hyperacidity, as with all drugs containing amaroids (bitter compoounds).

Contraindications: Occlusion of the biliary or intestinal tract, acute gallbladder inflammation or gallbladder disease. Contraindicated in individuals with known allergy to members of the Asteraceae Compositae family.

Qualities: Cold 2nd degree, dry 2nd degree

Typical dosage: 20–40 ml per week

Terminalia arjuna

Common names: Arjuna

Family: Combretaceae

Part used: Bark

Description: Terminalia arjuna has been widely used in the traditional Ayurvedic system of medicine as a cardioprotectant and for acute and chronic renal diseases supporting its ethnopharmacological use.

Constituents: Triterpenoids (arjunin, arjunic acid, arjunolic acid, arjungenin, and terminic acid), glycosides (arjunin, arjunoside I, arjunoside II, arjunaphthanoloside and terminoside A), sitosterol; flavonoids (arjunolone, arjunone, bicalein, luteolin, gallic acid, ethyl gallate, quercetin, kempferol, pelorgonidin, oligomeric and proanthocyanidins), tannins and minerals.

Primary actions: Anti-inflammatory, Antiarrhythmic, Cardioprotective.

All actions: Anti-inflammatory, Antibacterial, Anticancer, Antihyperlipidemic, Antihypertensive, Antioxidant, Antiviral (systemically), Cardioprotective, Cardiotonic, Cytoprotective, Gastroprotective, Wound healing/Vulnerary.

Indications:

- Angina pectoris, Chemotherapy; to minimise the side effects of, Congestive heart failure, Diabetes, Dyslipidaemia, Dysuria, Hypertension, Metabolic syndrome, Myocardial ischaemia, Ulcer; gastrointestinal, Wounds (topically).
- **Other uses:** Arjuna is indicated in chronic cardiovascular diseases including chronic, stable angina, mild congestive heart failure, weakness of the heart, hypercholesterolemia, hypertension and metabolic syndrome. Improvement of cardiac muscle function and subsequent improved pumping activity of the heart seems to be the primary benefit of arjuna. It is thought the saponin glycosides might be responsible for inotropic effects of arjuna, while the flavonoids and OPCs provide free radical antioxidant activity and vascular strengthening.

Cautions: Minor adverse reactions include mild gastritis, headache and constipation.

Contraindications: Traditionally contraindicated during pregnancy.

Qualities: The Taste (Rasa) is astringent and bitter, the Energy (Virya) is cooling, the post-digestive effect (Vipaka) is pungent, the Quality (Guna) is light and dry, the target tissue (Dhatu) is blood, bone and reproductive tissues, the Channels (Srotas) are circulatory and reproductive. It affects all Dosa and purifies excess pitta from the blood.

Typical dosage: 20–40 ml per week

Thuja occidentalis

Synonym or related species: Biota occidentalis

Common names: Thuja, white cedar, arbor-vitae (American)

Family: Cupressaceae

Part used: Leaves (actually young flattened branches)

Description: Thuja is a native European tree widely used in homeopathy. Thuja's antiviral action and immunomodulating potential, including stimulation of cytokines and antibody production and activation of macrophages and other immune cells, have been evaluated in vitro and in vivo. A low dose formulation containing thuja with echinacea and baptisia has been shown to be beneficial in reducing symptoms of the common cold.

Constituents: Essential oil (terpenic ketones – mostly thujone, also isothujone, thujane, camphor, fenchone, alpha-pinene, borneol), mucilage as thuja polysaccharides and other polysaccharides, flavonoids (thujin, beta-sitosterol, kaempferol, quercetin), a lectin, plicatic acid, thujaplicin, alpha-thujaplicin, tannins.

Primary actions: Antibacterial, Antiviral (systemically), Depurative/Alterative.

All actions: Antibacterial, Antiviral (systemically), Astringent, Counter-irritant, Depurative/Alterative, Emmenagogue, Expectorant (stimulating).

Indications:

- Amenorrhoea, Arthritis, Bronchitis, Cardiac debility, Common cold, Cystitis, Enuresis, Infection; throat, Osteoarthritis, Ovarian cyst, Psoriasis, Rheumatism, Rheumatoid arthritis, Warts, Warts (topically).

- **BHP:** Bronchial catarrh, enuresis, cystitis, psoriasis, amenorrhoea, rheumatism. Has been used in uterine carcinomas. Topically: warts, particularly genital and anal. Specific indications: bronchitis with cardiac weakness, warts (oral and topical). Reported to be of value as anticarcinomatous agent. Counteracts ill effects of smallpox vaccination.

Cautions: Use with caution in patients with underlying defects in hepatic haem synthesis. High doses should be avoided with epilepsy, also with acute and chronic airway obstruction, due to stimulating effect on smooth muscles. May cause headache when taken in high doses.

Contraindications: Contraindicated in pregnancy – may cause abortion due to reflex uterine contractions. Contraindicated during lactation due to potential toxicity of essential oil.

Qualities: Cool, dry

Typical dosage: 10–20 ml per week

Thymus vulgaris

Common names: Thyme

Family: Lamiaceae

Part used: Leaves and flowering tops

Description: Traditionally used for bronchitis and cough with viscous sputum, and associated hoarseness; expectorant in cough associated with cold. Mucolytic and expectorant in cough associated with the common cold. Suitable for children.

Constituents: Essential oil containing phenols (thymol and carvacrol), labiate tannins polymethoxyflavones, triterpenes and polysaccharides.

Primary actions: Antimicrobial, Antiseptic (respiratory tract), Expectorant (relaxing).

All actions: Anthelmintic, Antiasthmatic, Antidiarrhoeal, Antifungal, Antimicrobial, Antiparasitic, Antiseptic (respiratory tract), Antispasmodic (respiratory tract), Antitussive, Antiviral (systemically), Astringent, Bitter tonic, Carminative, Expectorant (relaxing).

Indications:

- Asthma, Bronchitis, Cough, Diarrhoea, Dyspepsia, Enuresis, Gastritis, Infection; respiratory tract, Infection; throat, Inflammation; oral cavity, Laryngitis, Pertussis, Sore throat (gargle), Tonsillitis, Tracheitis.

- **BHP:** Dyspepsia, chronic gastritis, bronchitis, pertussis, asthma, diarrhoea in children, enuresis in children, laryngitis and tonsillitis (gargle).

Specific indications: pertussis, bronchitis.

- **Commission E:** For symptoms of bronchitis and whooping cough, and catarrhs of upper respiratory tract.

- **ESCOP:** Catarrh of the upper respiratory tract, bronchial catarrh and supportive treatment of pertussis. Stomatitis and halitosis.

- **WHO:** Orally to treat dyspepsia and other gastrointestinal disturbances; coughs due to colds, bronchitis and pertussis; and laryngitis and tonsillitis (as a gargle). Topical applications of thyme extract have been used in the treatment of minor wounds, the common cold, disorders of the oral cavity, and as an antibacterial agent in oral hygiene.

Cautions: Thyme essential oil consisting of 48% p-cymene and 24% thymol (0.25% essential oil in the feed over two weeks and during first four days of pregnancy, n=15, number of embryos: 126) showed no influence on the growth and development of mouse embryos in vivo (Domaracky et al., 2006).

Contraindications: Do not administer to patients with a known sensitivity to plants in the Lamiaceae (Labiatae) family.

Qualities: Dry 3rd degree, hot 3rd degree

Typical dosage: 15–40 ml per week

Tilia cordata

Common names: Lime tree, linden

Family: Tiliaceae

Part used: Flowers

Description: Infusions of the flowers make a pleasant-tasting tea for promoting sweating in the case of common cold, chronic coughing and catarrh. Traditionally used as relaxant and to treat headaches, indigestion and diarrhoea and to relieve anxiety-related indigestion with heart palpitation.

Constituents: Mucilage polysaccharides, tannins, flavonoids (rutin, hyperoside, quercitrin, isoquercitrin), glycosides (astragalin), phenolic acids (caffeic, p-coumaric, chlorogenic), essential oil containing alkanes and monoterpenes.

Primary actions: Diaphoretic, Nervine tonic, Vasodilator.

All actions: Antifungal, Antipyretic, Antispasmodic/ Spasmolytic, Anxiolytic, Diaphoretic, Diuretic, Nervine tonic, Sedative, Vasodilator.

Indications:

- Anxiety, Arteriosclerosis, Common cold, Epilepsy, Fever, Hypertension, Migraine, Myocardial ischaemia, Nervous tension.

- **BHP:** Migraine, hysteria, arteriosclerotic hypertension, and feverish colds. Specific indications: raised arterial pressure associated with arteriosclerosis and nervous tension.

- **BHC:** upper respiratory catarrh, common colds, irritable coughs, hypertension, restlessness.

109

- **Commission E:** Colds and cold-related coughs.

Cautions: Avoid in patients with known allergy to tilia.

Contraindications: None known.

Qualities: Dry, secondary cooling effect, warm

Typical dosage: 15–30 ml per week

Trametes versicolor

Synonym or related species: Coriolus versicolor

Common names: Turkey tail PSK, PSP

Family: Polyporaceae

Part used: Dried and whole fruiting bodies.

Description: PSP has proven beneficial to survival and quality of life not only for cancer patients, but also for patients with hepatitis, hyperlipidemia, and other chronic diseases. PSP activates immune cells, increases the expressions of cytokines and chemokines such as tumor necrosis factor-α (TNF-α), interleukins (IL-1β and IL-6), histamine, and prostaglandin E, enhances dendritic and T-cell infiltration into tumors, and ameliorates the adverse events associated with chemotherapy.

Constituents: The main bioactives in the mushroom are two proteoglycans: polysaccharide–K, (PSK or krestin) and polysaccharide–P, (PSP). Other major isolated compounds include verisicolor polysaccharide (VPS), heteropolysaccharide, β-1,4-glucan, proteins, polypeptides, amino acids, deoxycoriolic acids, nucleotides, coriolan, triterpenoids, coriolins, phenolic acids, polyphenols, active hexose correlated compounds, ergosta-7,22-dien-3β-ylpalmitate, ergosta-7,22-dien-3β-ol, betulic acid, 4-hydroxy benzoic acid, 3-methoxy-4-hydroxy benzoic acid, 3, 5-dimethoxyl-4-hydroxy benzoic acid, 2-furoic acid, nicotinic acid, lipid compounds, vitamins, mineral and trace elements, among many other minor compounds.

Primary actions: Anticancer, Chemoprotective, Immunomodulator.

All actions: Analgesic, Anti-inflammatory, Antibacterial, Anticancer, Anticatarrhal, Antidiabetic, Antifungal, Antimicrobial, Antinociceptive, Antiseptic (GIT), Antiviral (systemically), Chemoprotective, Hepatoprotective, Immunomodulator.

Indications:

- Cancer; including prevention/supportive treatment, Hepatitis, Immune deficiency, Infection; gastrointestinal system, Infection; respiratory tract.

Qualities: Slightly sweet, cool.

Typical dosage: 3–6 g daily

Tribulus terrestris

Common names: Tribulus, calthrops, puncture vine, Bai Ji Li

Family: Zygophyllaceae

Part used: Aerial parts

Description: Traditionally used in China as a component in formulations for the liver, kidney, cardiovascular system and immune systems. In Ayurveda, the plant and fruit have been used to treat spermatorrhoea, gonorrhoea, impotence, uterine disorders after parturition, cystitis, painful urination, kidney stones and gout. It is claimed that the tribulus from Eastern Europe and Iran is more effective for sexual health. Now popular for erectile dysfunction, low sperm count or motility, low libido in men, and poor ovulation rates (steroidal saponins may interact with the hypothalamus or pituitary to re-establish ovulation) or menopausal symptoms (hot flushes, sweating, insomnia and depression) in women. Also used to improve fertility and to treat fluid retention, abdominal distension and cardiovascular diseases. Animal studies suggest a benefit in liver disease, hyperglycaemia and hyperlipidaemia.

Constituents: Tribulus from Eastern Europe and Iran contains steroidal saponins (protodioscin, prototribestin, pseudoprotodioscin, dioscin, tribestin and tribulosin) and flavonoids, including rutin. Protodioscin and prototribestin are the dominant saponins. Tribulus from India and Vietnam contain tribulosin as the dominant saponin, small amounts of protodioscin, and lack prototribestin and tribestin. Levels also depend on the plant part. In Eastern Europe the leaf is the main part while the fruit is used in India.

Primary actions: Antihyperlipidemic, Aphrodisiac, Hepatotonic.

All actions: Anti-inflammatory, Antibacterial, Antihyperlipidemic, Aphrodisiac, Hepatotonic, Hypoglycaemic.

Indications:

- Cardiovascular disease prevention, Depression, Dyslipidaemia, Erectile dysfunction, Impotence, Infertility, Insomnia, Liver insufficiency, Menopausal symptoms, Ovulation; eratic, Sexual weakness, Sperm count; low.

Contraindications: Contraindicated in pregnancy due to traditional use as an abortifacient. Avoid use in patients with androgen-sensitive tumours.

Drug interactions: Tribulus leaf extracts standardised to protodioscin may reduce hot flushes in postmenopausal women. Tribulus fruit is used in the treatment of urinary stones in traditional Indian medicine. There are no indications that tribulus interferes with the effect of oral contraceptives or postmenopausal hormonal therapy.

Typical dosage: Liquid extract equivalent to 5–7 g daily.

Trifolium pratense

Common names: Red clover, trifoil

Family: Fabaceae

Part used: Flowerheads

Description: Red clover is a traditional alterative mainly used for inflammatory skin disorders. Due to its content of isoflavone, it has also been developed as a phyto-oestrogen supplement (Promensil).

Constituents: Most chemical research is in agricultural contexts for leaf, not flower. Flowerheads contain essential oil, fatty acids, flavonoids, flavonols, isoflavones, p-coumaric acid, phenolic acids, quercetin glucosides, salicylic acid, sitosterol, starch. Red clover contains four major isoflavones: biochanin A and formononetin, with a very small amount of genistein and daidzein. Around 97% of the total isoflavone content in red clover leaves are formononetin and biochanin. The level is around 82% in flowers (Saviranta et al., 2008). Formononetin is metabolised into daidzein and equol. Across different maturity stages the leaves are the most important source of isoflavones. The level is highest in young leaves and reduces as the plant matures. The total content of formononetin and biochanin is up to 27-fold higher in leaves compared with flowers. Flowering buds harvested in early summer contain on average about 4 mg/g total isoflavones. Young flowers contains about 1.8 mg/g, larger flowers later in summer about 0.8 mg/g, while the flowers at the end of summer contains about 2.2 mg/g isoflavones.

Primary actions: Anti-inflammatory, Depurative/ Alterative, Expectorant (general).

All actions: Anti-inflammatory, Anticancer, Depurative/Alterative, Expectorant (general), Selective oestrogen receptor modulator (SERM).

Indications:

- Acne, Bronchitis, Cough, Eczema, Menopausal symptoms, Psoriasis.
- **BHP:** Chronic skin disease, pertussis. Specific indications: eczema, psoriasis.
- **Other uses:** Chronic skin disorders including acne, eczema, psoriasis, cough, bronchitis. Extracts of the red clover leaf are promoted for the relief of menopausal symptoms, especially hot flushes, although a 2007 Cochrane review of isoflavones concluded that there was no convincing evidence that isoflavones are efficacious. The recommended thereapeutic dosage of isoflavones for menopausal symptoms is 40 mg isoflavones daily.

Cautions: Use with caution during pregnancy. Patients with endometriosis, uterine fibroids, or other conditions that are aggravated by increased oestrogen levels should be monitored closely. Do not administer concentrated isoflavone extracts to patients with oestrogen-sensitive cancers without medical supervision.

It would be demanding to reach an intake of 40 mg isoflavones from drinking red clover flower tea. Assuming a midsummer harvest, the isoflavone content is not likely to be more than about 2 mg/g total isoflavones. This would entail ingesting 20 g dried red clover daily, the equivalent of about 10 heaped tablespoons of red clover flowers (unmilled).

Contraindications: None known.

Drug interactions: Isoflavones are selective oestrogen modulators (SERMs) and mostly interact with oestrogen receptor ER-β. In premenopausal women, with high endogenous oestrogen levels, isoflavones may exert antioestrogenic activity by competitive inhibition, preventing oestrogen from binding to the oestrogen receptor. Coadministration with an oral contraceptive is unlikely to cause clinically significant interactions. In menopausal women isoflavones may produce a surrogate oestrogen effect. Coadministration with postmenopausal hormone therapy is unlikely to cause clinically significant interactions.

Qualities: Cooling potential, neutral

Typical dosage: 20–40 ml per week

Trigonella foenum-graecum

Synonym or related species: Buceras foenum-graecum

Common names: Fenugreek

Family: Fabaceae

Part used: Ripe dried seed

Description: Diosgenin (steroidal sapogenin) is used abundantly in medicinal herbs such as *Dioscorea villosa* and *Trigonella foenum-graecum*. Diosgenin is utilised as a raw material for the production of steroidal drugs in the pharmaceutical industry. Due to its wide range of pharmacological activities, it has been used in the treatment of cancers, hyperlipidemia, inflammation, and infections. Numerous studies have reported that diosgenin is useful in the prevention and treatment of neurological diseases. Trigonella can lower triglycerides and LDL levels and increases HDL levels in diabetic subjects. The dose of the seed is quite high. Up to 50 g of powdered fenugreek seed is used for diabetes and dyslipidaemia. The dose of the standardised extract (Libifem and Testofen, Gencor Pacific Ltd., 50% saponins) is 600 mg daily for the treatment of poor libido in women and men. Another standardised extract (Furocyst, 40% furostanolic saponins) is 1000 mg each/day for the treatment of PCOS.

Constituents: Mucilage (galactomannans), lipids, proteins, protease inhibitors, steroidal saponins, aglycone (diosgenin and its epimer yamogenin), alkaloid (trigonelline), steroidal peptide (foenugraecin).

Primary actions: Antihyperlipidemic, Galactagogue, Hypoglycaemic.

All actions: Antihyperlipidemic, Antinociceptive, Demulcent, Emollient, Galactagogue, Hypoglycaemic, Laxative.

Indications:

- Anorexia, Convalescence, Diabetes, Dyslipidaemia, Dyspepsia, Gastritis, Lactation; poor, Libido; low, Menopausal symptoms, Obesity, Polycystic ovarian syndrome.
- **BHP:** Dyspepsia, anorexia, gastritis,

convalescence. Topically: furunculosis, myalgia, lymphadenitis, gout, wounds, crural ulcer. Specific indications: general debility and anorexia of convalescence.

- **Commission E:** Loss of appetite (internal use), local inflammation (poultice).

- **ESCOP:** Internal use: Adjuvant therapy in diabetes mellitus, anorexia, as an adjunct to a low fat diet in the treatment of mild to moderate hypercholesterolaemia. External use: Furunculosis, ulcers, and eczema.

- **WHO:** As an adjunct for the management of hypercholesterolaemia, and hyperglycaemia in cases of diabetes mellitus. Prevention and treatment of mountain sickness. Internally for loss of appetite, and externally as a poultice for local inflammations. Treatment of pain, and weakness and oedema of the legs.

Drug interactions: In vitro and in vivo observations suggested that fenugreek does not have substantial effect on the metabolic activity of CYP2D6 and CYP3A4.

Results of pharmacodynamics and pharmacokinetics studies suggested that simultaneous administration of fenugreek or *N. sativa* with amlodipine improves the pharmacological response of amlodipine in hypertensive rats, though there was no remarkable change in pharmacokinetic parameters (Alam et al., 2020).

Reference:

Alam MA, Bin Jardan YA, Raish M, Al-Mohizea AM, Ahad A, Al-Jenoobi FI (2020) Effect of Nigella sativa and Fenugreek on the pharmacokinetics and pharmacodynamics of amlodipine, in hypertensive rats. Curr Drug Metab

Qualities: Pungent, warm

Typical dosage: 15–30 ml per week

Trillium erectum

Synonym or related species: Trillium pendulum

Common names: Beth root, birth root

Family: Liliaceae

Part used: Root

Description: Disturbance through logging and other forest developments have large impacts on *T. erectum* and most other *Trillium* spp. populations. Endangered in Illinois, threatened in Rhode Island, and Exploitable/Vulnerable in New York. Use alternative herb if possible: *Alchemilla vulgaris, Lamium album* or *Capsella bursa-pastoris* as indicated.

Constituents: Diosgenin, fixed oil, tannin, steroidal saponin (trillarin).

Primary actions: Antihaemorrhagic (uterine), Hypothalamic-pituitary-ovarian (HPO) regulator, Uterine tonic.

All actions: Antihaemorrhagic (uterine), Astringent, Hypothalamic-pituitary-ovarian (HPO) regulator, Selective oestrogen receptor modulator (SERM), Uterine tonic.

Indications:

- Cystic hyperplasia, Depression, Haematuria, Haemorrhage; postpartum, Leucorrhoea, Leucorrhoea and vaginitis (douche), Menopause, Menorrhagia, Metrorrhagia, Uterine bleeding; dysfunctional.

- **BHP:** Metrorrhagia, menorrhagia, haematuria, haemoptysis, leucorrhoea (douche), indolent ulcers (poultice/ointment). Specific indication: menopausal menorrhagia associated with depression.

Cautions: Due to the high tannin content, constipation may occur after long-term administration. At risk species: use sparingly or find a suitable alternative.

Contraindications: None known

Qualities: Moist, neutral

Typical dosage: 10–30 ml per week

Turnera diffusa

Common names: Damiana

Family: Turneraceae

Part used: Leaves and stems

Description: Antianxiety, antiaromatase, antibacterial including antimycobacterial, antidiabetic, antioxidant, adapatogenic, antiobesity, antispasmodic, cytotoxic, gastroprotective, hepatoprotective, and aphrodisiac activities. Most of these activities have so far been investigated only in chemical, cell based, or animal assays. Turnera is shown to have phosphodiesterase-5 (PDE-5) inhibiting properties which may explain its use in erectile dysfunction and libido.

Constituents: Turnera spp. may contain flavonoids, maltol glucoside, phenolics, cyanogenic glycosides, monoterpenoids, sesquiterpenoids, triterpenoids, the polyterpene ficaprenol-11, fatty acids, and caffeine.

Primary actions: Antidepressant, Nervine tonic, Stomachic.

All actions: Antidepressant, Male tonic, Nervine tonic, Stomachic.

Indications:

- Anxiety, Constipation, Depression, Dyspepsia; nervous, Fibroids, Nervous tension, Stress.

- **BHP:** Depression, nervous dyspepsia, atonic constipation, and coital inadequacy. Specific indication: anxiety neurosis with a predominant sexual factor.

Cautions: Arbutin is a mandatory component of *Turnera diffusa*.

The concentration of arbutin in the medicine must be no more than 25 mg/kg or 25mg/L or 0.0025% unless used on the hair.

Contraindications: Traditionally contraindicated for people with an overactive sympathetic nervous system

Qualities: Dry, neutral

Typical dosage: 20–40 ml per week

Tussilago farfara

Common names: Coltsfoot

Family: Asteraceae

Description: Described by Priest & Priest as a diffusive expectorant, sedative and demulcent: suitable for debilitated and chronic respiratory conditions, especially where there is diathesis (predisposition).

The mucilage is main active component responsible for its use in pulmonary disorder. Unfortunately, coltsfoot also contains pyrrolizidine alkaloids (Pas). During hepatic biotransformation, toxic PA metabolites are produced, which can cause hepatic veno-occlusive disease. The lungs may also be affected leading to pulmonary arterial hypertension.

A systemic review of case reports of possible pyrrolizidine alkaloid related harm from ingestion of comfrey, coltsfoot or borage identified 11 appropriate case reports, none of which involved borage. Nine reports were assessed for causality and indicated some degree of association between the material ingested and the adverse event. Some cases may have wrongly attributed the adverse event to comfrey or coltsfoot when other plants with established toxicity may have been the culprit (Avila et al., 2020).

References: Avila, C., et al., *A systematic review and quality assessment of case reports of adverse events for borage (Borago officinalis), coltsfoot (Tussilago farfara) and comfrey (Symphytum officinale).* Fitoterapia, 2020. 142: p. 104519.

Part used: Leaf, flower

Constituents: Pyrrolizidine-type alkaloids including senkrikine, senecionine (saturated) and tussilagine (saturated). Caffeic, caffeoyltartaric, ferulic, gallic, malic and other acids. Mucilage (7%), flavonoids including kaempherol and quercetin and their glycosides, tannins (up to 17%), bitter glycosides, phytosterols, triterpenes including tussilagone (sesquiterpene) and volatile oil. Tussilagine is a potent cardiovascular and respiratory stimulant.

Primary actions: Expectorant, antitussive, anticatarral.

All actions: Expectorant, antitussive, anticatarral, demulcent.

Indications:

- Asthma, Bronchitis, Emphysema, Silicosis, Pertussis.
- **BHP:** Asthma, bronchitis, laryngitis, pertussis. Specific indication: Chronic spasmodic bronchial cough. Combines well with Marrubium vulgare and Verbascum thapsus in irritating cough.

Cautions: In Australasia comfrey, coltsfoot and borage cannot be legally prescribed for internal use. In Germany and the Netherlands short-term use of a prescribed dose is recommended (up to six weeks use at dose levels of 1 µg/day), while the European Medicines Agency recommends two weeks as the maximum duration of use while insufficient safety data is established regarding a herbal medicine.

Pregnancy/Lactation: Not recommended in pregnancy or lactation.

Contraindications: Not recommended for children.

Dosages: Tincture 1:5: 2–8 ml three times daily.

Extract equivalent to not more than1 µg/day PAs daily for up to six weeks.

Ulmus fulva

Synonym or related species: Ulmus rubra

Common names: Slippery elm, red elm

Family: Ulmaceae

Part used: Inner bark

Description: The inner bark of slippery elm is used in several popular herbal tea blends including Essiac®. Also used in throat lozenges. Traditionally used for its demulcent properties for inflammatory digestive, respiratory, and urinary disorder, and topically for skin diseases and for healing wounds.

Constituents: Contains a mixture of water-soluble and water-insoluble fibre including mucilages, gums, pectin, lignin, insoluble hemicelluloses

Primary actions: Demulcent, Laxative, Mucilaginous.

All actions: Antidiarrhoeal, Demulcent, Demulcent (urinary), Emollient, Expectorant (general), Laxative, Mucilaginous.

Indications:

- Allergies/Sensitivities, Boils (poultice), Candidiasis, Colic, Colitis, Constipation, Cough, Crohn's disease, Cystitis, Diarrhoea, Digestive complaints, Diverticulitis, Dyslipidaemia, Flatulence, Gastric reflux, Gastritis, Gastrointestinal catarrh, Gastrointestinal tract dysbiosis, Hyperactivity, Indigestion, Infection; gastrointestinal system, Inflammation; gastrointestinal tract, Inflammatory bowel disease, Ulcer; gastrointestinal, Ulcerative colitis.
- **Other uses:** Soluble fibre is often described as mucilaginous or slippery as it has the capacity to carry lots of water and thereby form a gel; this may also reduce cholesterol and glucose absorption from the gut. The insoluble fibre (roughage) is more resistant to digestion and is fermented by bacteria to produce special fatty acids for the health of the gut wall. Both fibres are needed for a healthy digestive system. Slippery elm also acts as a pre-biotic.

Cautions: Take with adequate water.

Contraindications: Intestinal obstruction.

Drug interactions: Slippery elm forms an inert

barrier over the gastrointestinal lining, therefore it may alter the rate and/or extent of absorption of drugs that have a narrow therapeutic window (e.g. digoxin, warfarin, phenytoin, barbituates, lithium); separate doses by at least two hours.

Typical dosage: 1–3 teaspoon powder as required.

Uncaria tomentosa

Common names: Cat's claw

Family: Rubiaceae

Part used: Root or stem bark

Description: Although there are no randomised controlled trials or published human outcome studies on PubMed, some conditions reportedly improved by U. tomentosa include osteoarthritis, rheumatoid arthritis, prostatitis, viral illnesses and cancer (acting as a non-specific immunomodulanting agent) and it may also have potential as an immunomodulating adaptogen in cellular aging. Its use in arthritis may be due to a possible inhibition of TNF-alpha. Pharmacological studies are described according to antibacterial, anticancer, antiHIV, antidiabetic, antibacterial, anti-inflammatory, antioxidant, antiviral, cytotoxicity, immunostimulation, vascular, hypotensive, mutagenicity and well as AChE inhibitory, antileishmanial, β3 adrenergic receptor agonistic, phosphatase inhibitory, analgesic, spermicidal, vasopressin antagonists, progesterone antagonists, neuroprotective properties.

Constituents: There are two chemotypes of *Uncaria tomentosa* with different alkaloid patterns occurring in nature. The roots of one type contain pentacyclic oxindoles and the other contains tetracyclic oxindoles. This difference should be considered when the plant is to be used for medicinal applications. Tetracyclic oxindole alkaloids act on the central nervous system, whereas pentacyclic oxindole alkaloids affect the cellular immune system. Recent studies have shown that the tetracyclic alkaloids exert antagonistic effects on the action of the pentacyclic alkaloids. Mixtures of these two types of drugs are therefore unsuitable for medicinal uses. Pentacyclic oxindole alkaloids stimulate endothelial cells in vitro to produce a lymphocyte-proliferation-regulating factor. Tetracyclic oxindole alkaloids act as antagonists.

Primary actions: Anti-inflammatory, Anticancer, Immunomodulator.

All actions: Anti-inflammatory, Anticancer, Antioxidant, Antiviral (systemically), Immunomodulator, Wound healing/Vulnerary.

Indications:

- Arthritis, Asthma, Autoimmune disease, Cancer; including prevention/supportive treatment, Chronic fatigue syndrome, Convalescence, Crohn's disease, Debility, Depression, Diverticulitis, Gastritis, Haemorrhoids (topically), Hayfever, Herpes (topically), Immune deficiency, Infection; fungal, Infection; systemic, Ulcer;

gastrointestinal, Wounds (topically).

- **WHO:** Symptomatic treatment of arthritis, rheumatism and gastric ulcers. May be an immunostimulant and increase the number of white blood cells.

Cautions: Safety during lactation and in children has not yet been established; use only under the supervision of a healthcare provider. Adverse effects include indigestion, constipation, diarrhoea, lymphocytosis, erythrocytosis, and aggravation of acne.

Drug interactions: May increase HIV protease inhibitors levels (case report).

Qualities: Warm

Typical dosage: 30–80 ml per week

Urtica dioica folia

Common names: Nettle leaf, stinging nettle

Family: Urticaceae

Part used: Aerial parts

Description: Despite the use of nettle in folk veterinary medicine being well documented, *U. dioica* is today an underestimated and frequently neglected plant, considered by the contemporary agriculture as a weed to be eliminated. Stinging nettle has been used by nursing mothers orally as a postpartum herb, as a tonic for treating anemia, and as a galactogogue. Ingredient in 'Ankaferd'. Ankaferd has been traditionally used in Anatolia as a haemostatic agent. Ankaferd contains a standardised combination of *Glycyrrhiza glabra, Thymus vulgaris, Alpinia officinarum, Vitis vinifera,* and *Urtica dioica.* Ankaferd is used in inflammation and bleeding of gastrointestinal and bronchial mucosal membranes and cutaneous bleeding and also in abdominal, thoracic, dental and oropharyngeal, and pelvic surgeries. Extracts of nettle leaf are used as an anti-inflammatory remedy for rheumatoid arthritis. The antiproliferative and apoptotic effects of *U. dioica* have been demonstrated on different human cancers.

Constituents: Minerals, amines (histamine, acetycholine, serotinin), flavonol glycosides, phenolic acids, scopolten, tannins, chlorophyll, xanthophyll, vitamins, enzymes.

Primary actions: Antirheumatic, Diuretic, Styptic/ Haemostatic.

All actions: Antirheumatic, Astringent, Diuretic, Galactagogue, Hypoglycaemic, Nutritive.

Indications:

- Arthritis, Eczema, Gout, Urinary gravel.

- **BHP:** Uterine haemorrhage, cutaneous eruptions, infantile and psychogenic eczema, epistaxis, melaena. Specific indication: nervous eczema.

- **Commission E:** Irrigation therapy for inflammatory diseases of the lower urinary tract and prevention and treatment of kidney gravel. Also approved for rheumatic ailments.

- **ESCOP:** Adjuvant in the symptomatic treatment of arthritis, arthroses and/or rheumatic conditions. Nettle leaf is also used as a diuretic, but there is limited clinical evidence to confirm this effect.

Cautions: Do not administer during pregnancy or lactation without professional supervision. The fresh herb may cause irritation if handled (hairs act like miniature syringes, injecting histamine and acetylcholine into skin); people with known sensitivities or allergies to stinging nettle should use this herb cautiously.

Contraindications: None known

Qualities: Dry 3rd degree, hot 3rd degree

Typical dosage: 15–40 ml per week

Urtica dioica radix

Synonym or related species: Urtica gracilis

Common names: Nettle root

Family: Urticaceae

Part used: Root and rhizome

Description: Nettle root is widely used to treat benign prostatic hypertrophy (BPH), allergies, arthritis, and inflammation. Often combined with *Serenoa repens* in the treatment of lower urinary tract symptoms and benigh hyperplasia of the prostate.

Constituents: Polysaccharides, a lectin (UDA), phenolics (lignans, coumarins), sterols and their glycosides.

Primary actions: Antihyperprostatic.

All actions: Antihyperprostatic.

Indications:

- Arthritis, Benign prostatic hyperplasia, Prostatitis, Rheumatism.
- **WHO:** Symptomatic treatment of lower urinary tract disorders (nocturia, polyuria, urinary retention) resulting from early BPH stages, in cases where diagnosis of prostate cancer is negative. As a diuretic and for the treatment of rheumatism and sciatica.

Qualities: Dry 3rd degree, hot 3rd degree

Typical dosage: 30–60 ml per week

Usnea spp.

Synonym or related species: U. barbata, U. florida, U. hirta, U. plicata

Common names: Old man's beard, songluo

Family: Parmeliaceae

Part used: Thallus

Description: The common name, Old Man's Beard, refers to how usnea hangs from tree limbs looking like a beard. Usnea has a long history in both TCM and Western herbal medicine. Generally used as a lozenge or mouth wash for inflammation of the oral cavity, skin creams, and vaginal douches, it is also used internally for bronchitis.

Constituents: Benzofurans including the antibacterial usnic acid.

Primary actions: Anticatarrhal, Antifungal, Antifungal (topically), Antimicrobial.

All actions: Analgesic, Anti-inflammatory, Anticancer, Anticatarrhal, Antifungal, Antifungal (topically), Antimicrobial, Antiparasitic, Antipyretic, Antiviral (topically).

Indications:

- Bronchitis, Candidiasis, Cough, Fever, Headache, Infection; fungal, Infection; genitourinary tract, Infection; respiratory tract, Leucorrhoea.
- **Commission E:** Mild inflammation of the oral and pharyngeal mucosa. Taken as a lozenge.

Cautions: May cause contact dermatitis.

The FDA has warned about liver damage from the use of usnic acid for weight loss. Some products were found to contain other compounds including phenylpropanolamine, caffeine, yohimbine hydrochloride, and diiodothyronine, however there has been one case report of fulminant liver failure due to consumption of 500 mg usnic acid daily for two weeks for weight loss.

Usnea lichen preparations containing equivalent concentrations of usnic acid produced greater toxicity than pure usnic acid.

Contraindications: Do not use internally during pregnancy. Safety in lactation has not been established. Do not use internally long-term for chronic conditions.

Qualities: Bitter, sweet. Cooling, drying.

Typical dosage: 50–100 ml per week

Vaccinium myrtillus

Common names: Bilberry, blueberry

Family: Ericaceae

Part used: Ripe fruit, dried or fresh

Description: *Vaccinium myrtillus* is one of the richest natural sources of anthocyanins which give berries their red/purple/blue coloration. Anthocyanins are reported to play an important role in the prevention of metabolic disease and CVD as well as cancer and other conditions. Although there is evidence to support the use of bilberry supplementation as part of a healthy diet, the potential benefits from the use of bilberry supplementation in patients with T2DM or CVD needs to be clarified in clinical trials. Ingredient in Samital with *Macleaya cordata* and *Echinacea angustifolia* used for oral mucositis induced by chemo-radiotherapy. A number of pilot trials in oncological patients demonstrated that SAMITAL has good clinical efficacy and tolerability as evidenced by its significant effects in terms of reduction of mucositis, pain and a general improvement in patient quality of life. British Royal Air Force pilots reported that the ingestion of bilberry jam just prior to missions seemed to improve their vision. Poor-quality studies during the 1960s and 1970s purportedly supported these claims. The hypothesis that *V. myrtillus* anthocyanosides improves normal night vision is not supported by evidence from rigorous clinical studies.

Constituents: Tannins, invert sugar, fruit acids, flavonol glycosides (including astragalin, hyperoside, isoquercitrin and quercitrin), phenolic acids, pectics, triterpenes, polyphenols (anthocyanosides).

Primary actions: Antioedematous, Cytoprotective, Vasoprotective.

All actions: Anti-inflammatory, Antigalactagogue, Antioedematous, Antioxidant, Antiplatelet, Astringent, Cytoprotective, Vasoprotective.

Indications:

- Capillary fragility, Cataract and diabetic complications, Circulation; peripheral; impaired, Diabetic neuropathy, Diabetic retinopathy, Gums; bleeding, Night blindness, Nose bleeds, Retinal blood flow disorders, Retinal damage, Senile macular degeneration, Varicose veins, Varicose veins (topically), Venous insufficiency, Visual fatigue.

- **Commission E:** Non-specific acute diarrhoea, and as local therapy for mild inflammation of the mucous membranes of mouth and throat.

- **ESCOP:** Internal use: Symptomatic treatment of problems related to varicose veins. External use: Topical treatment of mild inflammation of the mucous membranes of the mouth and throat.

Contraindications: None known

Drug interactions: Antiplatelet activity may theoretically potentiate the action of warfarin (low risk).

Qualities: Cold, dry

Typical dosage: 20–40 ml per week. 320–480 mg/day (standard extracts) of bilberry fruit containing 36% of anthocyanins.

Valeriana officinalis

Synonym or related species: Valeriana edulis (Mexican valerian)

Common names: Valerian, heliotrope, Mexican valerian (*V. edulis*) has stronger sedative properties.

Family: Valerianaceae

Part used: Roots, rhizome

Description: Valerian is among the most widely used herbal medicines in the world. Despite its use as a sedative and hypnotic for sleep, stress and anxiety, the research is not very supporting. Earlier studies were positive; however more recent studies are much less convincing. Compared to diazepam, acute administration of valerian did not have mood-altering or psychomotor or cognitive effects in young healthy volunteers. One study found that 450 mg valerian at bedtime did not improve sleep as measured by the PSQI. Another study found that 300 mg did not improve sleep in a sample of older women with insomnia. It is likely that valerian is more effective when combined with other herbal medicines such as fixed combination Ze 91019 containing *V. officinalis*

and *Humulus lupulus*. NSF-3, a combination of standardised extracts of *V. officinalis*, *Passiflora incarnate* and *Humulus lupulus* is a safe and effective short-term alternative to zolpidem for primary insomnia. Ze 185, a fixed combination of *V. officinalis*, *Passiflora incarnate*, *Verbena officinalis* and *Petasites hybridus* (butterbur) extracts, significantly attenuated the subjective emotional stress response during an acute stress situation, without affecting biological stress responses. Valarian has also been shown to have anti-obsessive properties in a pilot study. Mexican valerian may be a more potent alternative. Valerian root and its preparations seem to improve sleep structure with a gradual onset of efficacy rather than to exert a general sedating effect. After single intake valerian root changed mainly subjective perception of sleep, while sleep EEG changes were more pronounced after several days of intake. These observations are in concordance with clinical experiences showing a gradual improvement of symptoms over 2–4 weeks. Valerian root probably exerts its effects in pathological conditions rather than in healthy volunteers.

Constituents: Iridoids known as valepotriates (valtrates, didrovaltrates and isovaltrates), essential oil containing monoterpenes (mainly bornyl acetate), cyclopentane sesquiterpenoids including valerinic acid. Chemical analysis of the hydroalcoholic extract of *V. edulis* indicated that this extract contains 0.26% of dihydroisovaltrate as the main valepotriate, and that it does not contain valerenic acid.

Primary actions: Antispasmodic/Spasmolytic, Anxiolytic, Sedative.

All actions: Antiepileptic, Antispasmodic (muscles), Anxiolytic, Carminative, Hypnotic, Nervine tonic, Sedative.

Indications:

- Anxiety, Colic; childhood, Colic; intestinal, Cramps; muscular spasm; muscular tension, Dysmenorrhoea, Excitability, Hyperactivity, Hypertension, Insomnia, Migraine, Nervous tension, Premenstrual syndrome, Restlessness.

- **BHP:** Hysterical states, excitability, insomnia, hypochondriasis, migraine, cramp, intestinal colic, rheumatic pains, and dysmenorrhoea. Specific indication: conditions presenting as nervous excitability.

- **Commission E:** Restlessness and sleeping disorders based on nervous conditions.

- **ESCOP:** Relief of temporary mild nervous tension and/or difficulty in falling asleep.

- **WHO:** As a mild sedative and sleep-promoting agent. Used as a milder alternative or a possible substitute for stronger synthetic sedatives (e.g. benzodiazepines), in the treatment of states of nervous excitation and anxiety-induced sleep disturbances.

Cautions: Single doses not always effective. Continuous use for 1–2 weeks appears to produce best results. Avoid consuming alcoholic beverages or other sedatives in conjunction with valerian.

Contraindications: Do not administer to children under 3 years.

Drug interactions: May theoretically potentiate sedative medication.

Qualities: Dry 2nd degree, hot 1st degree

Typical dosage: 15–40 ml per week

Verbascum thapsus

Common names: Mullein, candlewick plant, flannel-leaf, bunny's ears

Family: Scrophulariaceae

Part used: Aerial parts

Description: Used to treat inflammed and irritated mucous membranes of the respiratory systems. Otikon, an ear drop formulation containing oily extracts of *Allium sativum, Verbascum thapsus, Calendula officinalis, Hypericum perfoliatum, Lavendula officinalis,* and vitamin E in olive oil taken five drops three times daily, has been shown to be effective as anaesthetic ear drops and may be an appropriate for the management of acute otitis media-associated ear pain in children.

Constituents: Triterpene saponins (verbascosaponin), mucilage, iridoid glycoside, flavonoids (including rutin and hesperidin), various phenolic acids.

Primary actions: Anticatarrhal, Demulcent, Expectorant (general).

All actions: Demulcent, Emollient, Expectorant (general), Wound healing/Vulnerary.

Indications:

- Bronchitis, Cough, Influenza, Jaundice, Otitis media, Tonsillitis, Tracheitis.
- **BHP:** Bronchitis, tracheitis, influenzal cold with respiratory catarrh. Topically as preparation in olive oil for inflamed mucosa. Specific indication: bronchitis with hard cough and soreness.
- **Commission E:** Flower extracts approved for respiratory catarrh.

Contraindications: None known

Qualities: Cool, moist, secondary drying effect

Typical dosage: 30–60 ml per week

Verbena officinalis

Common names: Vervain

Family: Verbenaceae

Part used: Aerial parts

Description: Mainly used for complaints of the oral and pharyngeal mucosa such as sore throat, and of the respiratory tract including cough and asthma. Also pain, spasms, states of exhaustion, nervous disorders, digestive and urinary disorders. The Commission E did not find evidence of efficacy and did not recommend its use. Pharmacological investigations have demonstrated antitussive and secrotolytic effects. Hot water extract shown to have significant luteinizing hormone screting and possibly FSH stimulating effects.

Constituents: Iridoid glycosides (e.g., verbenalin, hastatoside), verbascoside, flavonoids including luteolin, and the diglucuronides of apigenin and acecetin, and small amounts of beta-sitosterol, ursolic acid, lupeol and traces of an essential oil.

Primary actions: Antitussive, Anxiolytic, Nervine tonic.

All actions: Antidepressant, Astringent, Bitter tonic, Diaphoretic, Galactagogue, Nervine tonic, Sedative.

Indications:

- Anxiety, Cholecystitis, Debility, Depression, Dysmenorrhoea, Fever, Gingivitis, Jaundice, Migraine.
- **BHP:** Depression, melancholia, hysteria, generalised seizures, cholecystalgia, jaundice, early stages of fevers. Specific indications: depression and debility of convalescence after fevers, especially influenza.

Cautions: None known

Qualities: Dry 2nd degree, hot 2nd degree

Typical dosage: 20–40 ml per week

Viburnum opulus

Common names: Cramp bark

Family: Caprifoliaceae

Part used: Bark

Description: V. opulus and V. prunifolium are mainly used for cramps, including menstrual cramps and muscle cramping associated with arthritis. Also used by Native Americans for swollen glands, mumps and eye disorders, and as a diuretic. Sedative action on the uterus.

Constituents: Bitter glycoside viburnin, valerianic acid, tannins, coumarins, resin.

Primary actions: Antispasmodic (muscles), Antispasmodic (uterus), Antispasmodic/Spasmolytic.

All actions: Antispasmodic (muscles), Antispasmodic (uterus), Antispasmodic/Spasmolytic, Astringent, Sedative.

Indications:

- Colic; intestinal, Cramps; muscular spasm; muscular tension, Dysmenorrhoea, Dysmenorrhoea; spasmodic, Endometriosis, Enuresis, Menopause; Menorrhagia, Miscarriage; threatened, Myalgia, Ovarian and uterine pains, Uterine bleeding; dysfunctional, Uterine contractions.
- **BHP:** Spasmodic muscular cramping, uterine dysfunction, menopausal metrorrhagia, threatened miscarriage, partus praeparator and infantile enuresis. Specific indications: cramps, ovarian

and uterine pains.

- **Other uses:** Partus praeparator, infantile enuresis.

Contraindications: None known

Qualities: Cool, dry

Typical dosage: 10–30 ml per week

Viburnum prunifolium

Common names: Black haw, Sweet viburnum

Family: Caprifoliaceae

Part used: Stem bark

Description: V. opulus and V. prunifolium are mainly used for cramps; including menstrual cramps and muscle cramping associated with arthritis. Especially indicated for spasmodic dysmenorrhoea. Sedative action on the uterus.

Constituents: Biflavones, iridoid glucosides, triterpenes and triterpenic acids, coumarins including scopoletin, scopolin, and aesculetin, organic acids, including acetic, capronic, caprylic, citric, isovaleric, linoleic, malic, myristic, oleic, oxalic, palmitic, valeric, and salicylic acids, and salicin, hydroxycinnamic acid derivatives, such as caffeic, chlorogenic, and isochlorogenic acids. Others include arbutin, beta-sitosterin, bitter principle, essential oil, tannins, pentosanes, and traces of alkaloids.

All actions: Antiasthmatic, Antispasmodic (muscles), Antispasmodic (uterus), Astringent.

Indications:

- Asthma, Dysmenorrhoea, Miscarriage; threatened, Ovarian and uterine pains, Uterine contractions.
- **BHP:** Dysmenorrhoea, false labour pains, threatened miscarriage, asthma. Specific indication: threatened abortion, especially with rise in arterial tension.

Cautions: Avoid using in gastric or enteric poisoning incidents, due to antispasmodic activity. Nausea and vomiting have been reported at high doses.

Contraindications: None known

Qualities: Cool, dry

Typical dosage: 10–30 ml per week

Vinca minor

Common names: Periwinkle, lesser or common periwinkle

Family: Apocynaceae

Part used: Aerial parts

Description: Vinpocetine is a synthetic ethyl-ester derivative of the alkaloid apovincamine from *Vinca minor* leaves. Vinpocetine is a selective inhibitor of phosphodiesterase type 1 that has potential neurological effects through inhibition of voltage-gated sodium channel and reduction of neuronal calcium influx. Vinpocetine has noteworthy antioxidant, anti-inflammatory, and anti-apoptotic effects with inhibitory effect on glial and astrocyte cells during and following ischemic stroke. Vinpocetine is effective as adjuvant therapy in the management of epilepsy.

Constituents: Monoterpene indole alkaloids (vincamine, pervincamine), bitter principle (vincine), phenolic compounds.

Primary actions: Antihypertensive, Nootropic, Sedative.

All actions: Antihypertensive, Astringent, Nootropic, Sedative.

Indications:

- Cerebrovascular disease, Depression, Headache, Hypertension, Leucorrhoea, Memory and concentration; poor, Retinal blood flow disorders, Stroke; recovery after, Tinnitus, Vertigo.
- **Other uses:** Dizziness from Meniere's disease.

Contraindications: Contraindicated in pregnancy.

Qualities: Warm

Typical dosage: 30–50 ml per week

Viola tricolor

Common names: Heartsease, wild pansy, viola

Family: Violaceae

Part used: Dried aerial parts

Description: Wild pansy preparations were used during the Middle Ages mainly as an topical and internal remedy for various skin ailments including impetigo, acne, psoriasis and pruritus. Other uses include respiratory disorders and as a diuretic in urinary tract disorders.

Constituents: Salicylates, saponins, alkaloids, flavonoids (including anthocyanidins, rutin and violaquercitrin), tannins, mucilage.

Primary actions: Antirheumatic, Depurative/Alterative, Expectorant (general).

All actions: Anti-inflammatory, Antirheumatic, Depurative/Alterative, Diuretic, Expectorant (general), Laxative.

Indications:

- Bronchitis, Capillary fragility, Cystitis, Dysuria, Eczema, Pertussis, Rheumatism, Urticaria.
- **BHP:** Pertussis, acute bronchitis, cystitis, polyuria and dysuria capillary fragility, and cutaneous affections. Specific indication: eczema and skin eruptions with serous exudate, particularly when associated with rheumatic symptoms.

Contraindications: None known

Qualities: Moist, neutral

Typical dosage: 20–40 ml per week

Viscum album

Common names: Mistletoe

Family: Loranthaceae

Part used: Aerial parts

Description: *Viscum album* has a long traditional history as an adjunctive therapy in cancer treatment in German-speaking countries. Besides antitumoral and quality of life-promoting activities, *V. album* reduces side effects of modern conventional anticancer therapies and exerts immunomodulatory activities. Preclinical studies have demonstrated cytotoxic, apoptosis-inducing, and immunomodulatory effects. Many clinical studies indicate a supportive efficacy of mistletoe extracts in tumor patients, even though methodological quality may be low. Mistletoe products for cancer support incude Helixor®, Iscador®, Iscador Qu®, Lektinol™, Cefalektin®, Eurixor®, ABNOBAviscum®, Abnoba-viscum Quercus. Mistletoe cancer therapy is appropriate for almost all cancers and can be given any time – before or after surgery, as well as before, during, or after radiation, chemotherapy, hormonal, or antibody therapies. The mistletoe extract is injected subcutaneously. Outside the Germanic countries, mistletoe is traditionally used for nervous tension and cardiovascular disorders.

Primary actions: Anticancer, Antihypertensive, Sedative.

All actions: Antiatherosclerotic, Anticancer, Antihypertensive, Sedative.

Indications:

* Arteriosclerosis, Cancer; including prevention/ supportive treatment, Headache, Hypertension, Nervous tachycardia, Nervous tension.
* **BHP:** High blood pressure, arteriosclerosis, nervous tachycardia, hypertensive headache, chorea, hysteria. Specific indication: arterial hypertension.

Contraindications: Avoid during pregnancy, except for the last six weeks.

Qualities: Cold, moist

Typical dosage: 20–40 ml per week

Vitex agnus-castus

Common names: Chaste tree, chasteberry, Man Jing Zi

Family: Verbenaceae

Part used: Ripe fruit (dried or fresh)

Description: Vitex agnus-castus has been shown to be effective in the treatment of menopausal symptoms, premenstrual syndrome (PMS), premenstrual dysphoric disorder, dysmenorrhoea, luteal phase defects, premature ovarian failure, and infertility in both men and women. Dopaminergic compounds in vitex help to treat cyclical mastalgia as well as other symptoms of the premenstrual syndrome.

Constituents: Essential oil (cinelole, limonene, pinene), luteolin-like flavonoids, iridoid glycosides (agnuside, aucubin), eurostoside, some triterpenoids.

Primary actions: Antihyperprolactinaemic, Hypothalamic-pituitary-ovarian (HPO) regulator,

Selective oestrogen receptor modulator (SERM).

All actions: Antiandrogenic, Antihyperprolactinaemic, Carminative, Dopaminergic, Galactagogue, Hypothalamic-pituitary-ovarian (HPO) regulator, Menstrual cycle regulator, Selective oestrogen receptor modulator (SERM), Uterine tonic.

Indications:

* Acne, Adenomyosis, Amenorrhoea, Benign breast disease, Cystic hyperplasia, Depression, Depression; postnatal, Dysmenorrhoea, Endometriosis, Fibroids, Follicular cyst, Infertility, Insomnia, Lactation; poor, Latent hyperprolactinaemia, Luteal phase complaints, Mastalgia, Menopausal symptoms, Menopause, Menopause; Menorrhagia, Menstrual irregularity, Migraine, Miscarriage; repeated, Miscarriage; threatened, Oligomenorrhoea, Ovarian cyst, Ovulation; eratic, Ovulation; painful, Premature ovarian failure, Premenstrual syndrome, Uterine bleeding; dysfunctional, Weight loss; to assist.
* **Commission E:** Menstrual irregularities, PMS, mastodynia.
* **ESCOP:** Premenstrual syndrome including symptoms such as mastodynia or mastalgia. Menstrual cycle disorders such as polymenorrhoea, oligomenorrhoea or amenorrhoea.

Cautions: Not traditionally recommended during pregnancy; use cautiously and only in early stages, for insufficient corpus luteal function. Use with caution in women under 20 years as hypothalamic-pituitary-ovarian axis is easily disrupted. For this reason, it is recommended that treatment with Vitex is commenced in the early part of the follicular phase of the menstrual cycle (often given as 2–3 ml on rising, starting day one of menstrual cycle). Avoid using with progesterone drugs, OCP or HRT. May aggravate pure spasmodic dysmenorrhoea. Usually stopped postmenopausally: not indicated for classical oestrogen deficiency symptoms of menopause. Avoid use in people with oestrogen or progesterone sensitive tumours until safety established. Gastrointestinal disturbances, nausea, skin conditions and headaches have been reported as adverse effects.

Contraindications: None known

Drug interactions: Chaste tree has antihyperprolactinaemic properties and may contain compounds with affinity for the oestrogen receptor beta (ER-β). There is no evidence of interaction with oral contraceptives or postmenopausal hormone therapy. Chaste tree may be used for symptoms of PMS in women using oral contraceptives, but it is generally not recommended for the treatment of menopausal symptoms. Oestrogenic effects unlikely and unsubstantiated.

Qualities: Cooling potential, dry, neutral, warming potential

Typical dosage: 5–20 ml per week

Vitis vinifera

Common names: Grape vine, grapeseed extract

Family: Vitaceae

Part used: Seeds, skins of fruit, leaves

Description: Rich in oligomeric procyanidins. Use as an alternative to *Pinus pinaster* extract. Clinical studies have found grape seed alone or in combination with other natural products to be beneficial in leg ulcers, radiation creams, inflammation in obesity and gingivitis.

Constituents: Nonhydrolysable tannins (aka procyanidins, oligomeric procyanidins [OPCs], proanthocyanidins, leucoanthocyanidins, polyphenols), anthocyanins, organic acids, tannins, other phenolic compounds, potassium bitartrates, tartrates.

Primary actions: Antioedematous, Vasoprotective, Venotonic.

All actions: Anti-inflammatory, Antioedematous, Antioxidant, Antiplatelet, Astringent, Diuretic, Vasoprotective, Venotonic.

Indications:

- Allergies/Sensitivities, Capillary fragility, Cellulitis, Connective tissue disorders, Diabetic neuropathy, Diabetic retinopathy, Dysmenorrhoea; congestive, Gums; bleeding, Intestinal worms, Radiation; side effects of, Retinal damage, Rhinitis, Varicose veins, Venous insufficiency, Weight loss; to assist, Wounds.

Cautions: Dispense liquid extracts separately due to high tannin content.

Contraindications: None known

Qualities: Cold, dry

Typical dosage: 20–40 ml per week

Withania somnifera

Common names: Ashwaghanda, withania, winter cherry

Family: Solanaceae

Part used: Root

Description: Clinical studies have shown beneficial effects in infertility in men, sexual function, chemotherapy-induced fatigue, cognitive dysfunction, memory, stress, anxiety, poor sleep, schizophrenia, obsessive compulsive disorder, pain relief in arthritis, subclinical hypothyroidism, and as an adjunct during resistance training.

Constituents: Alkaloids (including withasomnine), saponins, steroidal lactones (withanolides).

Primary actions: Adaptogen, Anticancer, Anxiolytic.

All actions: Adaptogen, Anti-inflammatory, Antiarrhythmic, Anticancer, Antihyperlipidemic, Anxiolytic, Bladder tonic, Chemoprotective, Hypoglycaemic, Immunomodulator, Nervine tonic, Sedative, Tonic.

Indications:

- Anaemia, Anorexia, Cancer; including prevention/ supportive treatment, Chemotherapy; to minimise the side effects of, Chronic fatigue syndrome, Connective tissue disorders, Convalescence, Debility, Depression, Emaciation, Exhaustion, Hypertension, Immune deficiency, Impotence, Inflammation, Menopause, Nervous exhaustion, Premenstrual syndrome, Stress.

Cautions: Use with caution in peptic ulcer disease. High doses may cause gastrointestinal disturbances, vomiting and diarrhoea. Caution when administering to patients with known sensitivity to the Solanaceae family.

Contraindications: The results from a study of a withania hot water extract, administered to rats over a period of eight months, suggest that withania may not be harmful during pregnancy. The withania-treated animals produced litters with higher birth weight compared to the control group, suggesting healthier infant rats in this group. No toxicity was observed during the study. In other animal experiments, no foetal abnormalities were found in mice fed a withania root extract for four weeks.

Drug interactions: Use with caution in patients taking immunosuppressant medication.

Qualities: Warm

Typical dosage: 40–90 ml per week

Zanthoxylum clava-herculis

Common names: Prickly ash

Family: Rutaceae

Part used: Bark

Description: Native Americans used the powdered inner bark packed into a cavity for toothache. An infusion was used externally for swollen joints. It was also used for sore throat, dyspepsia, dysentery, kidney disorders and as a circulatory stimulant. The alkaloid chelerythrine exhibited potent activity against strains of methicillin-resistant *Staphylococcus aureus* (MRSA), which were highly resistant to clinically useful antibiotics via multidrug efflux mechanisms. Cannabinoid receptors, CB1 and CB2, are therapeutic targets in the treatment of anxiety, obesity, movement disorders, glaucoma, and pain. Preliminary results suggest the presence of a high-affinity phytocannabinoid in zanthoxylum.

Constituents: Isoquinoline alkaloids including magnoflorine and an isobutyl polyeneamide known as neoherculin (gives characteristic tingle on tongue also noticed when tasting other herbal extracts containing isobutylamides, e.g., echinacea).

Primary actions: Antipyretic, Antirheumatic, Circulatory stimulant.

All actions: Antimicrobial, Antipyretic, Antirheumatic, Antiseptic, Carminative, Circulatory stimulant, Diaphoretic, Diuretic, Sialogogue.

Indications:

- Chilblains; unbroken (topically), Circulation;

peripheral; impaired, Cramps; muscular spasm; muscular tension, Intermittent claudication, Raynaud's syndrome, Rheumatism.

- **BHP:** Cramps, intermittent claudication, Raynaud's syndrome, chronic rheumatic conditions. Specific indication: peripheral circulatory insufficiency associated with rheumatic symptoms.

Contraindications: BHC recommends that prickly ash not be used during pregnancy due to presence of alkaloids.

Qualities: Dry, warm

Typical dosage: 10–30 ml per week

Zea mays

Common names: Corn silk, maize

Family: Poaceae

Part used: Styles and stigma harvested before fertilisation

Description: Corn silk is made from stigmas, the yellowish thread like strands from the female flower of maize. It is a waste material from corn cultivation and available in abundance. It is used in the treatment of cystitis, edema, kidney stones, diuretic, prostate disorder, and urinary infections as well as bed-wetting. It soothes and relaxes the lining of the bladder and urinary tubules, hence reducing irritation and increasing urine secretion.

Constituents: Essential oil (with carvacrol and other terpenes), unidentified saponins, glavonoids, bitter substances, polyphenols, sugars, mucilage, potassium salts.

Primary actions: Anti-inflammatory (urinary), Demulcent (urinary), Diuretic.

All actions: Anti-inflammatory (urinary), Demulcent (urinary), Diuretic.

Indications:

- Cystitis, Enuresis, Prostatitis, Urethritis, Urinary gravel.
- **BHP:** Cystitis, urethritis, nocturnal enuresis, and prostatitis. Specific indications: acute or chronic inflammation of the urinary system.
- **Other uses:** Nocturnal enuresis, urinary tract infection.

Contraindications: None known

Qualities: Cool, drying potential, moistening potential

Typical dosage: 20–40 ml per week

Zingiber officinale

Common names: Ginger, Sheng Jiang (fresh), Gan Jiang (dried)

Family: Zingiberaceae

Part used: Rhizome

Description: The rhizomes of *Zingiber officinale* have been used since ancient times as a traditional remedy for gastrointestinal complaints. Ginger (and its constituents) acts peripherally, within the gastrointestinal tract, by increasing the gastric tone and motility due to anticholinenergic and antiserotonergic actions. It is also reported to increase gastric emptying. This combination of functions explains the widely accepted ability of ginger to relieve symptoms of functional gastrointestinal disorders, such as dyspepsia, abdominal pain, and nausea, which is often associated with decreased gastric motility. Ginger extract and its constituents 6-gingerols, 6-shogoals and zhingerol reduce inflammatory mediators such as inflammatory cytokines and chemokines due to their effects on NF-κB activation, cyclooxygenase 2 reduction and serotonin receptor inhibition. Several clinical studies have found ginger beneficial in reducing nausea, including nausea induced by motion sickness and chemotherapy. Others have examined dysmenorrhoea, arthritis and ulcerative colitis.

Constituents: Oleoresin containing sesquiterpenes including zingiberene, the pungent phenolic compounds gingerols and shogaols and galanolactones

Primary actions: Anti-inflammatory, Antiemetic, Expectorant (general).

All actions: Analgesic, Anti-inflammatory, Anti-inflammatory (topically), Antiemetic, Antiplatelet, Antipyretic, Bitter tonic, Carminative, Chemoprotective, Choleretic, Demulcent, Diaphoretic, Expectorant (general), Galactogogue.

Indications:

- Anorexia, Arteriosclerosis, Arthritis, Circulation; peripheral; impaired, Colic; childhood, Colic; intestinal, Digestive complaints, Dysmenorrhoea, Dyspepsia; flatulent, Endometriosis, Fever, Halitosis, Hypochlorhydria, Mammary abscess (poultice), Mastitis, Morning sickness, Nausea, Osteoarthritis, Poor breast milk volume.
- **BHP:** Colic, flatulent dyspepsia. Specific indication: flatulent intestinal colic.
- **Commission E:** Dyspepsia and prevention of motion sickness.
- **ESCOP:** Prophylaxis of the nausea and vomiting of motion sickness and as a postoperative anti-emetic for minor day-case surgical procedures.
- **WHO:** The prophylaxis of nausea and vomiting associated with motion sickness, postoperative nausea, pernicious vomiting in pregnancy, and seasickness. The treatment of dyspepsia, flatulence, and other stomach complaints and as an anti-inflammatory agent in the treatment of migraine headache and rheumatic and muscular disorders.

Cautions: Do not administer during pregnancy or in patients with peptic ulceration without professional supervision. It is recommended that high doses be avoided in pregnancy (maximum of 2000 mg/day).

Use with caution in people with gastric ulcers or reflux. Mild gastrointestinal disturbances, heartburn, bloating and spice allergies have been reported.

Contraindications: Not recommended for children under 6 years.

Drug interactions: Dabigatran

Co-administration of cinnamon/ginger with dabigatran should be avoided (case report). The American Heart Association recommend that direct-acting oral anticoagulants (DOACs) rather than warfarin in patients with non-valvular atrial fibrillation.

A case where self-administration of ginger and cinnamon together with dabigatran in an 80-year-old man caused fatal bleeding. The history of recent combination of herbal products (ginger and cinnamon) with DOACs (dabigatran) and the presence of diffuse haemorrhage of the mucosal membrane of the upper gastrointestinal tract raised the possibility of a herb–drug interaction leading to severe gastrointestinal bleeding.

Qualities: Acrid, hot

Typical dosage: 5–20 ml per week

Ziziphus jujuba var. spinosa

Synonym or related species: Z. jujuba, Z. vulgaris, Z. spinosa

Common names: Zizyphus, sour Chinese date, jujube, Da Zao, Suan Zao Ren

Family: Rhamnaceae

Part used: Seed, ripe fruit

Description: Zizyphus is a nervine tonic used for anxiety and sleep disorders. It is also used to treat digestive disorders and gastric ulcers. PHY906 containing *Glycyrrhiza uralensis, Paeonia lactiflora, Scutellaria baicalensis* and *Ziziphus jujube* is a very well researched formulation as adjunctive therapy in cancer.

Constituents: 0.1% saponins including jujubosides A, B, C and acetyljujuboside B., betulic acid, essential oil, fixed oil, jujubosides, minerals, mucilage, oligomeric procyanidins (OPCs), proanthocyanidins, saponins, triterpenoids, vitamins, ziziphin, zizyphic acid.

Primary actions: Anxiolytic, Nervine tonic, Sedative

All actions: Anticonvulsant, Antihydrotic, Anxiolytic, Digestive tonic, Hypnotic, Nutritive, Relaxant, Sedative, Stomachic.

Indications:

- Anxiety, Depression, Hypertension, Insomnia, Irritability, Nervous exhaustion, Nervous tension, Neurasthenia, Night sweats, Palpitations, Restlessness, Stress, Sweating; excessive.

- **WHO:** Treatment of insomnia due to irritability. To promote weight gain, improve muscular strength, and as an immunostimulant to increase physical stamina.

Cautions: In TCM, the use of zizyphus is cautioned

in patients with severe diarrhoea or excess heat. May increase effects of other sedatives and hypnotics. Use with caution during pregnancy or lactation. Fever, chills and joint pain have been reported.

Contraindications: Conditions of excess dampness such as symptoms of epigastric distension and bloating.

Qualities: Neutral, sour, sweet

Typical dosage: 30–90 ml per week

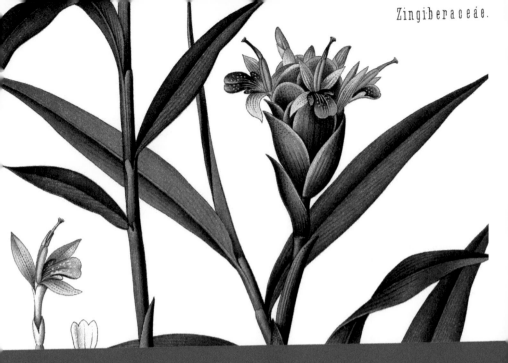

Therapeutic Actions

Phytotherapy Desk Reference

AMPK-activator
Primary herbs
- Gynostemma pentaphyllum (Jiaogulan, xiancao)

Adaptogen
Primary herbs
- Asparagus racemosus (Shatavari (Sanskrit), satavari (Hindi), satmuli (Bengali))
- Astragalus membranaceus (milk vetch, huang qi (Chinese), ogi (Japanese))
- Atractylodes macrocephala (Atractylodes, bai zhu)
- Bryonia dioica (Bryony)
- Codonopsis pilosula (Dang shen, codonopsis)
- Eleutherococcus senticosus (Eleuthero, eleutherokokk, Siberian ginseng)
- Gynostemma pentaphyllum (Jiaogulan, xiancao)
- Panax ginseng (Ginseng, ren shen)
- Panax quinquefolium (American ginseng)
- Rehmannia glutinosa (Rehmannia, sheng di huang (uncured), shu di huang (cured), Chinese foxglove)
- Rhodiola rosea (Golden root, rose root, arctic root)
- Schisandra chinensis (Bei-Wuweizi, Chinese magnolia vine, Wu Wei Zi)
- Withania somnifera (Ashwaghanda, winter cherry)

Additional herbs
- Andrographis paniculata (Andrographis, kalmegh)
- Bacopa monnieri (Bacopa, brahmi)
- Centaurium erythraea (Centaury)
- Centella asiatica (Gotu kola, brahmi, Indian pennywort)
- Crocus sativus (Saffron)
- Dulacia inopiflora (Muira puama)
- Glycyrrhiza spp. (Licorice, Liquorice, Gan Cao)

Aldose reductase inhibitor
Primary herbs
- Glycyrrhiza spp. (Licorice, Liquorice, Gan Cao)
- Scutellaria baicalensis (Baikal skullcap, baical skullcap, Chinese skullcap, Huang qin (Mandarin), ogon (Japanese))

Anaesthetising (mucous membranes)
Primary herbs
- Piper methysticum (Kava)

Analgesic
Primary herbs
- Anemone pulsatilla (Pulsatilla)
- Boswellia serrata (Boswellia, olibanum, frankincense)
- Capsicum spp. (Chilli, capsicum, pepper, paprika, cayenne)
- Eschscholzia californica (Californian poppy)
- Harpagophytum procumbens (Devil's claw)

- Macropiper excelsum (Kawakawa, New Zealand peppertree)
- Salix spp. (Willow bark, white willow)

Additional herbs
- Arnica montana (Arnica)
- Baptisia tinctoria (Wild indigo)
- Centaurium erythraea (Centaury)
- Commiphora myrrha (Myrrh)
- Corydalis ambigua (Corydalis)
- Epilobium parviflorum (Willow herb)
- Isatis tinctoria (Isatis, ban lan gen, woad, Chinese indigo)
- Ocimum tenuiflorum (Tulsi, Holy basil)
- Paeonia lactiflora (Peony, white peony, Bai Shao)
- Piper methysticum (Kava)
- Salvia rosmarinus (Rosemary)
- Scutellaria lateriflora (Blue skulcap)
- Smilax ornata (Sarsaparilla)
- Solidago virgaurea (Goldenrod)
- Syzygium aromaticum (Cloves)
- Tanacetum parthenium (Feverfew)
- Trametes versicolor (Turkey tail PSK, PSP)
- Usnea spp. (Old man's beard, songluo)
- Zingiber officinale (Ginger, Sheng Jiang (fresh), Gan Jiang (dried))

Anodyne
Primary herbs
- Piscidia piscipula (Jamaican dogwood)
- Plantago major (Plantain, broad-leaved plantain, Che Qian Zi)

Additional herbs
- Anemone pulsatilla (Pulsatilla)
- Corydalis ambigua (Corydalis)
- Humulus lupulus (Hops)
- Nigella sativa (Black cumin)
- Passiflora incarnata (Passion flower)
- Piper methysticum (Kava)
- Salix spp. (Willow bark, white willow)
- Scrophularia nodosa (Figwort)

Antacid
Primary herbs
- Filipendula ulmaria (Meadowsweet)

Anthelmintic
Primary herbs
- Annona muricata (Graviola, soursop, guanábana)
- Artemisia absinthium (Wormwood, absinthe)
- Artemisia vulgaris (Mugwort)
- Chelidonium majus (Greater celandine)
- Juglans nigra (Black walnut)
- Syzygium aromaticum (Cloves)

Additional herbs

- Allium sativum (Garlic)
- Artemisia annua (Sweet Annie, Chinese wormwood, qing hao)
- Chamaelirium luteum (False unicorn root, helonias)
- Euphorbia hirta (Euphorbia)
- Handroanthus impetiginosus (Pau d'arco, lapacho (Spanish))
- Inula helenium (Elecampane)
- Juglans cinerea (Butternut bark, white walnut, lemon walnut)
- Macropiper excelsum (Kawakawa, New Zealand peppertree)
- Momordica charantia (Bitter melon, bitter gourd, African or wild cucumber)
- Nigella sativa (Black cumin)
- Peumus boldus (Boldo)
- Thymus vulgaris (Thyme)

Anti-inflammatory

Primary herbs

- Actaea racemosa (Black cohosh, squawroot, snakeroot)
- Aesculus hippocastanum (Horse chestnut)
- Agrimonia eupatoria (Agrimony)
- Albizia lebbeck (Albizia, sirisha)
- Alchemilla vulgaris (Lady's mantle)
- Aloe ferox (Aloe vera (gel), bitter aloes (resin))
- Alpinia galanga (Greater galangal, Thai ginger)
- Angelica polymorpha (Dong quai, dang gui, Chinese angelica)
- Apium graveolens (Celery seed, karafs)
- Arctium lappa (Burdock)
- Arnica montana (Arnica)
- Berberis aquifolium (Oregon grape, mountain grape)
- Betula pendula (Silver birch)
- Boswellia serrata (Boswellia, olibanum, frankincense)
- Bupleurum falcatum (Bupleurum, sickle-leaved hare's ear)
- Calendula officinalis (Calendula, marigold)
- Caulophyllum thalictroides (Blue cohosh)
- Centaurium erythraea (Centaury)
- Cnicus benedictus (Blessed or holy thistle)
- Codonopsis pilosula (Dang shen, codonopsis)
- Commiphora myrrha (Myrrh)
- Cryptolepis sanguinolenta (Yellow dye root, delboi)
- Curcuma longa (Turmeric)
- Dioscorea spp. (Wild yam)
- Dipsacus asper (Teasel root)
- Echinacea spp. (Echinacea)
- Epilobium parviflorum (Willow herb)

- Eupatorium perfoliatum (Boneset, feverwort)
- Euphrasia officinalis (Eyebright)
- Filipendula ulmaria (Meadowsweet)
- Glycyrrhiza spp. (Licorice, Liquorice, Gan Cao)
- Guaiacum officinale (Guaiacum)
- Gynostemma pentaphyllum (Jiaogulan, xiancao)
- Hamamelis virginiana (Witch hazel)
- Handroanthus impetiginosus (Pau d'arco, lapacho (Spanish))
- Harpagophytum procumbens (Devil's claw)
- Hemidesmus indicus (Anantamul, Indian sarsparilla)
- Houttuynia cordata (Yu Xing Cao, chameleon plant, fish mint)
- Isatis tinctoria (Isatis, ban lan gen, woad, Chinese indigo)
- Isodon rubescens (Dong ling cao, Chinese sage bush, rabdosia)
- Ligustrum lucidum (Glossy privet, nu zhen zi, joteishi)
- Perilla frutescens (Perilla, su zi, shisu)
- Plantago major (Plantain, broad-leaved plantain, Che Qian Zi)
- Rehmannia glutinosa (Rehmannia, sheng di huang (uncured), shu di huang (cured), Chinese foxglove)
- Rhodiola rosea (Golden root, rose root, arctic root)
- Ruscus aculeatus (Butcher's broom, box holly)
- Scrophularia nodosa (Figwort)
- Serenoa repens (Saw palmetto, cabbage palm, dwarf palmetto)
- Smilax ornata (Sarsaparilla)
- Stellaria media (Chickweed, starweed)
- Syzygium aromaticum (Cloves)
- Tanacetum parthenium (Feverfew)
- Terminalia arjuna (Arjuna)
- Trifolium pratense (Red clover, trifoil)
- Uncaria tomentosa (Cat's claw)
- Zingiber officinale (Ginger, Sheng Jiang (fresh), Gan Jiang (dried))

Additional herbs

- Andrographis paniculata (kalmegh)
- Artemisia annua (Sweet Annie, Chinese wormwood, qing hao)
- Asparagus racemosus (Shatavari (Sanskrit), satavari (Hindi), satmuli (Bengali))
- Atractylodes macrocephala (Atractylodes, bai zhu)
- Berberis vulgaris (Barberry)
- Bidens tripartita (Burr marigold, water agrimony, gui zhen cao, longbacao)
- Bistorta officinalis (Bistort, common bistort, European bistort or meadow bistort)
- Capsella bursa-pastoris (Shepherd's purse)
- Carica papaya (Paw paw, papaya)

- Cinnamomum verum (Cinnamon, cassia bark, rou gui)
- Coptis chinensis (Huanglian (China), makino (Japan))
- Cordyceps militaris (Cordyceps, orange catapillar fungus, dong chong xia cao (China), hyakurakusou (Japan))
- Crateva magna (Varuna)
- Crocus sativus (Saffron)
- Ephedra sinensis (Ma-huang)
- Epimedium sagittatum (Horny goat weed, barrenwort, yin yang huo, Inyokaku)
- Foeniculum vulgare (Fennel)
- Fucus vesiculosus (Bladderwrack)
- Ginkgo biloba (Maidenhair)
- Glechoma hederacea (Ground ivy)
- Grindelia camporum (Gum weed)
- Gymnema sylvestre (Gumar, meshashringi)
- Hypericum perforatum (St John's wort)
- Hyssopus officinalis (Hyssop)
- Juglans nigra (Black walnut)
- Leonurus cardiaca (Motherwort)
- Leptospermum scoparium (Manuka, tea tree)
- Macropiper excelsum (Kawakawa, New Zealand peppertree)
- Magnolia officinalis (Magnolia, Hou po)
- Marrubium vulgare (White horehound)
- Matricaria chamomilla (Chamomile, German chamomile)
- Nigella sativa (Black cumin)
- Paeonia lactiflora (Peony, white peony, Bai Shao)
- Panax ginseng (Ginseng, Ren Shen)
- Panax notoginseng (Tienchi ginseng (san qi, tian qi – Mandarin) Yunnan bayou)
- Picrorhiza kurroa (Kutki)
- Pinus pinaster (Maritime bark)
- Piscidia piscipula (Jamaican dogwood)
- Plantago lanceolata (Ribwort, narrow-leaved plantain)
- Plectranthus barbatus (Coleus, makandi)
- Poria cocos (Hoelen, China root, sclerotium of tuckahoe, fu ling (Mandarin) and bukuryo (Japanese))
- Pseudowintera colorata (Horopito)
- Pueraria lobata (Kudzu)
- Punica granatum (Pomegranate)
- Quercus robur (Oak bark)
- Rhamnus frangula (Alder buckthorn)
- Rheum palmatum (Da Huang, Chinese rhubarb)
- Rumex crispus (Yellow dock, curled dock)
- Salix spp. (Willow bark, white willow)
- Salvia rosmarinus (Rosemary)

- Scutellaria baicalensis (Baikal skullcap, baical skullcap, Chinese skullcap, Huang qin (Mandarin), ogon (Japanese))
- Silybum marianum (St Mary's thistle, milk thistle, silymarin)
- Solidago virgaurea (Goldenrod)
- Stachys officinalis (Wood betony)
- Trametes versicolor (Turkey tail PSK, PSP)
- Tribulus terrestris (Tribulus, calthrops, puncture vine, Bai Ji Li)
- Usnea spp. (Old man's beard, songluo)
- Vaccinium myrtillus (Bilberry, blueberry)
- Viola tricolor (Heartsease, wild pansy, viola)
- Vitis vinifera (Grape vine, grapeseed extract)
- Withania somnifera (Ashwaghanda, winter cherry)

Anti-inflammatory (GIT)

Primary herbs

- Althaea officinalis (Marshmallow, white mallow)
- Matricaria chamomilla (Chamomile, German chamomile)
- Pseudowintera colorata (Horopito)
- Symphytum officinale (Comfrey)

Additional herbs

- Alpinia galanga (Greater galangal, Thai ginger)
- Berberis aquifolium (Oregon grape, mountain grape)
- Berberis vulgaris (Barberry)
- Boswellia serrata (Boswellia, olibanum, frankincense)
- Calendula officinalis (Calendula, marigold)
- Dioscorea spp. (Wild yam)
- Filipendula ulmaria (Meadowsweet)
- Glycyrrhiza spp. (Licorice, Liquorice, Gan Cao)
- Rheum palmatum (Da Huang, Chinese rhubarb)
- Stellaria media (Chickweed, starweed)

Anti-inflammatory (musculoskeletal)

Primary herbs

- Rosa canina (Rosehip, dog rose)
- Salix spp. (Willow bark, white willow)

Additional herbs

- Apium graveolens (Celery seed, karafs)
- Arnica montana (Arnica)
- Artemisia annua (Sweet Annie, Chinese wormwood, qing hao)
- Boswellia serrata (Boswellia, olibanum, frankincense)
- Curcuma longa (Turmeric)
- Harpagophytum procumbens (Devil's claw)
- Solidago virgaurea (Goldenrod)

Anti-inflammatory (topically)

Primary herbs

- Phytolacca americana (Poke root, pokeweed)
- Symphytum officinale (Comfrey)
- Zingiber officinale (Ginger, Sheng Jiang (fresh), Gan Jiang (dried))

Anti-inflammatory (urinary)

Primary herbs

- Crateva magna (Varuna)
- Elymus repens (Couch grass)
- Solidago virgaurea (Goldenrod)
- Zea mays (Corn silk, maize)

Additional herbs

- Agrimonia eupatoria (Agrimony)
- Althaea officinalis (Marshmallow, white mallow)
- Apium graveolens (Celery seed, karafs)
- Arctostaphylos uva-ursi (Bearberry)
- Betula pendula (Silver birch)
- Glycyrrhiza spp. (Licorice, Liquorice, Gan Cao)
- Plantago lanceolata (Ribwort, narrow-leaved plantain)
- Rheum palmatum (Da Huang, Chinese rhubarb)

Antiacteylcholinesterase

Primary herbs

- Crocus sativus (Saffron)

Antiaddictive

Primary herbs

- Pueraria lobata (Kudzu)

Antiageing

Primary herbs

- Codonopsis pilosula (Dang shen, codonopsis)
- Cordyceps militaris (Cordyceps, orange catapillar fungus, dong chong xia cao (China), hyakurakusou (Japan))
- Epimedium sagittatum (Horny goat weed, barrenwort, yin yang huo, Inyokaku)
- Ligustrum lucidum (Glossy privet, nu zhen zi, joteishi)
- Panax quinquefolium (American ginseng)

Antiallergic

Primary herbs

- Albizia lebbeck (Albizia, sirisha)
- Hemidesmus indicus (Anantamul, Indian sarsparilla)
- Perilla frutescens (Perilla, su zi, shisu)
- Picrorhiza kurroa (Kutki)
- Scutellaria baicalensis (Baikal skullcap, baical skullcap, Chinese skullcap, Huang qin (Mandarin), ogon (Japanese))
- Tanacetum parthenium (Feverfew)

Additional herbs

- Alpinia galanga (Greater galangal, Thai ginger)
- Crocus sativus (Saffron)
- Houttuynia cordata (Yu Xing Cao, chameleon plant, fish mint)
- Matricaria chamomilla (Chamomile, German chamomile)
- Paeonia lactiflora (Peony, white peony, Bai Shao)
- Plectranthus barbatus (Coleus, makandi)
- Pseudowintera colorata (Horopito)

Antiandrogenic

Primary herbs

- Serenoa repens (Saw palmetto, cabbage palm, dwarf palmetto)

Additional herbs

- Actaea racemosa (Black cohosh, squawroot, snakeroot)
- Camellia sinensis (Green tea (green, black or oolong according to processing))
- Ganoderma lucidum (Reishi, lingzhi)
- Glycyrrhiza spp. (Licorice, Liquorice, Gan Cao)
- Paeonia lactiflora (Peony, white peony, Bai Shao)
- Vitex agnus-castus (Chaste tree, chasteberry, Man Jing Zi)

Antiangina

Primary herbs

- Inula racemosa (Inula)
- Plectranthus barbatus (Coleus, makandi)

Additional herbs

- Curcuma longa (Turmeric)

Antiarrhythmic

Primary herbs

- Angelica polymorpha (Dong quai, dang gui, Chinese angelica)
- Convallaria majalis (Lily of the valley)
- Corydalis ambigua (Corydalis)
- Salvia miltiorrhiza (Dan shen (Mandarin), red root sage)
- Terminalia arjuna (Arjuna)

Additional herbs

- Coptis chinensis (Huanglian (China), makino (Japan))
- Crataegus monogyna (Hawthorn)
- Harpagophytum procumbens (Devil's claw)
- Leonurus cardiaca (Motherwort)
- Panax ginseng (Ginseng, Ren Shen)
- Panax notoginseng (Tienchi ginseng (san qi, tian qi – Mandarin) Yunnan bayou)
- Pueraria lobata (Kudzu)
- Withania somnifera (Ashwaghanda, winter cherry)

Antiasthmatic

Primary herbs

- Drosera spp. (Sundew)
- Ephedra sinensis (Ma-huang)
- Euphorbia hirta (Euphorbia)
- Grindelia camporum (Gum weed)
- Justicia adhatoda (Basak, vasaka, Malabar nut)
- Lobelia inflata (Indian tobacco)
- Plectranthus barbatus (Coleus, makandi)
- Viburnum prunifolium (Black haw, Sweet viburnum)

Additional herbs

- Albizia lebbeck (Albizia, sirisha)
- Boswellia serrata (Boswellia, olibanum, frankincense)
- Curcuma longa (Turmeric)
- Glycyrrhiza spp. (Licorice, Liquorice, Gan Cao)
- Inula helenium (Elecampane)
- Nigella sativa (Black cumin)
- Panax ginseng (Ginseng, Ren Shen)
- Picrorhiza kurroa (Kutki)
- Scutellaria baicalensis (Baikal skullcap, baical skullcap, Chinese skullcap, Huang qin (Mandarin), ogon (Japanese))
- Thymus vulgaris (Thyme)

Antiatherosclerotic

Primary herbs

- Allium sativum (Garlic)
- Ganoderma lucidum (Reishi, lingzhi)
- Hemidesmus indicus (Anantamul, Indian sarsparilla)
- Magnolia officinalis (Magnolia, Hou po)
- Salvia rosmarinus (Rosemary)
- Silybum marianum (St Mary's thistle, milk thistle, silymarin)
- Viscum album (Mistletoe)

Antibacterial

Primary herbs

- Coptis chinensis (Huanglian (China), makino (Japan))
- Cryptolepis sanguinolenta (Yellow dye root, delboi)
- Isodon rubescens (Dong ling cao, Chinese sage bush, rabdosia)
- Juglans nigra (Black walnut)
- Lycopus spp. (Bugleweed, gypsy wort)
- Pelargonium sidoides (African geranium, umckaloabo)
- Solidago virgaurea (Goldenrod)
- Thuja occidentalis (Thuja, white cedar, arbor-vitae (American))

Additional herbs

- Alpinia galanga (Greater galangal, Thai ginger)
- Annona muricata (Graviola, soursop, guanábana)
- Artemisia vulgaris (Mugwort)
- Asparagus racemosus (Shatavari (Sanskrit), satavari (Hindi), satmuli (Bengali))
- Ballota nigra (Black horehound)
- Berberis aristata (Daruharidra, Daruhaldi, Darvi, Chitra, Indian barberry)
- Berberis vulgaris (Barberry)
- Bidens tripartita (Burr marigold, water agrimony, gui zhen cao, longbacao)
- Camellia sinensis (Green tea (green, black or oolong according to processing))
- Citrus reticulata (Chen pi, mandarin, tangerine)
- Cordyceps militaris (Cordyceps, orange catapillar fungus, dong chong xia cao (China), hyakurakusou (Japan))
- Drosera spp. (Sundew)
- Epilobium parviflorum (Willow herb)
- Hedera helix (Ivy leaf, English ivy)
- Houttuynia cordata (Yu Xing Cao, chameleon plant, fish mint)
- Leptospermum scoparium (Manuka, tea tree)
- Lomatium dissectum (Fern-leaf biscuit root, tohza, desert parsley)
- Mentha x piperita (Peppermint, Bo He)
- Nigella sativa (Black cumin)
- Perilla frutescens (Perilla, su zi, shisu)
- Plantago lanceolata (Ribwort, narrow-leaved plantain)
- Pseudowintera colorata (Horopito)
- Salvia miltiorrhiza (Dan shen (Mandarin), red root sage)
- Syzygium aromaticum (Cloves)
- Terminalia arjuna (Arjuna)
- Trametes versicolor (Turkey tail PSK, PSP)
- Tribulus terrestris (Tribulus, calthrops, puncture vine, Bai Ji Li)

Anticancer

Primary herbs

- Albizia lebbeck (Albizia, sirisha)
- Annona muricata (Graviola, soursop, guanábana)
- Artemisia annua (Sweet Annie, Chinese wormwood, qing hao)
- Astragalus membranaceus (milk vetch, huang qi (Chinese), ogi (Japanese))
- Atractylodes macrocephala (Atractylodes, bai zhu)
- Berberis aristata (Daruharidra, Daruhaldi, Darvi, Chitra, Indian barberry)
- Boswellia serrata (Boswellia, olibanum, frankincense)
- Coptis chinensis (Huang lian, makino)

- Cordyceps militaris (Cordyceps, orange catapillar fungus, dong chong xia cao (China), hyakurakusou (Japan))
- Curcuma longa (Turmeric)
- Eleuterococcus senticosus (Eleuthero, eleutherokokk, Siberian ginseng)
- Ganoderma lucidum (Reishi, lingzhi)
- Handroanthus impetiginosus (Pau d'arco, lapacho (Spanish))
- Isodon rubescens (Dong ling cao, Chinese sage bush, rabdosia)
- Nigella sativa (Black cumin)
- Trametes versicolor (Turkey tail PSK, PSP)
- Uncaria tomentosa (Cat's claw)
- Viscum album (Mistletoe)
- Withania somnifera (Ashwaghanda, winter cherry)

Additional herbs

- Actaea racemosa (Black cohosh, squawroot, snakeroot)
- Alpinia galanga (Greater galangal, Thai ginger)
- Angelica polymorpha (Dong quai, dang gui, Chinese angelica)
- Asparagus racemosus (Shatavari (Sanskrit), satavari (Hindi), satmuli (Bengali))
- Carica papaya (Paw paw, papaya)
- Codonopsis pilosula (Dang shen, codonopsis)
- Crocus sativus (Saffron)
- Cryptolepis sanguinolenta (Yellow dye root, delboi)
- Epimedium sagittatum (Horny goat weed, barrenwort, yin yang huo, Inyokaku)
- Fucus vesiculosus (Bladderwrack)
- Gymnema sylvestre (Gumar, meshashringi)
- Hemidesmus indicus (Anantamul, Indian sarsparilla)
- Isatis tinctoria (Isatis, ban lan gen, woad, Chinese indigo)
- Ligustrum lucidum (Glossy privet, nu zhen zi, joteishi)
- Magnolia officinalis (Magnolia, Hou po)
- Panax ginseng (Ginseng, Ren Shen)
- Panax quinquefolium (American ginseng)
- Perilla frutescens (Perilla, su zi, shisu)
- Petroselinum crispum (Parsley root)
- Picrorhiza kurroa (Kutki)
- Pinus pinaster (Maritime bark)
- Plectranthus barbatus (Coleus, makandi)
- Pueraria lobata (Kudzu)
- Punica granatum (Pomegranate)
- Rhodiola rosea (Golden root, rose root, arctic root)
- Ruta graveolens (Rue)
- Salvia miltiorrhiza (Dan shen (Mandarin), red root sage)
- Salvia rosmarinus (Rosemary)

- Schisandra chinensis (Bei-Wuweizi, Schisandra, Chinese magnolia vine, Wu Wei Zi)
- Terminalia arjuna (Arjuna)
- Trifolium pratense (Red clover, trifoil)
- Usnea spp. (Old man's beard, songluo)

Anticatarrhal

Primary herbs

- Angelica archangelica (European angelica, angelica)
- Bistorta officinalis (Bistort, common bistort, European bistort or meadow bistort)
- Citrus reticulata (Chen pi, mandarin, tangerine)
- Euphrasia officinalis (Eyebright)
- Glechoma hederacea (Ground ivy)
- Grindelia camporum (Gum weed)
- Hedera helix (Ivy leaf, English ivy)
- Plantago lanceolata (Ribwort, narrow-leaved plantain)
- Sambucus nigra (Elder, elderflower, elderberry, sambuco)
- Tussilago farfara (Coltsfoot)
- Usnea spp. (Old man's beard, songluo)
- Verbascum thapsus (Mullein, candlewick plant, flannel-leaf, bunny's ears)

Additional herbs

- Isodon rubescens (Dong ling cao, Chinese sage bush, rabdosia)
- Solidago virgaurea (Goldenrod)
- Trametes versicolor (Turkey tail PSK, PSP)

Anticonvulsant

Primary herbs

- Crocus sativus (Saffron)
- Nigella sativa (Black cumin)
- Paeonia lactiflora (Peony, white peony, Bai Shao)
- Scutellaria lateriflora (Blue skulcap)
- Ziziphus jujuba var. spinosa (Zizyphus, sour Chinese date, jujube, Da Zao, Suan Zao Ren)

Antidepressant

Primary herbs

- Cola spp. (Kola nut, cola nut)
- Crocus sativus (Saffron)
- Hypericum perforatum (St John's wort)
- Lavandula angustifolia (Lavender)
- Magnolia officinalis (Magnolia, Hou po)
- Turnera diffusa (Damiana)

Additional herbs

- Annona muricata (Graviola, soursop, guanábana)
- Asparagus racemosus (Shatavari (Sanskrit), satavari (Hindi), satmuli (Bengali))
- Avena sativa (green) (Oats, green oats, oat straw)
- Avena sativa (seed) (Oats, groats, oatmeal)

- Cnicus benedictus (Blessed or holy thistle)
- Dulacia inopiflora (Muira puama)
- Epimedium sagittatum (Horny goat weed, barrenwort, yin yang huo, Inyokaku)
- Rhodiola rosea (Golden root, rose root, arctic root)
- Verbena officinalis (Vervain)

Antidiabetic

Primary herbs

- Annona muricata (Graviola, soursop, guanábana)
- Bidens tripartita (Burr marigold, water agrimony, gui zhen cao, longbacao)
- Centaurium erythraea (Centaury)
- Cinnamomum verum (Cinnamon, cassia bark, rou gui)
- Galega officinalis (Goat's rue)
- Gymnema sylvestre (Gumar, meshashringi)
- Nigella sativa (Black cumin)
- Ocimum tenuiflorum (Tulsi, Holy basil)
- Stevia rebaudiana (Stevia)

Additional herbs

- Agrimonia eupatoria (Agrimony)
- Alpinia galanga (Greater galangal, Thai ginger)
- Anethum graveolens (Dill)
- Codonopsis pilosula (Dang shen, codonopsis)
- Coptis chinensis (Huanglian (China), makino (Japan))
- Cryptolepis sanguinolenta (Yellow dye root, delboi)
- Fucus vesiculosus (Bladderwrack)
- Ganoderma lucidum (Reishi, lingzhi)
- Hemidesmus indicus (Anantamul, Indian sarsparilla)
- Houttuynia cordata (Yu Xing Cao, chameleon plant, fish mint)
- Ligustrum lucidum (Glossy privet, nu zhen zi, joteishi)
- Perilla frutescens (Perilla, su zi, shisu)
- Pueraria lobata (Kudzu)
- Punica granatum (Pomegranate)
- Salvia rosmarinus (Rosemary)
- Schisandra chinensis (Bei-Wuweizi, Schisandra, Chinese magnolia vine, Wu Wei Zi)
- Trametes versicolor (Turkey tail PSK, PSP)

Antidiarrhoeal

Primary herbs

- Agrimonia eupatoria (Agrimony)
- Bistorta officinalis (Bistort, common bistort, European bistort or meadow bistort)
- Geranium maculatum (Cranesbill)
- Glechoma hederacea (Ground ivy)
- Myrica cerifera (Bayberry, candleberry, wax myrtle)

Additional herbs

- Agathosma betulina (Buchu)
- Alchemilla vulgaris (Lady's mantle)
- Andrographis paniculata (Andrographis, kalmegh)
- Asparagus racemosus (Shatavari (Sanskrit), satavari (Hindi), satmuli (Bengali))
- Atractylodes macrocephala (Atractylodes, bai zhu)
- Berberis aquifolium (Oregon grape, mountain grape)
- Bidens tripartita (Burr marigold, water agrimony, gui zhen cao, longbacao)
- Cinnamomum verum (Cinnamon, cassia bark, rou gui)
- Codonopsis pilosula (Dang shen, codonopsis)
- Coptis chinensis (Huanglian (China), makino (Japan))
- Echinacea spp. (Echinacea)
- Epilobium parviflorum (Willow herb)
- Filipendula ulmaria (Meadowsweet)
- Hamamelis virginiana (Witch hazel)
- Harpagophytum procumbens (Devil's claw)
- Matricaria chamomilla (Chamomile, German chamomile)
- Poria cocos (Hoelen, China root, sclerotium of tuckahoe, fu ling (Mandarin) and bukuryo (Japanese))
- Punica granatum (Pomegranate)
- Rosa canina (Rosehip, dog rose)
- Rubus idaeus (Raspberry leaf)
- Thymus vulgaris (Thyme)
- Ulmus fulva (Slippery elm, red elm)

Antiemetic

Primary herbs

- Ballota nigra (Black horehound)
- Mentha x piperita (Peppermint, Bo He)
- Zingiber officinale (Ginger, Sheng Jiang (fresh), Gan Jiang (dried))

Additional herbs

- Alpinia galanga (Greater galangal, Thai ginger)
- Berberis aquifolium (Oregon grape, mountain grape)
- Berberis vulgaris (Barberry)
- Chelidonium majus (Greater celandine)
- Chionanthus virginicus (Fringe tree, old man's beard)
- Cinnamomum verum (Cinnamon, cassia bark, rou gui)
- Poria cocos (Hoelen, China root, sclerotium of tuckahoe, fu ling (Mandarin) and bukuryo (Japanese))
- Scutellaria baicalensis (Baikal skullcap, baical skullcap, Chinese skullcap, Huang qin (Mandarin), ogon (Japanese))

Antiepileptic

Primary herbs

- Bacopa monnieri (Bacopa, brahmi)
- Crocus sativus (Saffron)
- Paeonia lactiflora (Peony, white peony, Bai Shao)
- Piper methysticum (Kava)
- Valeriana officinalis (Valerian, heliotrope, Mexican valerian (V. edulis))

Antifibrotic

Primary herbs

- Centaurium erythraea (Centaury)
- Centella asiatica (Gotu kola, brahmi, Indian pennywort)
- Salvia miltiorrhiza (Dan shen (Mandarin), red root sage)
- Scutellaria baicalensis (Baikal skullcap, baical skullcap, Chinese skullcap, Huang qin (Mandarin), ogon (Japanese))

Antifungal

Primary herbs

- Grindelia camporum (Gum weed)
- Pseudowintera colorata (Horopito)
- Usnea spp. (Old man's beard, songluo)

Additional herbs

- Allium sativum (Garlic)
- Alpinia galanga (Greater galangal, Thai ginger)
- Annona muricata (Graviola, soursop, guanábana)
- Artemisia vulgaris (Mugwort)
- Ballota nigra (Black horehound)
- Berberis aquifolium (Oregon grape, mountain grape)
- Citrus reticulata (Chen pi, mandarin, tangerine)
- Cnicus benedictus (Blessed or holy thistle)
- Coptis chinensis (Huanglian (China), makino (Japan))
- Cordyceps militaris (Cordyceps, orange catapillar fungus, dong chong xia cao (China), hyakurakusou (Japan))
- Dipsacus asper (Teasel root)
- Epilobium parviflorum (Willow herb)
- Handroanthus impetiginosus (Pau d'arco, lapacho (Spanish))
- Hedera helix (Ivy leaf, English ivy)
- Houttuynia cordata (Yu Xing Cao, chameleon plant, fish mint)
- Juglans nigra (Black walnut)
- Leptospermum scoparium (Manuka, tea tree)
- Rhamnus frangula (Alder buckthorn)
- Solidago virgaurea (Goldenrod)
- Syzygium aromaticum (Cloves)
- Thymus vulgaris (Thyme)
- Tilia cordata (Lime tree, linden)
- Trametes versicolor (Turkey tail PSK, PSP)

Antifungal (topically)

Primary herbs

- Usnea spp. (Old man's beard, songluo)

Additional herbs

- Artemisia vulgaris (Mugwort)
- Calendula officinalis (Calendula, marigold)
- Pseudowintera colorata (Horopito)
- Salvia officinalis (Sage)
- Syzygium aromaticum (Cloves)

Antigalactagogue

Primary herbs

- Salvia officinalis (Sage)

Additional herbs

- Vaccinium myrtillus (Bilberry, blueberry)

Antihaemorrhagic (uterine)

Primary herbs

- Alchemilla vulgaris (Lady's mantle)
- Capsella bursa-pastoris (Shepherd's purse)
- Lamium album (White dead nettle)
- Panax notoginseng (Tienchi ginseng (san qi, tian qi – Mandarin) Yunnan bayou)
- Trillium erectum (Beth root, birth root)

Additional herbs

- Achillea millefolium (Yarrow)
- Mitchella repens (Partridgeberry)
- Rehmannia glutinosa (Rehmannia, sheng di huang (uncured), shu di huang (cured), Chinese foxglove)

Antihydrotic

Primary herbs

- Salvia officinalis (Sage)

Additional herbs

- Salix spp. (Willow bark, white willow)
- Ziziphus jujuba var. spinosa (Zizyphus, sour Chinese date, jujube, Da Zao, Suan Zao Ren)

Antihyperlipidemic

Primary herbs

- Allium sativum (Garlic)
- Berberis aristata (Daruharidra, Daruhaldi, Darvi, Chitra, Indian barberry)
- Berberis vulgaris (Barberry)
- Cinnamomum verum (Cinnamon, cassia bark, rou gui)
- Coptis chinensis (Huanglian (China), makino (Japan))
- Curcuma longa (Turmeric)
- Cynara scolymus (Globe artichoke)
- Glycine max (Soy, soy germ, soy isoflavones

(genistein), phyto-oestrogens, tofu (bean curd))
- Momordica charantia (Bitter melon, bitter gourd, African or wild cucumber)
- Olea europaea (Olive tree)
- Panax notoginseng (Tienchi ginseng (san qi, tian qi – Mandarin) Yunnan bayou)
- Reynoutria multiflora (He Shou Wu, Fo-Ti)
- Silybum marianum (St Mary's thistle, milk thistle, silymarin)
- Tribulus terrestris (Tribulus, calthrops, puncture vine, Bai Ji Li)
- Trigonella foenum-graecum (Fenugreek)

Additional herbs
- Agrimonia eupatoria (Agrimony)
- Albizia lebbeck (Albizia, sirisha)
- Anethum graveolens (Dill)
- Calendula officinalis (Calendula, marigold)
- Camellia sinensis (Green tea (green, black or oolong according to processing))
- Cordyceps militaris (Cordyceps, orange catapillar fungus, dong chong xia cao (China), hyakurakusou (Japan))
- Crataegus monogyna (Hawthorn)
- Crocus sativus (Saffron)
- Dipsacus asper (Teasel root)
- Ganoderma lucidum (Reishi, lingzhi)
- Gymnema sylvestre (Gumar, meshashringi)
- Ligustrum lucidum (Glossy privet, nu zhen zi, joteishi)
- Pueraria lobata (Kudzu)
- Punica granatum (Pomegranate)
- Salvia officinalis (Sage)
- Salvia rosmarinus (Rosemary)
- Schisandra chinensis (Bei-Wuweizi, Schisandra, Chinese magnolia vine, Wu Wei Zi)
- Scutellaria baicalensis (Baikal skullcap, baical skullcap, Chinese skullcap, Huang qin (Mandarin), ogon (Japanese))
- Terminalia arjuna (Arjuna)
- Withania somnifera (Ashwaghanda, winter cherry)

Antihyperprolactinaemic
Primary herbs
- Paeonia lactiflora (Peony, white peony, Bai Shao)
- Vitex agnus-castus (Chaste tree, chasteberry, Man Jing Zi)

Additional herbs
- Glycyrrhiza spp. (Licorice, Liquorice, Gan Cao)

Antihyperprostatic
Primary herbs
- Epilobium parviflorum (Willow herb)
- Serenoa repens (Saw palmetto, cabbage palm)
- Urtica dioica radix (Nettle root)

Antihypertensive
Primary herbs
- Allium sativum (Garlic)
- Stevia rebaudiana (Stevia)
- Vinca minor (Periwinkle, lesser or common periwinkle)
- Viscum album (Mistletoe)

Additional herbs
- Achillea millefolium (Yarrow)
- Alpinia galanga (Greater galangal, Thai ginger)
- Annona muricata (Graviola, soursop, guanábana)
- Astragalus membranaceus (milk vetch, huang qi (Chinese), ogi (Japanese))
- Avena sativa (seed) (Oats, groats, oatmeal)
- Carica papaya (Paw paw, papaya)
- Centaurium erythraea (Centaury)
- Coptis chinensis (Huanglian (China), makino (Japan))
- Crataegus monogyna (Hawthorn)
- Crocus sativus (Saffron)
- Cryptolepis sanguinolenta (Yellow dye root, delboi)
- Ganoderma lucidum (Reishi, lingzhi)
- Gynostemma pentaphyllum (Jiaogulan, xiancao)
- Piper methysticum (Kava)
- Plectranthus barbatus (Coleus, makandi)
- Pueraria lobata (Kudzu)
- Rhodiola rosea (Golden root, rose root, arctic root)
- Ruta graveolens (Rue)
- Salvia rosmarinus (Rosemary)
- Silybum marianum (St Mary's thistle, milk thistle, silymarin)
- Terminalia arjuna (Arjuna)

Antihyperuricaemic
Primary herbs
- Camellia sinensis (Green tea (green, black or oolong according to processing))
- Pueraria lobata (Kudzu)

Antilithic
Primary herbs
- Crateva magna (Varuna)
- Equisetum arvense (Horsetail)
- Eutrochium purpureum (Gravel root, Joe Pye weed)
- Hydrangea arborescens (Hydrangea)
- Petroselinum crispum (Parsley root)

Additional herbs
- Alchemilla vulgaris (Lady's mantle)
- Althaea officinalis (Marshmallow, white mallow)
- Arctostaphylos uva-ursi (Bearberry)
- Elymus repens (Couch grass)

Antimicrobial
Primary herbs
- Allium sativum (Garlic)
- Arctostaphylos uva-ursi (Bearberry)
- Ballota nigra (Black horehound)
- Berberis aristata (Daruharidra, Daruhaldi, Darvi, Chitra, Indian barberry)
- Bidens tripartita (Burr marigold, water agrimony, gui zhen cao, longbacao)
- Calendula officinalis (Calendula, marigold)
- Cryptolepis sanguinolenta (Yellow dye root, delboi)
- Handroanthus impetiginosus (Pau d'arco, lapacho (Spanish))
- Houttuynia cordata (Yu Xing Cao, chameleon plant, fish mint)
- Hydrastis canadensis (Goldenseal)
- Isatis tinctoria (Isatis, ban lan gen, woad, Chinese indigo)
- Lomatium dissectum (Fern-leaf biscuit root, tohza, desert parsley)
- Lycopus spp. (Bugleweed, gypsy wort)
- Ocimum tenuiflorum (Tulsi, Holy basil)
- Propolis (Propolis)
- Punica granatum (Pomegranate)
- Quercus robur (Oak bark)
- Salvia rosmarinus (Rosemary)
- Scutellaria baicalensis (Baikal skullcap, baical skullcap, Chinese skullcap, Huang qin (Mandarin), ogon (Japanese))
- Thymus vulgaris (Thyme)
- Usnea spp. (Old man's beard, songluo)

Additional herbs
- Albizia lebbeck (Albizia, sirisha)
- Aloe ferox (Aloe vera (gel), bitter aloes (resin))
- Alpinia galanga (Greater galangal, Thai ginger)
- Althaea officinalis (Marshmallow, white mallow)
- Annona muricata (Graviola, soursop, guanábana)
- Arnica montana (Arnica)
- Baptisia tinctoria (Wild indigo)
- Berberis aquifolium (Oregon grape, mountain grape)
- Berberis vulgaris (Barberry)
- Camellia sinensis (Green tea (green, black or oolong according to processing))
- Cinnamomum verum (Cinnamon, cassia bark, rou gui)
- Citrus reticulata (Chen pi, mandarin, tangerine)
- Cnicus benedictus (Blessed or holy thistle)
- Cordyceps militaris (Cordyceps, orange catapillar fungus, dong chong xia cao (China), hyakurakusou (Japan))
- Crocus sativus (Saffron)
- Echinacea spp. (Echinacea)
- Euphorbia hirta (Euphorbia)
- Foeniculum vulgare (Fennel)
- Ganoderma lucidum (Reishi, lingzhi)
- Gymnema sylvestre (Gumar, meshashringi)
- Hemidesmus indicus (Anantamul, Indian sarsparilla)
- Inula helenium (Elecampane)
- Leptospermum scoparium (Manuka, tea tree)
- Macropiper excelsum (Kawakawa, New Zealand peppertree)
- Matricaria chamomilla (Chamomile, German chamomile)
- Melissa officinalis (Lemon balm, Melissa)
- Momordica charantia (Bitter melon, bitter gourd, African or wild cucumber)
- Nigella sativa (Black cumin)
- Piper methysticum (Kava)
- Rumex crispus (Yellow dock, curled dock)
- Ruta graveolens (Rue)
- Salvia miltiorrhiza (Dan shen (Mandarin), red root sage)
- Sambucus nigra (Elder, elderflower, elderberry, sambuco)
- Trametes versicolor (Turkey tail PSK, PSP)
- Zanthoxylum clava-herculis (Prickly ash)

Antinociceptive
Primary herbs
- Centella asiatica (Gotu kola, brahmi, Indian pennywort)
- Dipsacus asper (Teasel root)

Additional herbs
- Agrimonia eupatoria (Agrimony)
- Alpinia galanga (Greater galangal, Thai ginger)
- Epimedium sagittatum (Horny goat weed, barrenwort, yin yang huo, Inyokaku)
- Pueraria lobata (Kudzu)
- Syzygium aromaticum (Cloves)
- Trametes versicolor (Turkey tail PSK, PSP)
- Trigonella foenum-graecum (Fenugreek)

Antiobesity
Primary herbs
- Fucus vesiculosus (Bladderwrack)

Additional herbs
- Coptis chinensis (Huanglian (China), makino (Japan))
- Magnolia officinalis (Magnolia, Hou po)
- Momordica charantia (Bitter melon, bitter gourd, African or wild cucumber)
- Panax notoginseng (Tienchi ginseng (san qi, tian qi – Mandarin) Yunnan bayou)

- Plectranthus barbatus (Coleus, makandi)
- Silybum marianum (St Mary's thistle, milk thistle, silymarin)

Antioedematous

Primary herbs

- Aesculus hippocastanum (Horse chestnut)
- Pinus pinaster (Maritime bark)
- Ruscus aculeatus (Butcher's broom, box holly)
- Taraxacum officinale folia (Dandelion leaf, Pu Gong Ying)
- Vaccinium myrtillus (Bilberry, blueberry)
- Vitis vinifera (Grape vine, grapeseed extract)

Additional herbs

- Apium graveolens (Celery seed, karafs)
- Atractylodes macrocephala (Atractylodes, bai zhu)
- Betula pendula (Silver birch)

Antiosteoporotic

Primary herbs

- Epimedium sagittatum (Horny goat weed, barrenwort, yin yang huo, Inyokaku)

Additional herbs

- Atractylodes macrocephala (Atractylodes, bai zhu)
- Ligustrum lucidum (Glossy privet, nu zhen zi, joteishi)
- Pueraria lobata (Kudzu)

Antioxidant

Primary herbs

- Pinus pinaster (Maritime bark)

Additional herbs

- Allium sativum (Garlic)
- Andrographis paniculata (Andrographis, kalmegh)
- Astragalus membranaceus (milk vetch, huang qi (Chinese), ogi (Japanese))
- Bacopa monnieri (Bacopa, brahmi)
- Berberis aristata (Daruharidra, Daruhaldi, Darvi, Chitra, Indian barberry)
- Camellia sinensis (Green tea)
- Crataegus monogyna (Hawthorn)
- Crocus sativus (Saffron)
- Curcuma longa (Turmeric)
- Dulacia inopiflora (Muira puama)
- Epimedium sagittatum (Horny goat weed, barrenwort, yin yang huo, Inyokaku)
- Ginkgo biloba (Maidenhair)
- Glycine max (Soy, soy germ, soy isoflavones (genistein), phyto-oestrogens, tofu (bean curd))
- Olea europaea (Olive tree)
- Perilla frutescens (Perilla, su zi, shisu)
- Poria cocos (Hoelen, China root, sclerotium of tuckahoe, fu ling (Mandarin) and bukuryo (Japanese))

- Punica granatum (Pomegranate)
- Quercus robur (Oak bark)
- Reynoutria multiflora (He Shou Wu, Fo-Ti)
- Rhodiola rosea (Golden root, rose root, arctic root)
- Salvia rosmarinus (Rosemary)
- Schisandra chinensis (Bei-Wuweizi, Schisandra, Chinese magnolia vine, Wu Wei Zi)
- Scutellaria baicalensis (Baikal skullcap, baical skullcap, Chinese skullcap, Huang qin (Mandarin), ogon (Japanese))
- Silybum marianum (St Mary's thistle, milk thistle, silymarin)
- Syzygium aromaticum (Cloves)
- Terminalia arjuna (Arjuna)
- Uncaria tomentosa (Cat's claw)
- Vaccinium myrtillus (Bilberry, blueberry)
- Vitis vinifera (Grape vine, grapeseed extract)

Antiparasitic

Primary herbs

- Artemisia annua (Sweet Annie, Chinese wormwood, qing hao)
- Punica granatum (Pomegranate)
- Rhamnus purshiana (Cascara sagrada (sacred bark), Californian buckthorn)

Additional herbs

- Allium sativum (Garlic)
- Andrographis paniculata (Andrographis, kalmegh)
- Annona muricata (Graviola, soursop, guanábana)
- Artemisia absinthium (Wormwood, absinthe)
- Berberis vulgaris (Barberry)
- Commiphora myrrha (Myrrh)
- Coptis chinensis (Huanglian (China), makino (Japan))
- Cordyceps militaris (Cordyceps, orange catapillar fungus, dong chong xia cao (China), hyakurakusou (Japan))
- Cryptolepis sanguinolenta (Yellow dye root, delboi)
- Euphorbia hirta (Euphorbia)
- Hydrastis canadensis (Goldenseal)
- Pimpinella anisum (Aniseed)
- Syzygium aromaticum (Cloves)
- Thymus vulgaris (Thyme)
- Usnea spp. (Old man's beard, songluo)

Antiplatelet

Primary herbs

- Allium sativum (Garlic)
- Andrographis paniculata (Andrographis, kalmegh)
- Angelica polymorpha (Dong quai, dang gui, Chinese angelica)
- Crataegus monogyna (Hawthorn)
- Curcuma longa (Turmeric)

- Ginkgo biloba (Maidenhair)
- Leonurus cardiaca (Motherwort)
- Plectranthus barbatus (Coleus, makandi)
- Salix spp. (Willow bark, white willow)
- Salvia miltiorrhiza (Dan shen (Mandarin), red root sage)
- Scutellaria baicalensis (Baikal skullcap, baical skullcap, Chinese skullcap, Huang qin (Mandarin), ogon (Japanese))
- Vaccinium myrtillus (Bilberry, blueberry)
- Vitis vinifera (Grape vine, grapeseed extract)
- Zingiber officinale (Ginger, Sheng Jiang (fresh), Gan Jiang (dried))
- Antiproliferative

Additional herbs
- Leonurus cardiaca (Motherwort)

Antiprotozoal
Primary herbs
- Asparagus racemosus (Shatavari (Sanskrit), satavari (Hindi), satmuli (Bengali))

Antipruritic
Primary herbs
- Stellaria media (Chickweed, starweed)

Additional herbs
- Avena sativa (green) (Oats, green oats, oat straw)
- Avena sativa (seed) (Oats, groats, oatmeal)
- Smilax ornata (Sarsaparilla)

Antipsoriatic
Primary herbs
- Berberis aquifolium (Oregon grape, mountain grape)

Additional herbs
- Plectranthus barbatus (Coleus, makandi)

Antipyretic
Primary herbs
- Agathosma betulina (Buchu)
- Bryonia dioica (Bryony)
- Capsella bursa-pastoris (Shepherd's purse)
- Centaurium erythraea (Centaury)
- Eupatorium perfoliatum (Boneset, feverwort)
- Hyssopus officinalis (Hyssop)
- Mentha pulegium (Pennyroyal)
- Nepeta cataria (Catnip, catmint, Jing Jie)
- Sambucus nigra (Elder, elderflower, elderberry, sambuco)
- Zanthoxylum clava-herculis (Prickly ash)

Additional herbs
- Achillea millefolium (Yarrow)
- Alchemilla vulgaris (Lady's mantle)
- Andrographis paniculata (Andrographis, kalmegh)

- Artemisia absinthium (Wormwood, absinthe)
- Asclepias tuberosa (Pleurisy root, butterfly weed)
- Baptisia tinctoria (Wild indigo)
- Berberis aristata (Daruharidra, Daruhaldi, Darvi, Chitra, Indian barberry)
- Berberis vulgaris (Barberry)
- Bupleurum falcatum (Bupleurum, sickle-leaved hare's ear)
- Capsicum spp. (Chilli, capsicum, pepper, paprika, cayenne)
- Cryptolepis sanguinolenta (Yellow dye root, delboi)
- Inula helenium (Elecampane)
- Melissa officinalis (Lemon balm, Melissa)
- Rehmannia glutinosa (Rehmannia, sheng di huang (uncured), shu di huang (cured), Chinese foxglove)
- Salix spp. (Willow bark, white willow)
- Scutellaria baicalensis (Baikal skullcap, baical skullcap, Chinese skullcap, Huang qin (Mandarin), ogon (Japanese))
- Tilia cordata (Lime tree, linden)
- Usnea spp. (Old man's beard, songluo)
- Zingiber officinale (Ginger, Sheng Jiang (fresh), Gan Jiang (dried))

Antirheumatic
Primary herbs
- Apium graveolens (Celery seed, karafs)
- Betula pendula (Silver birch)
- Eutrochium purpureum (Gravel root, Joe Pye weed)
- Filipendula ulmaria (Meadowsweet)
- Fucus vesiculosus (Bladderwrack)
- Guaiacum officinale (Guaiacum)
- Juniperus communis (Juniper)
- Phytolacca americana (Poke root, pokeweed)
- Salix spp. (Willow bark, white willow)
- Smilax ornata (Sarsaparilla)
- Symphytum officinale (Comfrey)
- Taraxacum officinale folia (Dandelion leaf)
- Urtica dioica folia (Nettle leaf, stinging nettle)
- Viola tricolor (Heartsease, wild pansy, viola)
- Zanthoxylum clava-herculis (Prickly ash)

Additional herbs
- Actaea racemosa (Black cohosh, snakeroot)
- Bryonia dioica (Bryony)
- Cassia senna (Senna pod)
- Dioscorea spp. (Wild yam)
- Eupatorium perfoliatum (Boneset, feverwort)
- Lavandula angustifolia (Lavender)
- Petroselinum crispum (Parsley root)
- Stellaria media (Chickweed, starweed)
- Taraxacum officinale radix (Dandelion root)

Antiseptic

Primary herbs

- Baptisia tinctoria (Wild indigo)
- Cnicus benedictus (Blessed or holy thistle)
- Commiphora myrrha (Myrrh)
- Juniperus communis (Juniper)
- Syzygium aromaticum (Cloves)

Additional herbs

- Agathosma betulina (Buchu)
- Arctostaphylos uva-ursi (Bearberry)
- Arnica montana (Arnica)
- Bidens tripartita (Burr marigold, water agrimony, gui zhen cao, longbacao)
- Calendula officinalis (Calendula, marigold)
- Capsicum spp. (Chilli, capsicum, pepper, paprika, cayenne)
- Matricaria chamomilla (Chamomile, German chamomile)
- Plantago lanceolata (Ribwort, narrow-leaved plantain)
- Plantago major (Plantain, broad-leaved plantain, Che Qian Zi)
- Zanthoxylum clava-herculis (Prickly ash)

Antiseptic (GIT)

Primary herbs

- Allium sativum (Garlic)
- Berberis vulgaris (Barberry)
- Calendula officinalis (Calendula, marigold)
- Coptis chinensis (Huang lian)
- Hydrastis canadensis (Golden seal)

Additional herbs

- Achillea millefolium (Yarrow)
- Albizia lebbeck (Albizia, sirisha)
- Allium sativum (Garlic)
- Berberis vulgaris (Barberry)
- Echinacea spp. (Echinacea)
- Hamamelis virginiana (Witch hazel)
- Juniperus communis (Juniper)
- Picrorhiza kurroa (Kutki)
- Propolis (Propolis)
- Rheum palmatum (Da Huang, Chinese rhubarb)
- Scutellaria baicalensis (Baikal skullcap, baical skullcap, Chinese skullcap, Huang qin (Mandarin), ogon (Japanese))
- Trametes versicolor (Turkey tail PSK, PSP)

Antiseptic (respiratory tract)

Primary herbs

- Armoracia rusticana (Horseradish)
- Asclepias tuberosa (Pleurisy root, butterfly weed)
- Inula helenium (Elecampane)

- Salvia officinalis (Sage)
- Thymus vulgaris (Thyme)

Additional herbs

- Echinacea spp. (Echinacea)
- Picrorhiza kurroa (Kutki)

Antiseptic (topically)

Primary herbs

- Propolis (Propolis)

Additional herbs

- Calendula officinalis (Calendula, marigold)
- Echinacea spp. (Echinacea)
- Hydrastis canadensis (Goldenseal)
- Hypericum perforatum (St John's wort)

Antiseptic (urinary)

Primary herbs

- Arctostaphylos uva-ursi (Bearberry)
- Bidens tripartita (Burr marigold, water agrimony, gui zhen cao, longbacao)

Additional herbs

- Apium graveolens (Celery seed, karafs)
- Crateva magna (Varuna)
- Echinacea spp. (Echinacea)
- Filipendula ulmaria (Meadowsweet)
- Glycyrrhiza spp. (Licorice, Liquorice, Gan Cao)
- Serenoa repens (Saw palmetto, cabbage palm, dwarf palmetto)
- Solidago virgaurea (Goldenrod)

Antispasmodic (muscles)

Primary herbs

- Lavandula angustifolia (Lavender)
- Viburnum opulus (Cramp bark)
- Viburnum prunifolium (Black haw, Sweet viburnum)

Additional herbs

- Annona muricata (Graviola, soursop, guanábana)
- Apium graveolens (Celery seed, karafs)
- Corydalis ambigua (Corydalis)
- Dioscorea spp. (Wild yam)
- Glycyrrhiza spp. (Licorice, Liquorice, Gan Cao)
- Hemidesmus indicus (Anantamul, Indian sarsparilla)
- Leptospermum scoparium (Manuka, tea tree)
- Macropiper excelsum (Kawakawa, New Zealand peppertree)
- Melissa officinalis (Lemon balm, Melissa)
- Mentha x piperita (Peppermint, Bo He)
- Paeonia lactiflora (Peony, white peony, Bai Shao)
- Piper methysticum (Kava)
- Plectranthus barbatus (Coleus, makandi)
- Scutellaria lateriflora (Blue skulcap)

- Valeriana officinalis (Valerian, heliotrope, Mexican valerian (V. edulis))

Antispasmodic (respiratory tract)

Primary herbs

- Drosera spp. (Sundew)
- Ephedra sinensis (Ma-huang)
- Hedera helix (Ivy leaf, English ivy)
- Inula helenium (Elecampane)
- Inula racemosa (Inula)
- Justicia adhatoda (Basak, vasaka, Malabar nut)
- Lobelia inflata (Indian tobacco)
- Ocimum tenuiflorum (Tulsi, Holy basil)
- Prunus serotina (Wild cherry, black cherry)
- Tussilago farfara (Coltsfoot)

Additional herbs

- Alpinia galanga (Greater galangal, Thai ginger)
- Angelica archangelica (European angelica, angelica)
- Asclepias tuberosa (Pleurisy root, butterfly weed)
- Euphorbia hirta (Euphorbia)
- Glycyrrhiza spp. (Licorice, Liquorice, Gan Cao)
- Grindelia camporum (Gum weed)
- Marrubium vulgare (White horehound)
- Plantago lanceolata (Ribwort, narrow-leaved plantain)
- Plectranthus barbatus (Coleus, makandi)
- Thymus vulgaris (Thyme)

Antispasmodic (uterus)

Primary herbs

- Leonurus cardiaca (Motherwort)
- Ruta graveolens (Rue)
- Viburnum opulus (Cramp bark)
- Viburnum prunifolium (Black haw, Sweet viburnum)

Additional herbs

- Angelica polymorpha (Dong quai, dang gui, Chinese angelica)
- Cassia senna (Senna pod)
- Dioscorea spp. (Wild yam)
- Glycyrrhiza spp. (Licorice, Liquorice, Gan Cao)
- Inula racemosa (Inula)
- Mitchella repens (Partridgeberry)
- Paeonia lactiflora (Peony, white peony, Bai Shao)

Antispasmodic/Spasmolytic

Primary herbs

- Agathosma betulina (Buchu)
- Aletris farinosa (True unicorn root, white colic root)
- Anemone pulsatilla (Pulsatilla)
- Asparagus racemosus (Shatavari (Sanskrit), satavari (Hindi), satmuli (Bengali))

- Dioscorea spp. (Wild yam)
- Lobelia inflata (Indian tobacco)
- Matricaria chamomilla (Chamomile, German chamomile)
- Valeriana officinalis (Valerian, heliotrope, Mexican valerian (V. edulis))
- Viburnum opulus (Cramp bark)

Additional herbs

- Actaea racemosa (Black cohosh, squawroot, snakeroot)
- Ballota nigra (Black horehound)
- Eschscholzia californica (Californian poppy)
- Magnolia officinalis (Magnolia, Hou po)
- Petroselinum crispum (Parsley root)
- Piper methysticum (Kava)
- Piscidia piscipula (Jamaican dogwood)
- Rubus idaeus (Raspberry leaf)
- Ruta graveolens (Rue)
- Solidago virgaurea (Goldenrod)
- Tilia cordata (Lime tree, linden)

Antithyroid

Primary herbs

- Lycopus spp. (Bugleweed, gypsy wort)

Antitussive

Primary herbs

- Althaea officinalis (Marshmallow, white mallow)
- Ephedra sinensis (Ma-huang)
- Prunus serotina (Wild cherry, black cherry)
- Ruta graveolens (Rue)
- Tussilago farfara (Coltsfoot)
- Verbena officinalis (Vervain)

Additional herbs

- Actaea racemosa (Black cohosh, squawroot, snakeroot)
- Asparagus racemosus (Shatavari (Sanskrit), satavari (Hindi), satmuli (Bengali))
- Bupleurum falcatum (Bupleurum, sickle-leaved hare's ear)
- Crocus sativus (Saffron)
- Dioscorea spp. (Wild yam)
- Glycyrrhiza spp. (Licorice, Liquorice, Gan Cao)
- Humulus lupulus (Hops)
- Inula helenium (Elecampane)
- Piscidia piscipula (Jamaican dogwood)
- Schisandra chinensis (Bei-Wuweizi, Schisandra, Chinese magnolia vine, Wu Wei Zi)
- Stellaria media (Chickweed, starweed)
- Thymus vulgaris (Thyme)

Antiviral (systemically)

Primary herbs

- Andrographis paniculata (Andrographis, kalmegh)
- Baptisia tinctoria (Wild indigo)
- Hypericum perforatum (St John's wort)
- Hyssopus officinalis (Hyssop)
- Isatis tinctoria (Isatis, ban lan gen, woad, Chinese indigo)
- Lomatium dissectum (Fern-leaf biscuit root, tohza, desert parsley)
- Pelargonium sidoides (African geranium, umckaloabo (severe cough in Zulu))
- Phyllanthus spp. (Phyllanthus)
- Sambucus nigra (Elder, elderflower, elderberry, sambuco)
- Thuja occidentalis (Thuja, white cedar, arbor-vitae (American))

Additional herbs

- Allium sativum (Garlic)
- Annona muricata (Graviola, soursop, guanábana)
- Artemisia annua (Sweet Annie, Chinese wormwood, qing hao)
- Astragalus membranaceus (Astragalus, milk vetch, huang qi (Chinese), ogi (Japanese))
- Camellia sinensis (Green tea (green, black or oolong according to processing))
- Coptis chinensis (Huanglian (China), makino (Japan))
- Cordyceps militaris (Cordyceps, orange catapillar fungus, dong chong xia cao (China), hyakurakusou (Japan))
- Epimedium sagittatum (Horny goat weed, barrenwort, yin yang huo, Inyokaku)
- Ganoderma lucidum (Reishi, lingzhi)
- Handroanthus impetiginosus (Pau d'arco, lapacho (Spanish))
- Hedera helix (Ivy leaf, English ivy)
- Houttuynia cordata (Yu Xing Cao, chameleon plant, fish mint)
- Hydrastis canadensis (Goldenseal)
- Juglans nigra (Black walnut)
- Momordica charantia (Bitter melon, bitter gourd, African or wild cucumber)
- Pinus pinaster (Maritime bark)
- Poria cocos (Hoelen, China root, sclerotium of tuckahoe, fu ling (Mandarin) and bukuryo (Japanese))
- Propolis (Propolis)
- Punica granatum (Pomegranate)
- Rhamnus frangula (Alder buckthorn)
- Syzygium aromaticum (Cloves)
- Terminalia arjuna (Arjuna)
- Thymus vulgaris (Thyme)
- Trametes versicolor (Turkey tail PSK, PSP)
- Uncaria tomentosa (Cat's claw)

Antiviral (topically)

Primary herbs

- Melissa officinalis (Lemon balm, Melissa)

Additional herbs

- Coptis chinensis (Huanglian (China), makino (Japan))
- Glycyrrhiza spp. (Licorice, Liquorice, Gan Cao)
- Humulus lupulus (Hops)
- Hypericum perforatum (St John's wort)
- Salvia officinalis (Sage)
- Syzygium aromaticum (Cloves)
- Usnea spp. (Old man's beard, songluo)

Anxiolytic

Primary herbs

- Bacopa monnieri (Bacopa, brahmi)
- Eschscholzia californica (Californian poppy)
- Magnolia officinalis (Magnolia, Hou po)
- Passiflora incarnata (Passion flower)
- Piper methysticum (Kava)
- Scutellaria lateriflora (Blue skulcap)
- Stachys officinalis (Wood betony)
- Valeriana officinalis (Valerian, heliotrope, Mexican valerian (V. edulis))
- Verbena officinalis (Vervain)
- Withania somnifera (Ashwaghanda, winter cherry)
- Ziziphus jujuba var. spinosa (Zizyphus, sour Chinese date, jujube, Da Zao, Suan Zao Ren)

Additional herbs

- Angelica archangelica (European angelica, angelica)
- Asparagus racemosus (Shatavari (Sanskrit), satavari (Hindi), satmuli (Bengali))
- Ballota nigra (Black horehound)
- Baptisia tinctoria (Wild indigo)
- Crocus sativus (Saffron)
- Leptospermum scoparium (Manuka, tea tree)
- Matricaria chamomilla (Chamomile, German chamomile)
- Panax quinquefolium (American ginseng)
- Scutellaria baicalensis (Baikal skullcap, baical skullcap, Chinese skullcap, Huang qin (Mandarin), ogon (Japanese))
- Tilia cordata (Lime tree, linden)

Aphrodisiac

Primary herbs

- Tribulus terrestris (Tribulus, calthrops, puncture vine, Bai Ji Li)

Additional herbs

- Epimedium sagittatum (Horny goat weed, barrenwort, yin yang huo, Inyokaku)
- Panax quinquefolium (American ginseng)

Aromatic
Primary herbs

- Anethum graveolens (Dill)
- Foeniculum vulgare (Fennel)

Additional herbs

- Achillea millefolium (Yarrow)
- Angelica archangelica (European angelica, angelica)
- Mentha x piperita (Peppermint, Bo He)

Astringent
Primary herbs

- Bistorta officinalis (Bistort, common bistort, European bistort or meadow bistort)
- Collinsonia canadensis (Stone root)
- Commiphora myrrha (Myrrh)
- Euphrasia officinalis (Eyebright)
- Galium aparine (Clivers, cleavers)
- Geranium maculatum (Cranesbill)
- Glechoma hederacea (Ground ivy)
- Hamamelis virginiana (Witch hazel)
- Juglans nigra (Black walnut)
- Lamium album (White dead nettle)
- Myrica cerifera (Bayberry, candleberry, wax myrtle)
- Punica granatum (Pomegranate)
- Quercus robur (Oak bark)
- Rheum palmatum (Da Huang, Chinese rhubarb)
- Rosa canina (Rosehip, dog rose)
- Rumex crispus (Yellow dock, curled dock)

Additional herbs

- Agathosma betulina (Buchu)
- Albizia lebbeck (Albizia, sirisha)
- Alchemilla vulgaris (Lady's mantle)
- Annona muricata (Graviola, soursop, guanábana)
- Arctostaphylos uva-ursi (Bearberry)
- Bidens tripartita (Burr marigold, water agrimony, gui zhen cao, longbacao)
- Calendula officinalis (Calendula, marigold)
- Camellia sinensis (Green tea (green, black or oolong according to processing))
- Equisetum arvense (Horsetail)
- Filipendula ulmaria (Meadowsweet)
- Gymnema sylvestre (Gumar, meshashringi)
- Hypericum perforatum (St John's wort)
- Leptospermum scoparium (Manuka, tea tree)
- Mitchella repens (Partridgeberry)
- Nepeta cataria (Catnip, catmint, Jing Jie)

- Paeonia lactiflora (Peony, white peony, Bai Shao)
- Plantago lanceolata (Ribwort, narrow-leaved plantain)
- Plantago major (Plantain, broad-leaved plantain, Che Qian Zi)
- Prunus serotina (Wild cherry, black cherry)
- Pseudowintera colorata (Horopito)
- Rhamnus purshiana (Cascara sagrada (sacred bark), Californian buckthorn)
- Rubus idaeus (Raspberry leaf)
- Salix spp. (Willow bark, white willow)
- Syzygium aromaticum (Cloves)
- Thuja occidentalis (Thuja, white cedar, arbor-vitae (American))
- Thymus vulgaris (Thyme)
- Trillium erectum (Beth root, birth root)
- Urtica dioica folia (Nettle leaf, stinging nettle)
- Vaccinium myrtillus (Bilberry, blueberry)
- Verbena officinalis (Vervain)
- Viburnum opulus (Cramp bark)
- Viburnum prunifolium (Black haw, Sweet viburnum)
- Vinca minor (Periwinkle, lesser or common periwinkle)
- Vitis vinifera (Grape vine, grapeseed extract)

Bitter tonic
Primary herbs

- Agrimonia eupatoria (Agrimony)
- Aletris farinosa (True unicorn root, white colic root)
- Andrographis paniculata (Andrographis, kalmegh)
- Artemisia absinthium (Wormwood, absinthe)
- Artemisia annua (Sweet Annie, Chinese wormwood, qing hao)
- Artemisia vulgaris (Mugwort)
- Berberis vulgaris (Barberry)
- Chelidonium majus (Greater celandine)
- Chionanthus virginicus (Fringe tree, old man's beard)
- Cnicus benedictus (Blessed or holy thistle)
- Gentiana lutea (Gentian)
- Harpagophytum procumbens (Devil's claw)
- Humulus lupulus (Hops)
- Marrubium vulgare (White horehound)
- Reynoutria multiflora (He Shou Wu, Fo-Ti)
- Stachys officinalis (Wood betony)
- Taraxacum officinale radix (Dandelion root)

Additional herbs

- Achillea millefolium (Yarrow)
- Agathosma betulina (Buchu)
- Angelica archangelica (European angelica, angelica)

- Atractylodes macrocephala (Atractylodes, bai zhu)
- Berberis aquifolium (Oregon grape, mountain grape)
- Bidens tripartita (Burr marigold, water agrimony, gui zhen cao, longbacao)
- Bupleurum falcatum (Bupleurum, sickle-leaved hare's ear)
- Caulophyllum thalictroides (Blue cohosh)
- Coptis chinensis (Huanglian (China), makino (Japan))
- Corydalis ambigua (Corydalis)
- Cynara scolymus (Globe artichoke)
- Hydrastis canadensis (Goldenseal)
- Matricaria chamomilla (Chamomile, German chamomile)
- Momordica charantia (Bitter melon, bitter gourd, African or wild cucumber)
- Picrorhiza kurroa (Kutki)
- Taraxacum officinale folia (Dandelion leaf, Pu Gong Ying)
- Thymus vulgaris (Thyme)
- Verbena officinalis (Vervain)
- Zingiber officinale (Ginger, Sheng Jiang (fresh), Gan Jiang (dried))

Bladder tonic
Primary herbs
- Crateva magna (Varuna)
Additional herbs
- Withania somnifera (Ashwaghanda, winter cherry)

Blood sugar regulator
Primary herbs
- Avena sativa (seed) (Oats, groats, oatmeal)
- Codonopsis pilosula (Dang shen, codonopsis)
- Dipsacus asper (Teasel root)
- Glycyrrhiza spp. (Licorice, Liquorice, Gan Cao)
- Gymnema sylvestre (Gumar, meshashringi)
- Phyllanthus spp. (Phyllanthus)

Blood tonic
Primary herbs
- Angelica polymorpha (Dong quai, dang gui, Chinese angelica)
- Bidens tripartita (Burr marigold, water agrimony, gui zhen cao, longbacao)
- Codonopsis pilosula (Dang shen, codonopsis)

Bronchodilator
Primary herbs
- Drosera spp. (Sundew)
- Ephedra sinensis (Ma-huang)
- Euphorbia hirta (Euphorbia)
- Hedera helix (Ivy leaf, English ivy)

Additional herbs
- Inula racemosa (Inula)
- Justicia adhatoda (Basak, vasaka, Malabar nut)
- Nigella sativa (Black cumin)
- Plectranthus barbatus (Coleus, makandi)

Cardioprotective
Primary herbs
- Corydalis ambigua (Corydalis)
- Crataegus monogyna (Hawthorn)
- Inula racemosa (Inula)
- Olea europaea (Olive tree)
- Panax notoginseng (Tienchi ginseng (san qi, tian qi – Mandarin) Yunnan bayou)
- Pueraria lobata (Kudzu)
- Salvia miltiorrhiza (Dan shen (Mandarin), red root sage)
- Terminalia arjuna (Arjuna)

Additional herbs
- Andrographis paniculata (Andrographis, kalmegh)
- Coptis chinensis (Huanglian (China), makino (Japan))
- Epimedium sagittatum (Horny goat weed, barrenwort, yin yang huo, Inyokaku)
- Hemidesmus indicus (Anantamul, Indian sarsparilla)
- Magnolia officinalis (Magnolia, Hou po)
- Nigella sativa (Black cumin)
- Panax ginseng (Ginseng, Ren Shen)
- Panax quinquefolium (American ginseng)
- Rhodiola rosea (Golden root, rose root, arctic root)
- Salvia rosmarinus (Rosemary)
- Schisandra chinensis (Bei-Wuweizi, Schisandra, Chinese magnolia vine, Wu Wei Zi)
- Scutellaria baicalensis (Baikal skullcap, baical skullcap, Chinese skullcap, Huang qin (Mandarin), ogon (Japanese))

Cardiotonic
Primary herbs
- Convallaria majalis (Lily of the valley)
- Crataegus monogyna (Hawthorn)
- Leonurus cardiaca (Motherwort)
- Plectranthus barbatus (Coleus, makandi)

Additional herbs
- Albizia lebbeck (Albizia, sirisha)
- Angelica polymorpha (Dong quai, dang gui, Chinese angelica)
- Asparagus racemosus (Shatavari (Sanskrit), satavari (Hindi), satmuli (Bengali))
- Astragalus membranaceus (Astragalus, milk vetch, huang qi (Chinese), ogi (Japanese))
- Olea europaea (Olive tree)

- Panax ginseng (Ginseng, Ren Shen)
- Panax notoginseng (Tienchi ginseng (san qi, tian qi – Mandarin) Yunnan bayou)
- Terminalia arjuna (Arjuna)

Carminative

Primary herbs

- Anethum graveolens (Dill)
- Capsicum spp. (Chilli, capsicum, pepper, paprika, cayenne)
- Cinnamomum verum (Cinnamon, cassia bark, rou gui)
- Foeniculum vulgare (Fennel)
- Melissa officinalis (Lemon balm, Melissa)
- Mentha pulegium (Pennyroyal)
- Mentha x piperita (Peppermint, Bo He)
- Nepeta cataria (Catnip, catmint, Jing Jie)
- Petroselinum crispum (Parsley root)
- Pimpinella anisum (Aniseed)
- Salvia rosmarinus (Rosemary)

Additional herbs

- Alpinia galanga (Greater galangal, Thai ginger)
- Angelica archangelica (European angelica, angelica)
- Bidens tripartita (Burr marigold, water agrimony, gui zhen cao, longbacao)
- Hyssopus officinalis (Hyssop)
- Juniperus communis (Juniper)
- Lavandula angustifolia (Lavender)
- Macropiper excelsum (Kawakawa, New Zealand peppertree)
- Matricaria chamomilla (Chamomile, German chamomile)
- Nigella sativa (Black cumin)
- Salvia officinalis (Sage)
- Thymus vulgaris (Thyme)
- Valeriana officinalis (Valerian, heliotrope, Mexican valerian (V. edulis))
- Vitex agnus-castus (Chaste tree, chasteberry, Man Jing Zi)
- Zanthoxylum clava-herculis (Prickly ash)
- Zingiber officinale (Ginger, Sheng Jiang (fresh), Gan Jiang (dried))

Chemoprotective

Primary herbs

- Crocus sativus (Saffron)
- Echinacea spp. (Echinacea)
- Glycine max (Soy, soy germ, soy isoflavones (genistein), phyto-oestrogens, tofu (bean curd))
- Trametes versicolor (Turkey tail PSK, PSP)

Additional herbs

- Allium sativum (Garlic)
- Astragalus membranaceus (Astragalus, milk vetch, huang qi (Chinese), ogi (Japanese))
- Camellia sinensis (Green tea (green, black or oolong according to processing))
- Curcuma longa (Turmeric)
- Isodon rubescens (Dong ling cao, Chinese sage bush, rabdosia)
- Panax ginseng (Ginseng, Ren Shen)
- Phyllanthus spp. (Phyllanthus)
- Scutellaria baicalensis (Baikal skullcap, baical skullcap, Chinese skullcap, Huang qin (Mandarin), ogon (Japanese))
- Silybum marianum (St Mary's thistle, milk thistle, silymarin)
- Withania somnifera (Ashwaghanda, winter cherry)
- Zingiber officinale (Ginger, Sheng Jiang (fresh), Gan Jiang (dried))

Cholagogue

Primary herbs

- Chelidonium majus (Greater celandine)
- Chionanthus virginicus (Fringe tree, old man's beard)
- Gentiana lutea (Gentian)
- Iris versicolor (Blue flag)
- Juglans cinerea (Butternut bark, white walnut, lemon walnut)
- Peumus boldus (Boldo)
- Taraxacum officinale radix (Dandelion root)

Additional herbs

- Agathosma betulina (Buchu)
- Andrographis paniculata (Andrographis, kalmegh)
- Artemisia vulgaris (Mugwort)
- Berberis aquifolium (Oregon grape, mountain grape)
- Berberis vulgaris (Barberry)
- Betula pendula (Silver birch)
- Coptis chinensis (Huanglian (China), makino (Japan))
- Matricaria chamomilla (Chamomile, German chamomile)
- Rumex crispus (Yellow dock, curled dock)

Choleretic

Primary herbs

- Berberis vulgaris (Barberry)
- Fumaria officinalis (Fumitory)
- Hydrastis canadensis (Goldenseal)

Additional herbs

- Andrographis paniculata (Andrographis, kalmegh)
- Arctium lappa (Burdock)
- Calendula officinalis (Calendula, marigold)
- Curcuma longa (Turmeric)
- Cynara scolymus (Globe artichoke)

- Gentiana lutea (Gentian)
- Glycyrrhiza spp. (Licorice, Liquorice, Gan Cao)
- Hyssopus officinalis (Hyssop)
- Picrorhiza kurroa (Kutki)
- Silybum marianum (St Mary's thistle, milk thistle, silymarin)
- Zingiber officinale (Ginger, Sheng Jiang (fresh), Gan Jiang (dried))

Circulatory stimulant

Primary herbs

- Angelica archangelica (European angelica, angelica)
- Cola spp. (Kola nut, cola nut)
- Pseudowintera colorata (Horopito)
- Zanthoxylum clava-herculis (Prickly ash)

Additional herbs

- Armoracia rusticana (Horseradish)
- Macropiper excelsum (Kawakawa, New Zealand peppertree)

Connective tissue regenerator

Primary herbs

- Centella asiatica (Gotu kola, brahmi)

Additional herbs

- Centaurium erythraea (Centaury)

Counter irritant

Primary herbs

- Capsicum spp. (Chilli, capsicum, pepper, paprika, cayenne)

Additional herbs

- Arnica montana (Arnica)
- Capsicum spp. (Chilli, capsicum, pepper, paprika, cayenne)
- Thuja occidentalis (Thuja, white cedar, arbor-vitae (American))

Cytoprotective

Primary herbs

- Panax ginseng (Ginseng, Ren Shen)
- Silybum marianum (St Mary's thistle, milk thistle, silymarin)
- Symphytum officinale (Comfrey)
- Vaccinium myrtillus (Bilberry, blueberry)

Additional herbs

- Alchemilla vulgaris (Lady's mantle)
- Althaea officinalis (Marshmallow, white mallow)
- Berberis vulgaris (Barberry)
- Boswellia serrata (Boswellia, olibanum, frankincense)
- Camellia sinensis (Green tea (green, black or oolong according to processing))
- Commiphora myrrha (Myrrh)

- Crocus sativus (Saffron)
- Curcuma longa (Turmeric)
- Ginkgo biloba (Maidenhair)
- Glycyrrhiza spp. (Licorice, Liquorice, Gan Cao)
- Phyllanthus spp. (Phyllanthus)
- Terminalia arjuna (Arjuna)

Decongestant

Primary herbs

- Armoracia rusticana (Horseradish)

Additional herbs

- Capsicum spp. (Chilli, capsicum, pepper, paprika, cayenne)
- Crocus sativus (Saffron)
- Hydrastis canadensis (Goldenseal)

Demulcent

Primary herbs

- Elymus repens (Couch grass)
- Plantago lanceolata (Ribwort, narrow-leaved plantain)
- Plantago major (Plantain, broad-leaved plantain, Che Qian Zi)
- Symphytum officinale (Comfrey)
- Tussilago farfara (Coltsfoot)
- Ulmus fulva (Slippery elm, red elm)
- Verbascum thapsus (Mullein, candlewick plant, flannel-leaf, bunny's ears)

Additional herbs

- Agrimonia eupatoria (Agrimony)
- Althaea officinalis (Marshmallow, white mallow)
- Asparagus racemosus (Shatavari (Sanskrit), satavari (Hindi), satmuli (Bengali))
- Drosera spp. (Sundew)
- Glycyrrhiza spp. (Licorice, Liquorice, Gan Cao)
- Stellaria media (Chickweed, starweed)
- Trigonella foenum-graecum (Fenugreek)
- Zingiber officinale (Ginger, Sheng Jiang (fresh), Gan Jiang (dried))

Demulcent (urinary)

Primary herbs

- Zea mays (Corn silk, maize)

Additional herbs

- Agrimonia eupatoria (Agrimony)
- Alchemilla vulgaris (Lady's mantle)
- Ulmus fulva (Slippery elm, red elm)

Depurative/Alterative

Primary herbs

- Arctium lappa (Burdock)
- Collinsonia canadensis (Stone root)
- Hemidesmus indicus (Anantamul, Indian sarsparilla)

- Iris versicolor (Blue flag)
- Juglans cinerea (Butternut bark, white walnut, lemon walnut)
- Macropiper excelsum (Kawakawa, New Zealand peppertree)
- Rumex crispus (Yellow dock, curled dock)
- Scrophularia nodosa (Figwort)
- Smilax ornata (Sarsaparilla)
- Thuja occidentalis (Thuja, white cedar, arbor-vitae (American))
- Trifolium pratense (Red clover, trifoil)
- Viola tricolor (Heartsease, wild pansy, viola)

Additional herbs

- Berberis vulgaris (Barberry)
- Centella asiatica (Gotu kola, brahmi, Indian pennywort)
- Juglans nigra (Black walnut)
- Lamium album (White dead nettle)

Diaphoretic

Primary herbs

- Achillea millefolium (Yarrow)
- Asclepias tuberosa (Pleurisy root, butterfly weed)
- Eupatorium perfoliatum (Boneset, feverwort)
- Hyssopus officinalis (Hyssop)
- Lobelia inflata (Indian tobacco)
- Melissa officinalis (Lemon balm, Melissa)
- Mentha pulegium (Pennyroyal)
- Mentha x piperita (Peppermint, Bo He)
- Myrica cerifera (Bayberry, candleberry, wax myrtle)
- Nepeta cataria (Catnip, catmint, Jing Jie)
- Tilia cordata (Lime tree, linden)

Additional herbs

- Anemone pulsatilla (Pulsatilla)
- Angelica archangelica (European angelica, angelica)
- Bidens tripartita (Burr marigold, water agrimony, gui zhen cao, longbacao)
- Bryonia dioica (Bryony)
- Capsicum spp. (Chilli, capsicum, pepper, paprika, cayenne)
- Collinsonia canadensis (Stone root)
- Dioscorea spp. (Wild yam)
- Eschscholzia californica (Californian poppy)
- Filipendula ulmaria (Meadowsweet)
- Guaiacum officinale (Guaiacum)
- Hedera helix (Ivy leaf, English ivy)
- Hemidesmus indicus (Anantamul, Indian sarsparilla)
- Inula helenium (Elecampane)
- Macropiper excelsum (Kawakawa, New Zealand peppertree)

- Ruscus aculeatus (Butcher's broom, box holly)
- Sambucus nigra (Elder, elderflower, elderberry, sambuco)
- Smilax ornata (Sarsaparilla)
- Verbena officinalis (Vervain)
- Zanthoxylum clava-herculis (Prickly ash)
- Zingiber officinale (Ginger, Sheng Jiang (fresh), Gan Jiang (dried))

Digestive stimulant

Primary herbs

- Alpinia galanga (Greater galangal, Thai ginger)
- Armoracia rusticana (Horseradish)
- Gentiana lutea (Gentian)

Additional herbs

- Achillea millefolium (Yarrow)
- Nigella sativa (Black cumin)

Digestive tonic

Primary herbs

- Achillea millefolium (Yarrow)
- Angelica archangelica (European angelica, angelica)
- Atractylodes macrocephala (Atractylodes, bai zhu)
- Carica papaya (Paw paw, papaya)
- Citrus reticulata (Chen pi, mandarin, tangerine)
- Cynara scolymus (Globe artichoke)
- Dulacia inopiflora (Muira puama)
- Fumaria officinalis (Fumitory)
- Marrubium vulgare (White horehound)

Additional herbs

- Agathosma betulina (Buchu)
- Aletris farinosa (True unicorn root, white colic root)
- Alpinia galanga (Greater galangal, Thai ginger)
- Andrographis paniculata (Andrographis, kalmegh)
- Anethum graveolens (Dill)
- Artemisia annua (Sweet Annie, Chinese wormwood, qing hao)
- Artemisia vulgaris (Mugwort)
- Berberis vulgaris (Barberry)
- Bupleurum falcatum (Bupleurum, sickle-leaved hare's ear)
- Camellia sinensis (Green tea (green, black or oolong according to processing))
- Chamaelirium luteum (False unicorn root, helonias)
- Cnicus benedictus (Blessed or holy thistle)
- Gentiana lutea (Gentian)
- Harpagophytum procumbens (Devil's claw)
- Matricaria chamomilla (Chamomile, German chamomile)
- Momordica charantia (Bitter melon, bitter gourd, African or wild cucumber)
- Plectranthus barbatus (Coleus, makandi)

- Poria cocos (Hoelen, China root, sclerotium of tuckahoe, fu ling (Mandarin) and bukuryo (Japanese))
- Silybum marianum (St Mary's thistle, milk thistle, silymarin)
- Syzygium aromaticum (Cloves)
- Taraxacum officinale radix (Dandelion root)
- Ziziphus jujuba var. spinosa (Zizyphus, sour Chinese date, jujube, Da Zao, Suan Zao Ren)

Diuretic

Primary herbs

- Agathosma betulina (Buchu)
- Apium graveolens (Celery seed, karafs)
- Arctium lappa (Burdock)
- Arctostaphylos uva-ursi (Bearberry)
- Betula pendula (Silver birch)
- Convallaria majalis (Lily of the valley)
- Elymus repens (Couch grass)
- Equisetum arvense (Horsetail)
- Eutrochium purpureum (Gravel root, Joe Pye weed)
- Fumaria officinalis (Fumitory)
- Galium aparine (Clivers, cleavers)
- Guaiacum officinale (Guaiacum)
- Hydrangea arborescens (Hydrangea)
- Juniperus communis (Juniper)
- Macropiper excelsum (Kawakawa, New Zealand peppertree)
- Petroselinum crispum (Parsley root)
- Scrophularia nodosa (Figwort)
- Solidago virgaurea (Goldenrod)
- Taraxacum officinale folia (Dandelion leaf, Pu Gong Ying)
- Taraxacum officinale radix (Dandelion root)
- Urtica dioica folia (Nettle leaf, stinging nettle)
- Zea mays (Corn silk, maize)

Additional herbs

- Agrimonia eupatoria (Agrimony)
- Althaea officinalis (Marshmallow, white mallow)
- Angelica archangelica (European angelica, angelica)
- Asparagus racemosus (Shatavari (Sanskrit), satavari (Hindi), satmuli (Bengali))
- Astragalus membranaceus (Astragalus, milk vetch, huang qi (Chinese), ogi (Japanese))
- Atractylodes macrocephala (Atractylodes, bai zhu)
- Camellia sinensis (Green tea (green, black or oolong according to processing))
- Capsella bursa-pastoris (Shepherd's purse)
- Centaurium erythraea (Centaury)
- Chamaelirium luteum (False unicorn root, helonias)
- Cola spp. (Kola nut, cola nut)
- Collinsonia canadensis (Stone root)
- Cynara scolymus (Globe artichoke)
- Dioscorea spp. (Wild yam)
- Filipendula ulmaria (Meadowsweet)
- Foeniculum vulgare (Fennel)
- Glechoma hederacea (Ground ivy)
- Iris versicolor (Blue flag)
- Leptospermum scoparium (Manuka, tea tree)
- Ligustrum lucidum (Glossy privet, nu zhen zi, joteishi)
- Mitchella repens (Partridgeberry)
- Nigella sativa (Black cumin)
- Olea europaea (Olive tree)
- Peumus boldus (Boldo)
- Poria cocos (Hoelen, China root, sclerotium of tuckahoe, fu ling (Mandarin) and bukuryo (Japanese))
- Quercus robur (Oak bark)
- Ruscus aculeatus (Butcher's broom, box holly)
- Sambucus nigra (Elder, elderflower, elderberry, sambuco)
- Scutellaria baicalensis (Baikal skullcap, baical skullcap, Chinese skullcap, Huang qin (Mandarin), ogon (Japanese))
- Serenoa repens (Saw palmetto, cabbage palm, dwarf palmetto)
- Smilax ornata (Sarsaparilla)
- Tilia cordata (Lime tree, linden)
- Viola tricolor (Heartsease, wild pansy, viola)
- Vitis vinifera (Grape vine, grapeseed extract)
- Zanthoxylum clava-herculis (Prickly ash)

Dopaminergic

Primary herbs

- Vitex agnus-castus (Chaste tree, chasteberry, Man Jing Zi)

Emetic

Primary herbs

- Bryonia dioica (Bryony)
- Lobelia inflata (Indian tobacco)
- Myrica cerifera (Bayberry, candleberry, wax myrtle)

Emmenagogue

Primary herbs

- Achillea millefolium (Yarrow)
- Anemone pulsatilla (Pulsatilla)
- Artemisia vulgaris (Mugwort)
- Ruta graveolens (Rue)

Additional herbs

- Actaea racemosa (Black cohosh, squawroot, snakeroot)
- Alchemilla vulgaris (Lady's mantle)
- Apium graveolens (Celery seed, karafs)

- Calendula officinalis (Calendula, marigold)
- Cassia senna (Senna pod)
- Melissa officinalis (Lemon balm, Melissa)
- Mentha pulegium (Pennyroyal)
- Mitchella repens (Partridgeberry)
- Nigella sativa (Black cumin)
- Petroselinum crispum (Parsley root)
- Thuja occidentalis (Thuja, white cedar, arbor-vitae (American))

Emollient
Primary herbs
- Althaea officinalis (Marshmallow, white mallow)
- Avena sativa (seed) (Oats, groats, oatmeal)

Additional herbs
- Avena sativa (green) (Oats, green oats, oat straw)
- Stellaria media (Chickweed, starweed)
- Trigonella foenum-graecum (Fenugreek)
- Ulmus fulva (Slippery elm, red elm)
- Verbascum thapsus (Mullein, candlewick plant, flannel-leaf, bunny's ears)

Expectorant (general)
Primary herbs
- Asclepias tuberosa (Pleurisy root, butterfly weed)
- Glycyrrhiza spp. (Licorice, Liquorice, Gan Cao)
- Lobelia inflata (Indian tobacco)
- Plantago lanceolata (Ribwort, narrow-leaved plantain)
- Prunus serotina (Wild cherry, black cherry)
- Trifolium pratense (Red clover, trifoil)
- Tussilago farfara (Coltsfoot)
- Verbascum thapsus (Mullein, candlewick plant, flannel-leaf, bunny's ears)
- Viola tricolor (Heartsease, wild pansy, viola)
- Zingiber officinale (Ginger, Sheng Jiang (fresh), Gan Jiang (dried))

Additional herbs
- Alpinia galanga (Greater galangal, Thai ginger)
- Ganoderma lucidum (Reishi, lingzhi)
- Nigella sativa (Black cumin)
- Petroselinum crispum (Parsley root)
- Pimpinella anisum (Aniseed)
- Stellaria media (Chickweed, starweed)
- Ulmus fulva (Slippery elm, red elm)

Expectorant (relaxing)
Primary herbs
- Bryonia dioica (Bryony)
- Euphorbia hirta (Euphorbia)
- Marrubium vulgare (White horehound)
- Thymus vulgaris (Thyme)

Additional herbs
- Glycyrrhiza spp. (Licorice, Liquorice, Gan Cao)
- Justicia adhatoda (Basak, vasaka, Malabar nut)

Expectorant (stimulating)
Primary herbs
- Inula helenium (Elecampane)
- Lobelia inflata (Indian tobacco)
- Lomatium dissectum (Fern-leaf biscuit root, tohza, desert parsley)

Additional herbs
- Angelica archangelica (European angelica, angelica)
- Asclepias tuberosa (Pleurisy root, butterfly weed)
- Grindelia camporum (Gum weed)
- Thuja occidentalis (Thuja, white cedar, arbor-vitae (American))

Fibrinolytic
Primary herbs
- Allium sativum (Garlic)
- Centaurium erythraea (Centaury)
- Salvia miltiorrhiza (Dan shen (Mandarin), red root sage)

Galactagogue
Primary herbs
- Anethum graveolens (Dill)
- Foeniculum vulgare (Fennel)
- Galega officinalis (Goat's rue)
- Pimpinella anisum (Aniseed)
- Rubus idaeus (Raspberry leaf)
- Trigonella foenum-graecum (Fenugreek)
- Zingiber officinale (ginger)

Additional herbs
- Asparagus racemosus (Shatavari (Sanskrit), satavari (Hindi), satmuli (Bengali))
- Bidens tripartita (Burr marigold, water agrimony, gui zhen cao, longbacao)
- Humulus lupulus (Hops)
- Matricaria chamomilla (Chamomile, German chamomile)
- Mitchella repens (Partridgeberry)
- Nigella sativa (Black cumin)
- Urtica dioica folia (Nettle leaf, stinging nettle)
- Verbena officinalis (Vervain)
- Vitex agnus-castus (Chaste tree, chasteberry, Man Jing Zi)

Gastroprotective
Primary herbs
- Alpinia galanga (Greater galangal, Thai ginger)
- Propolis (Propolis)

Additional herbs

- Althaea officinalis (Marshmallow, white mallow)
- Angelica polymorpha (Dong quai, dang gui, Chinese angelica)
- Asparagus racemosus (Shatavari (Sanskrit), satavari (Hindi), satmuli (Bengali))
- Carica papaya (Paw paw, papaya)
- Centaurium erythraea (Centaury)
- Codonopsis pilosula (Dang shen, codonopsis)
- Filipendula ulmaria (Meadowsweet)
- Ganoderma lucidum (Reishi, lingzhi)
- Glycyrrhiza spp. (Licorice, Liquorice, Gan Cao)
- Hemidesmus indicus (Anantamul, Indian sarsparilla)
- Leptospermum scoparium (Manuka, tea tree)
- Marrubium vulgare (White horehound)
- Matricaria chamomilla (Chamomile, German chamomile)
- Melissa officinalis (Lemon balm, Melissa)
- Momordica charantia (Bitter melon, bitter gourd, African or wild cucumber)
- Pseudowintera colorata (Horopito)
- Rosa canina (Rosehip, dog rose)
- Scutellaria baicalensis (Baikal skullcap, baical skullcap, Chinese skullcap, Huang qin (Mandarin), ogon (Japanese))
- Syzygium aromaticum (Cloves)
- Terminalia arjuna (Arjuna)

Hepatoprotective

Primary herbs

- Artemisia absinthium (Wormwood, absinthe)
- Bupleurum falcatum (Bupleurum, sickle-leaved hare's ear)
- Cynara scolymus (Globe artichoke)
- Ganoderma lucidum (Reishi, lingzhi)
- Nigella sativa (Black cumin)
- Phyllanthus spp. (Phyllanthus)
- Picrorhiza kurroa (Kutki)
- Pueraria lobata (Kudzu)
- Salvia miltiorrhiza (Dan shen (Mandarin), red root sage)
- Silybum marianum (St Mary's thistle, milk thistle, silymarin)

Additional herbs

- Agrimonia eupatoria (Agrimony)
- Andrographis paniculata (Andrographis, kalmegh)
- Angelica polymorpha (Dong quai, dang gui, Chinese angelica)
- Asparagus racemosus (Shatavari (Sanskrit), satavari (Hindi), satmuli (Bengali))
- Berberis aristata (Daruharidra, Daruhaldi, Darvi, Chitra, Indian barberry)

- Bidens tripartita (Burr marigold, water agrimony, gui zhen cao, longbacao)
- Carica papaya (Paw paw, papaya)
- Centaurium erythraea (Centaury)
- Cinnamomum verum (Cinnamon, cassia bark, rou gui)
- Commiphora myrrha (Myrrh)
- Curcuma longa (Turmeric)
- Eleutherococcus senticosus (Eleuthero, eleutherokokk, Siberian ginseng)
- Epimedium sagittatum (Horny goat weed, barrenwort, yin yang huo, Inyokaku)
- Fumaria officinalis (Fumitory)
- Glechoma hederacea (Ground ivy)
- Glycyrrhiza spp. (Licorice, Liquorice, Gan Cao)
- Guaiacum officinale (Guaiacum)
- Gymnema sylvestre (Gumar, meshashringi)
- Hedera helix (Ivy leaf, English ivy)
- Hemidesmus indicus (Anantamul, Indian sarsparilla)
- Ligustrum lucidum (Glossy privet, nu zhen zi, joteishi)
- Panax ginseng (Ginseng, Ren Shen)
- Panax quinquefolium (American ginseng)
- Perilla frutescens (Perilla, su zi, shisu)
- Rhodiola rosea (Golden root, rose root, arctic root)
- Salvia rosmarinus (Rosemary)
- Schisandra chinensis (Bei-Wuweizi, Schisandra, Chinese magnolia vine, Wu Wei Zi)
- Smilax ornata (Sarsaparilla)
- Trametes versicolor (Turkey tail PSK, PSP)

Hepatotonic

Primary herbs

- Bupleurum falcatum (Bupleurum, sickle-leaved hare's ear)
- Chionanthus virginicus (Fringe tree, old man's beard)
- Peumus boldus (Boldo)
- Phyllanthus spp. (Phyllanthus)
- Schisandra chinensis (Bei-Wuweizi, Schisandra, Chinese magnolia vine, Wu Wei Zi)
- Tribulus terrestris (Tribulus, calthrops, puncture vine, Bai Ji Li)

Additional herbs

- Andrographis paniculata (Andrographis, kalmegh)
- Berberis aquifolium (Oregon grape, mountain grape)
- Berberis vulgaris (Barberry)
- Chelidonium majus (Greater celandine)
- Cynara scolymus (Globe artichoke)
- Ganoderma lucidum (Reishi, lingzhi)
- Panax ginseng (Ginseng, Ren Shen)

- Picrorhiza kurroa (Kutki)
- Salvia miltiorrhiza (Dan shen (Mandarin), red root sage)
- Silybum marianum (St Mary's thistle, milk thistle, silymarin)
- Taraxacum officinale radix (Dandelion root)

Hypnotic
Primary herbs
- Eschscholzia californica (Californian poppy)
- Passiflora incarnata (Passion flower)
- Piscidia piscipula (Jamaican dogwood)

Additional herbs
- Corydalis ambigua (Corydalis)
- Humulus lupulus (Hops)
- Piper methysticum (Kava)
- Valeriana officinalis (Valerian, heliotrope, Mexican valerian (V. edulis))
- Ziziphus jujuba var. spinosa (Zizyphus, sour Chinese date, jujube, Da Zao, Suan Zao Ren)

Hypoglycaemic
Primary herbs
- Galega officinalis (Goat's rue)
- Gymnema sylvestre (Gumar, meshashringi)
- Momordica charantia (Bitter melon, bitter gourd, African or wild cucumber)
- Trigonella foenum-graecum (Fenugreek)

Additional herbs
- Apium graveolens (Celery seed, karafs)
- Asparagus racemosus (Shatavari (Sanskrit), satavari (Hindi), satmuli (Bengali))
- Ballota nigra (Black horehound)
- Cordyceps militaris (Cordyceps, orange catapillar fungus, dong chong xia cao (China), hyakurakusou (Japan))
- Ligustrum lucidum (Glossy privet, nu zhen zi, joteishi)
- Panax ginseng (Ginseng, Ren Shen)
- Phyllanthus spp. (Phyllanthus)
- Salvia rosmarinus (Rosemary)
- Scutellaria baicalensis (Baikal skullcap, baical skullcap, Chinese skullcap, Huang qin (Mandarin), ogon (Japanese))
- Stevia rebaudiana (Stevia)
- Tribulus terrestris (Tribulus, calthrops, puncture vine, Bai Ji Li)
- Urtica dioica folia (Nettle leaf, stinging nettle)
- Withania somnifera (Ashwaghanda, winter cherry)

Hypothalamic-pituitary-ovarian (HPO) regulator
Primary herbs
- Chamaelirium luteum (False unicorn root, helonias)

- Paeonia lactiflora (Peony, white peony, Bai Shao)
- Trillium erectum (Beth root, birth root)
- Vitex agnus-castus (Chaste tree, chasteberry, Man Jing Zi)

Additional herbs
- Actaea racemosa (Black cohosh, squawroot, snakeroot)

Immunomodulator
Primary herbs
- Andrographis paniculata (Andrographis, kalmegh)
- Astragalus membranaceus (milk vetch, huang qi (Chinese), ogi (Japanese))
- Baptisia tinctoria (Wild indigo)
- Carica papaya (Paw paw, papaya)
- Codonopsis pilosula (Dang shen, codonopsis)
- Cordyceps militaris (Cordyceps, dong chong xia cao (China), hyakurakusou (Japan))
- Echinacea spp. (Echinacea)
- Eleutherococcus senticosus (Eleuthero, eleutherokokk, Siberian ginseng)
- Ganoderma lucidum (Reishi, lingzhi)
- Houttuynia cordata (Yu Xing Cao, chameleon plant, fish mint)
- Ligustrum lucidum (Glossy privet, nu zhen zi, joteishi)
- Panax ginseng (Ginseng, Ren Shen)
- Pelargonium sidoides (African geranium, umckaloabo (severe cough in Zulu))
- Phytolacca americana (Poke root, pokeweed)
- Picrorhiza kurroa (Kutki)
- Rehmannia glutinosa (Rehmannia, sheng di huang (uncured), shu di huang (cured), Chinese foxglove)
- Rhodiola rosea (Golden root, rose root, arctic root)
- Trametes versicolor (Turkey tail PSK, PSP)
- Uncaria tomentosa (Cat's claw)

Additional herbs
- Althaea officinalis (Marshmallow, white mallow)
- Angelica polymorpha (Dong quai, dang gui, Chinese angelica)
- Artemisia annua (Sweet Annie, Chinese wormwood, qing hao)
- Asparagus racemosus (Shatavari (Sanskrit), satavari (Hindi), satmuli (Bengali))
- Berberis aquifolium (Oregon grape, mountain grape)
- Bidens tripartita (Burr marigold, water agrimony, gui zhen cao, longbacao)
- Crocus sativus (Saffron)
- Epimedium sagittatum (Horny goat weed, barrenwort, yin yang huo, Inyokaku)
- Gynostemma pentaphyllum (Jiaogulan, xiancao)
- Lomatium dissectum (Fern-leaf biscuit root, tohza, desert parsley)

- Momordica charantia (Bitter melon, bitter gourd, African or wild cucumber)
- Nigella sativa (Black cumin)
- Paeonia lactiflora (Peony, white peony, Bai Shao)
- Panax quinquefolium (American ginseng)
- Plantago lanceolata (Ribwort, narrow-leaved plantain)
- Poria cocos (Hoelen, China root, sclerotium of tuckahoe, fu ling (Mandarin) and bukuryo (Japanese))
- Propolis (Propolis)
- Syzygium aromaticum (Cloves)
- Withania somnifera (Ashwaghanda, winter cherry)

LH-RH antagonist

Primary herbs

- Poria cocos (Hoelen, China root, sclerotium of tuckahoe, fu ling (Mandarin) and bukuryo (Japanese))

Laxative

Primary herbs

- Aloe ferox (Aloe vera (gel), bitter aloes (resin))
- Cassia senna (Senna pod)
- Iris versicolor (Blue flag)
- Juglans cinerea (Butternut bark, white walnut, lemon walnut)
- Peumus boldus (Boldo)
- Rhamnus frangula (Alder buckthorn)
- Rhamnus purshiana (Cascara sagrada (sacred bark), Californian buckthorn)
- Rheum palmatum (Da Huang, Chinese rhubarb)
- Rumex crispus (Yellow dock, curled dock)
- Ulmus fulva (Slippery elm, red elm)

Additional herbs

- Chelidonium majus (Greater celandine)
- Fumaria officinalis (Fumitory)
- Glycyrrhiza spp. (Licorice, Liquorice, Gan Cao)
- Macropiper excelsum (Kawakawa, New Zealand peppertree)
- Pimpinella anisum (Aniseed)
- Taraxacum officinale folia (Dandelion leaf, Pu Gong Ying)
- Taraxacum officinale radix (Dandelion root)
- Trigonella foenum-graecum (Fenugreek)
- Viola tricolor (Heartsease, wild pansy, viola)

Lipogenesis- and lipoxygenation-inhibitor

Primary herbs

- Berberis aquifolium (Oregon grape, mountain grape)
- Lipolytic

Additional herbs

- Plectranthus barbatus (Coleus, makandi)

Lithotryptic

Primary herbs

- Quercus robur (Oak bark)

Lymphatic

Primary herbs

- Galium aparine (Clivers, cleavers)
- Phytolacca americana (Poke root, pokeweed)

Additional herbs

- Baptisia tinctoria (Wild indigo)
- Calendula officinalis (Calendula, marigold)
- Echinacea spp. (Echinacea)
- Iris versicolor (Blue flag)
- Scrophularia nodosa (Figwort)

Male tonic

Primary herbs

- Cordyceps militaris (Cordyceps, orange catapillar fungus, dong chong xia cao (China), hyakurakusou (Japan))
- Epimedium sagittatum (Horny goat weed, barrenwort, yin yang huo, Inyokaku)
- Panax ginseng (Ginseng, Ren Shen)
- Turnera diffusa (Damiana)

Menstrual cycle regulator

Primary herbs

- Chamaelirium luteum (False unicorn root, helonias)
- Paeonia lactiflora (Peony, white peony, Bai Shao)

Additional herbs

- Alchemilla vulgaris (Lady's mantle)
- Vitex agnus-castus (Chaste tree, chasteberry, Man Jing Zi)

Migraine prophylactic

Primary herbs

- Tanacetum parthenium (Feverfew)

Mucilaginous

Primary herbs

- Ulmus fulva (Slippery elm, red elm)

Mucolytic

Primary herbs

- Justicia adhatoda (Basak, vasaka, Malabar nut)

Additional herbs

- Allium sativum (Garlic)

Mucous membrane tonic

Primary herbs

- Hydrastis canadensis (Goldenseal)

Additional herbs

- Bidens tripartita (Burr marigold, water agrimony, gui zhen cao, longbacao)
- Euphrasia officinalis (Eyebright)

Natriuretic

Primary herbs

- Equisetum arvense (Horsetail)

Nervine tonic

Primary herbs

- Avena sativa (green) (Oats, green oats, oat straw)
- Avena sativa (seed) (Oats, groats, oatmeal)
- Dulacia inopiflora (Muira puama)
- Reynoutria multiflora (He Shou Wu, Fo-Ti)
- Scutellaria lateriflora (Blue skulcap)
- Tilia cordata (Lime tree, linden)
- Turnera diffusa (Damiana)
- Verbena officinalis (Vervain)
- Ziziphus jujuba var. spinosa (Zizyphus, sour Chinese date, jujube, Da Zao, Suan Zao Ren)

Additional herbs

- Alchemilla vulgaris (Lady's mantle)
- Annona muricata (Graviola, soursop, guanábana)
- Bacopa monnieri (Bacopa, brahmi)
- Centaurium erythraea (Centaury)
- Centella asiatica (Gotu kola, brahmi, Indian pennywort)
- Dioscorea spp. (Wild yam)
- Hypericum perforatum (St John's wort)
- Schisandra chinensis (Bei-Wuweizi, Schisandra, Chinese magnolia vine, Wu Wei Zi)
- Valeriana officinalis (Valerian, heliotrope, Mexican valerian (V. edulis))
- Withania somnifera (Ashwaghanda, winter cherry)

Neuroprotective

Primary herbs

- Bacopa monnieri (Bacopa, brahmi)
- Cordyceps militaris (Cordyceps, orange catapillar fungus, dong chong xia cao (China), hyakurakusou (Japan))
- Crocus sativus (Saffron)
- Epimedium sagittatum (Horny goat weed, barrenwort, yin yang huo, Inyokaku)
- Schisandra chinensis (Bei-Wuweizi, Schisandra, Chinese magnolia vine, Wu Wei Zi)

Additional herbs

- Alpinia galanga (Greater galangal, Thai ginger)
- Asparagus racemosus (Shatavari (Sanskrit), satavari (Hindi), satmuli (Bengali))
- Atractylodes macrocephala (Atractylodes, bai zhu)
- Bidens tripartita (Burr marigold, water agrimony, gui zhen cao, longbacao)
- Codonopsis pilosula (Dang shen, codonopsis)
- Curcuma longa (Turmeric)
- Hemidesmus indicus (Anantamul, Indian sarsparilla)

- Magnolia officinalis (Magnolia, Hou po)
- Panax quinquefolium (American ginseng)
- Pueraria lobata (Kudzu)
- Salvia miltiorrhiza (Dan shen (Mandarin), red root sage)
- Scutellaria baicalensis (Baikal skullcap, baical skullcap, Chinese skullcap, Huang qin (Mandarin), ogon (Japanese))
- Silybum marianum (St Mary's thistle, milk thistle, silymarin)

Nootropic

Primary herbs

- Bacopa monnieri (Bacopa, brahmi)
- Dulacia inopiflora (Muira puama)
- Ginkgo biloba (Maidenhair)
- Panax quinquefolium (American ginseng)
- Vinca minor (Periwinkle, lesser or common periwinkle)

Additional herbs

- Eleutherococcus senticosus (Eleuthero, eleutherokokk, Siberian ginseng)
- Hemidesmus indicus (Anantamul, Indian sarsparilla)
- Paeonia lactiflora (Peony, white peony, Bai Shao)
- Rhodiola rosea (Golden root, rose root, arctic root)
- Salvia officinalis (Sage)
- Schisandra chinensis (Bei-Wuweizi, Schisandra, Chinese magnolia vine, Wu Wei Zi)

Nrf2-pathway activator

Primary herbs

- Astragalus membranaceus (milk vetch, huang qi (Chinese), ogi (Japanese))
- Commiphora myrrha (Myrrh)
- Inula racemosa (Inula)
- Magnolia officinalis (Magnolia, Hou po)

Nutritive

Primary herbs

- Avena sativa (seed) (Oats, groats, oatmeal)

Additional herbs

- Urtica dioica folia (Nettle leaf, stinging nettle)
- Ziziphus jujuba var. spinosa (Zizyphus, sour Chinese date, jujube, Da Zao, Suan Zao Ren)

Oxytocic

Primary herbs

- Capsella bursa-pastoris (Shepherd's purse)

Additional herbs

- Hydrastis canadensis (Goldenseal)
- Justicia adhatoda (Basak, vasaka, Malabar nut)

PAF inhibitor

Primary herbs

- Ginkgo biloba (Maidenhair)

PPARgamma agonist

Primary herbs

- Magnolia officinalis (Magnolia, Hou po)

Pancreatic trophorestorative

Primary herbs

- Gymnema sylvestre (Gumar, meshashringi)

Partus praeparator

Primary herbs

- Mitchella repens (Partridgeberry)
- Rubus idaeus (Raspberry leaf)

Additional herbs

- Cassia senna (Senna pod)

Phosphodiesterase-5 inhibitor

Primary herbs

- Epimedium sagittatum (Horny goat weed, barrenwort, yin yang huo, Inyokaku)

Photosensitising

Primary herbs

- Hypericum perforatum (St John's wort)

Postpartum tonic

Primary herbs

- Mitchella repens (Partridgeberry)

Purgative

Primary herbs

- Rhamnus purshiana (Cascara sagrada (sacred bark), Californian buckthorn)

Additional herbs

- Rheum palmatum (Da Huang, Chinese rhubarb)
- Rumex crispus (Yellow dock, curled dock)

Radiosensitiser

Primary herbs

- Panax quinquefolium (American ginseng)

Renal protective

Primary herbs

- Coptis chinensis (Huanglian (China), makino (Japan))
- Ligustrum lucidum (Glossy privet, nu zhen zi, joteishi)

Renal tonic

Primary herbs

- Astragalus membranaceus (milk vetch, huang qi (Chinese), ogi (Japanese))
- Bupleurum falcatum (Bupleurum, sickle-leaved hare's ear)

- Salvia miltiorrhiza (Dan shen (Mandarin), red root sage)
- Schisandra chinensis (Bei-Wuweizi, Schisandra, Chinese magnolia vine, Wu Wei Zi)

Reproductive tonic

Primary herbs

- Asparagus racemosus (Shatavari (Sanskrit), satavari (Hindi), satmuli (Bengali))
- Rubefacient

Additional herbs

- Pseudowintera colorata (Horopito)

Sedative

Primary herbs

- Avena sativa (green) (Oats, green oats, oat straw)
- Ballota nigra (Black horehound)
- Corydalis ambigua (Corydalis)
- Humulus lupulus (Hops)
- Lavandula angustifolia (Lavender)
- Leonurus cardiaca (Motherwort)
- Passiflora incarnata (Passion flower)
- Piper methysticum (Kava)
- Piscidia piscipula (Jamaican dogwood)
- Salvia rosmarinus (Rosemary)
- Scutellaria lateriflora (Blue skulcap)
- Stachys officinalis (Wood betony)
- Valeriana officinalis (Valerian, heliotrope, Mexican valerian (V. edulis))
- Vinca minor (Periwinkle, lesser or common periwinkle)
- Viscum album (Mistletoe)
- Ziziphus jujuba var. spinosa (Zizyphus, sour Chinese date, jujube, Da Zao, Suan Zao Ren)

Additional herbs

- Actaea racemosa (Black cohosh, squawroot, snakeroot)
- Anemone pulsatilla (Pulsatilla)
- Annona muricata (Graviola, soursop, guanábana)
- Bacopa monnieri (Bacopa, brahmi)
- Baptisia tinctoria (Wild indigo)
- Eschscholzia californica (Californian poppy)
- Ganoderma lucidum (Reishi, lingzhi)
- Hyssopus officinalis (Hyssop)
- Leptospermum scoparium (Manuka, tea tree)
- Lobelia inflata (Indian tobacco)
- Matricaria chamomilla (Chamomile, German chamomile)
- Melissa officinalis (Lemon balm, Melissa)
- Nepeta cataria (Catnip, catmint, Jing Jie)
- Nigella sativa (Black cumin)
- Paeonia lactiflora (Peony, white peony, Bai Shao)
- Peumus boldus (Boldo)

- Prunus serotina (Wild cherry, black cherry)
- Scutellaria baicalensis (Baikal skullcap, baical skullcap, Chinese skullcap, Huang qin (Mandarin), ogon (Japanese))
- Tilia cordata (Lime tree, linden)
- Verbena officinalis (Vervain)
- Viburnum opulus (Cramp bark)
- Withania somnifera (Ashwaghanda, winter cherry)

Selective oestrogen receptor modulator (SERM)

Primary herbs

- Actaea racemosa (Black cohosh, squawroot, snakeroot)
- Dioscorea spp. (Wild yam)
- Glycine max (Soy, soy germ, soy isoflavones (genistein), phyto-oestrogens, tofu (bean curd))
- Humulus lupulus (Hops)
- Pimpinella anisum (Aniseed)
- Vitex agnus-castus (Chaste tree, chasteberry, Man Jing Zi)

Additional herbs

- Alchemilla vulgaris (Lady's mantle)
- Chamaelirium luteum (False unicorn root, helonias)
- Foeniculum vulgare (Fennel)
- Glycyrrhiza spp. (Licorice, Liquorice, Gan Cao)
- Inula racemosa (Inula)
- Paeonia lactiflora (Peony, white peony, Bai Shao)
- Panax ginseng (Ginseng, Ren Shen)
- Pueraria lobata (Kudzu)
- Trifolium pratense (Red clover, trifoil)
- Trillium erectum (Beth root, birth root)

Sexual tonic

Primary herbs

- Asparagus racemosus (Shatavari (Sanskrit), satavari (Hindi), satmuli (Bengali))
- Cordyceps militaris (Cordyceps, orange catapillar fungus, dong chong xia cao (China), hyakurakusou (Japan))
- Epimedium sagittatum (Horny goat weed, barrenwort, yin yang huo, Inyokaku)

Sialogogue

Primary herbs

- Echinacea spp. (Echinacea)
- Gentiana lutea (Gentian)
- Lobelia inflata (Indian tobacco)
- Plectranthus barbatus (Coleus, makandi)
- Zanthoxylum clava-herculis (Prickly ash)

Stimulant

Primary herbs

- Cola spp. (Kola nut, cola nut)

Stomachic

Primary herbs

- Turnera diffusa (Damiana)

Additional herbs

- Artemisia vulgaris (Mugwort)
- Cnicus benedictus (Blessed or holy thistle)
- Collinsonia canadensis (Stone root)
- Dioscorea spp. (Wild yam)
- Filipendula ulmaria (Meadowsweet)
- Fumaria officinalis (Fumitory)
- Glechoma hederacea (Ground ivy)
- Hydrastis canadensis (Goldenseal)
- Juniperus communis (Juniper)
- Melissa officinalis (Lemon balm, Melissa)
- Rheum palmatum (Da Huang, Chinese rhubarb)
- Rosa canina (Rosehip, dog rose)
- Ziziphus jujuba var. spinosa (Chinese date, jujube, Da Zao, Suan Zao Ren)

Styptic/Haemostatic

Primary herbs

- Symphytum officinale (Comfrey)
- Rheum palmatum (Da Huang, Chinese rhubarb)
- Urtica dioica folia (Nettle leaf, stinging nettle)

Additional herbs

- Achillea millefolium (Yarrow)
- Alchemilla vulgaris (Lady's mantle)
- Bidens tripartita (Burr marigold, water agrimony, gui zhen cao, longbacao)
- Bistorta officinalis (Bistort, common bistort, European bistort or meadow bistort)
- Calendula officinalis (Calendula, marigold)
- Dioscorea spp. (Wild yam)

Taste improver

Primary herbs

- Glycyrrhiza spp. (Licorice, Liquorice, Gan Cao)
- Stevia rebaudiana (Stevia)

Thyroid stimulant

Primary herbs

- Fucus vesiculosus (Bladderwrack)
- Plectranthus barbatus (Coleus, makandi)

Tonic

Primary herbs

- Dipsacus asper (Teasel root)
- Ligustrum lucidum (Glossy privet, nu zhen zi, joteishi)
- Magnolia officinalis (Magnolia, Hou po)
- Panax quinquefolium (American ginseng)

Additional herbs

- Astragalus membranaceus (milk vetch, huang qi (Chinese), ogi (Japanese))
- Avena sativa (green) (Oats, green oats, oat straw)
- Avena sativa (seed) (Oats, groats, oatmeal)
- Bupleurum falcatum (Bupleurum, sickle-leaved hare's ear)
- Eleutherococcus senticosus (Eleuthero, eleutherokokk, Siberian ginseng)
- Epimedium sagittatum (Horny goat weed, barrenwort, yin yang huo, Inyokaku)
- Fumaria officinalis (Fumitory)
- Ganoderma lucidum (Reishi, lingzhi)
- Gynostemma pentaphyllum (Jiaogulan, xiancao)
- Panax ginseng (Ginseng, Ren Shen)
- Rumex crispus (Yellow dock, curled dock)
- Schisandra chinensis (Bei-Wuweizi, Schisandra, Chinese magnolia vine, Wu Wei Zi)
- Smilax ornata (Sarsaparilla)
- Withania somnifera (Ashwaghanda, winter cherry)

Uterine tonic

Primary herbs

- Actaea racemosa (Black cohosh, squawroot, snakeroot)
- Aletris farinosa (True unicorn root, white colic root)
- Angelica polymorpha (Dong quai, dang gui, Chinese angelica)
- Caulophyllum thalictroides (Blue cohosh)
- Chamaelirium luteum (False unicorn root, helonias)
- Mitchella repens (Partridgeberry)
- Rubus idaeus (Raspberry leaf)
- Trillium erectum (Beth root, birth root)

Additional herbs

- Alchemilla vulgaris (Lady's mantle)
- Cassia senna (Senna pod)
- Hydrastis canadensis (Goldenseal)
- Nigella sativa (Black cumin)
- Ruta graveolens (Rue)
- Schisandra chinensis (Bei-Wuweizi, Schisandra, Chinese magnolia vine, Wu Wei Zi)
- Vitex agnus-castus (Chaste tree, chasteberry, Man Jing Zi)

Vasodilator

Primary herbs

- Crataegus monogyna (Hawthorn)
- Olea europaea (Olive tree)
- Tilia cordata (Lime tree, linden)

Additional herbs

- Actaea racemosa (Black cohosh, squawroot, snakeroot)
- Alchemilla vulgaris (Lady's mantle)

- Allium sativum (Garlic)
- Angelica archangelica (European angelica, angelica)
- Centaurium erythraea (Centaury)
- Cryptolepis sanguinolenta (Yellow dye root, delboi)
- Echinacea spp. (Echinacea)
- Epimedium sagittatum (Horny goat weed, barrenwort, yin yang huo, Inyokaku)
- Ginkgo biloba (Maidenhair)
- Harpagophytum procumbens (Devil's claw)
- Plectranthus barbatus (Coleus, makandi)
- Pueraria lobata (Kudzu)
- Salvia miltiorrhiza (Dan shen (Mandarin), red root sage)
- Stevia rebaudiana (Stevia)

Vasoprotective

Primary herbs

- Ginkgo biloba (Maidenhair)
- Pinus pinaster (Maritime bark)
- Vaccinium myrtillus (Bilberry, blueberry)
- Vitis vinifera (Grape vine, grapeseed extract)

Additional herbs

- Cryptolepis sanguinolenta (Yellow dye root, delboi)
- Pueraria lobata (Kudzu)

Venotonic

Primary herbs

- Aesculus hippocastanum (Horse chestnut)
- Centella asiatica (Gotu kola, brahmi, Indian pennywort)
- Collinsonia canadensis (Stone root)
- Ginkgo biloba (Maidenhair)
- Hamamelis virginiana (Witch hazel)
- Ruscus aculeatus (Butcher's broom, box holly)
- Vitis vinifera (Grape vine, grapeseed extract)

Additional herbs

- Arnica montana (Arnica)
- Centaurium erythraea (Centaury)
- Dioscorea spp. (Wild yam)

Wound healing/Vulnerary

Primary herbs

- Alchemilla vulgaris (Lady's mantle)
- Aloe ferox (Aloe vera (gel), bitter aloes (resin))
- Arnica montana (Arnica)
- Calendula officinalis (Calendula, marigold)
- Carica papaya (Paw paw, papaya)
- Geranium maculatum (Cranesbill)
- Lamium album (White dead nettle)
- Matricaria chamomilla (Chamomile, German chamomile)
- Stellaria media (Chickweed, starweed)

- Symphytum officinale (Comfrey)

Additional herbs

- Althaea officinalis (Marshmallow, white mallow)
- Astragalus membranaceus (milk vetch, huang qi (Chinese), ogi (Japanese))
- Bidens tripartita (Burr marigold, water agrimony, gui zhen cao, longbacao)
- Centaurium erythraea (Centaury)
- Centella asiatica (Gotu kola, brahmi, Indian pennywort)
- Cnicus benedictus (Blessed or holy thistle)
- Dipsacus asper (Teasel root)
- Echinacea spp. (Echinacea)
- Glechoma hederacea (Ground ivy)
- Hedera helix (Ivy leaf, English ivy)
- Hypericum perforatum (St John's wort)
- Mitchella repens (Partridgeberry)
- Plantago lanceolata (Ribwort, narrow-leaved plantain)
- Propolis (Propolis)
- Salvia miltiorrhiza (Dan shen (Mandarin), red root sage)
- Terminalia arjuna (Arjuna)
- Uncaria tomentosa (Cat's claw)
- Verbascum thapsus (Mullein, candlewick plant, flannel-leaf, bunny's ears)

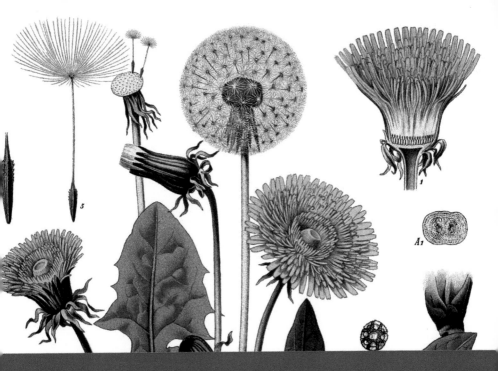

Therapeutic
Indications

Phytotherapy Desk Reference

Acne

- Arctium lappa (Burdock)
- Berberis vulgaris (Barberry)
- Bidens tripartita (Burr marigold, water agrimony, gui zhen cao, longbacao)
- Calendula officinalis (Calendula, marigold)
- Carica papaya (Paw paw, papaya)
- Commiphora myrrha (Myrrh)
- Echinacea spp. (Echinacea)
- Galium aparine (Clivers, cleavers)
- Houttuynia cordata (Yu Xing Cao, chameleon plant, fish mint)
- Paeonia lactiflora (Peony, white peony, Bai Shao)
- Phytolacca americana (Poke root, pokeweed)
- Salvia miltiorrhiza (Dan shen, red root sage)
- Scutellaria baicalensis (Baikal skullcap, baical skullcap, Chinese skullcap, Huang qin
- Trifolium pratense (Red clover, trifoil)
- Vitex agnus-castus (Chaste tree, chasteberry, Man Jing Zi)

Acne (topically)

- Berberis aquifolium (Oregon mountain grape)
- Calendula officinalis (Calendula, marigold)
- Commiphora myrrha (Myrrh)
- Echinacea spp. (Echinacea)
- Glycyrrhiza spp. (Licorice, Liquorice, Gan Cao)
- Paeonia lactiflora (Peony, white peony, Bai Shao)
- Phytolacca americana (Poke root, pokeweed)

Addison's disease

- Glycyrrhiza spp. (Licorice, Liquorice, Gan Cao)

Adenomyosis

- Aletris farinosa (True unicorn root, white colic root)
- Angelica polymorpha (Dong quai, dang gui, Chinese angelica)
- Chamaelirium luteum (False unicorn root, helonias)
- Paeonia lactiflora (Peony, white peony, Bai Shao)
- Vitex agnus-castus (Chaste tree, chasteberry, Man Jing Zi)

Age–related macular degeneration

- Crocus sativus (Saffron)
- Ligustrum lucidum (Glossy privet, nu zhen zi, joteishi)

Alcoholism

- Pueraria lobata (Kudzu)

Allergies/Sensitivities

- Albizia lebbeck (Albizia, sirisha)
- Angelica polymorpha (Dong quai, dang gui, Chinese angelica)
- Cynara scolymus (Globe artichoke)
- Ephedra sinensis (Ma-huang)
- Gentiana lutea (Gentian)

- Glycine max (Soy, soy germ, soy isoflavones (genistein), phyto-oestrogens, tofu (bean curd))
- Handroanthus impetiginosus (Pau d'arco, lapacho)
- Hemidesmus indicus (Anantamul, Indian sarsparilla)
- Matricaria chamomilla (Chamomile, German chamomile)
- Nigella sativa (Black cumin)
- Perilla frutescens (Perilla, su zi, shisu)
- Picrorhiza kurroa (Kutki)
- Plantago lanceolata (Ribwort, narrow-leaved plantain)
- Rehmannia glutinosa (Rehmannia, sheng di huang (uncured), shu di huang (cured), Chinese foxglove)
- Scutellaria baicalensis (Baikal skullcap, baical skullcap, Chinese skullcap, Huang qin (Mandarin), ogon (Japanese))
- Silybum marianum (St Mary's thistle, milk thistle, silymarin)
- Tanacetum parthenium (Feverfew)
- Ulmus fulva (Slippery elm, red elm)
- Vitis vinifera (Grape vine, grapeseed extract)

Alopecia neurotica (topical)

- Arnica montana (Arnica)
- Salvia rosmarinus (Rosemary)

Alzheimer's disease

- Bacopa monnieri (Bacopa, brahmi)
- Curcuma longa (Turmeric)
- Ginkgo biloba (Maidenhair)

Amenorrhoea

- Achillea millefolium (Yarrow)
- Alchemilla vulgaris (Lady's mantle)
- Aletris farinosa (True unicorn root, white colic root)
- Anemone pulsatilla (Pulsatilla)
- Angelica polymorpha (Dong quai, dang gui, Chinese angelica)
- Caulophyllum thalictroides (Blue cohosh)
- Chamaelirium luteum (False unicorn root, helonias)
- Leonurus cardiaca (Motherwort)
- Mitchella repens (Partridgeberry)
- Nigella sativa (Black cumin)
- Paeonia lactiflora (Peony, white peony, Bai Shao)
- Rehmannia glutinosa (Rehmannia, sheng di huang (uncured), shu di huang (cured), Chinese foxglove)
- Rhodiola rosea (Golden root, rose root, arctic root)
- Thuja occidentalis (Thuja, white cedar, arbor-vitae)
- Vitex agnus-castus (Chaste tree, chasteberry, Man Jing Zi)

Anaemia

- Angelica polymorpha (Dong quai, dang gui, Chinese angelica)
- Codonopsis pilosula (Dang shen, codonopsis)

- Crocus sativus (Saffron)
- Rehmannia glutinosa (Rehmannia, sheng di huang (uncured), shu di huang (cured), Chinese foxglove)
- Withania somnifera (Ashwaghanda, winter cherry)

Androgen excess

- Glycyrrhiza spp. (Licorice, Liquorice, Gan Cao)
- Paeonia lactiflora (Peony, white peony, Bai Shao)

Angina pectoris

- Angelica polymorpha (Dong quai, dang gui, Chinese angelica)
- Crataegus monogyna (Hawthorn)
- Inula racemosa (Inula)
- Paeonia lactiflora (Peony, white peony, Bai Shao)
- Panax ginseng (Ginseng, Ren Shen)
- Panax notoginseng (Tienchi ginseng (san qi, tian qi – Mandarin) Yunnan bayou)
- Plectranthus barbatus (Coleus, makandi)
- Pueraria lobata (Kudzu)
- Salvia miltiorrhiza (Dan shen (Mandarin), red root sage)
- Terminalia arjuna (Arjuna)

Anorexia

- Achillea millefolium (Yarrow)
- Agrimonia eupatoria (Agrimony)
- Aletris farinosa (True unicorn root, white colic root)
- Angelica archangelica (angelica)
- Arctium lappa (Burdock)
- Artemisia absinthium (Wormwood, absinthe)
- Artemisia vulgaris (Mugwort)
- Atractylodes macrocephala (Atractylodes, bai zhu)
- Centaurium erythraea (Centaury)
- Citrus reticulata (Chen pi, mandarin, tangerine)
- Cnicus benedictus (Blessed or holy thistle)
- Codonopsis pilosula (Dang shen, codonopsis)
- Cynara scolymus (Globe artichoke)
- Foeniculum vulgare (Fennel)
- Gentiana lutea (Gentian)
- Harpagophytum procumbens (Devil's claw)
- Hydrastis canadensis (Goldenseal)
- Hypericum perforatum (St John's wort)
- Marrubium vulgare (White horehound)
- Matricaria chamomilla (Chamomile, German chamomile)
- Nigella sativa (Black cumin)
- Plectranthus barbatus (Coleus, makandi)
- Taraxacum officinale radix (Dandelion root)
- Trigonella foenum-graecum (Fenugreek)
- Withania somnifera (Ashwaghanda, winter cherry)
- Zingiber officinale (Ginger, Sheng Jiang (fresh))

Anxiety

- Avena sativa (green) (Oats, green oats, oat straw)
- Avena sativa (seed) (Oats, groats, oatmeal)
- Bacopa monnieri (Bacopa, brahmi)
- Ballota nigra (Black horehound)
- Eschscholzia californica (Californian poppy)
- Harpagophytum procumbens (Devil's claw)
- Humulus lupulus (Hops)
- Hypericum perforatum (St John's wort)
- Lavandula angustifolia (Lavender)
- Leptospermum scoparium (Manuka, tea tree)
- Magnolia officinalis (Magnolia, Hou po)
- Matricaria chamomilla (Chamomile, German chamomile)
- Melissa officinalis (Lemon balm, Melissa)
- Panax quinquefolium (American ginseng)
- Passiflora incarnata (Passion flower)
- Piper methysticum (Kava)
- Poria cocos (Hoelen, China root, sclerotium of tuckahoe, fu ling (Mandarin) and bukuryo (Japanese))
- Rhodiola rosea (Golden root, rose root, arctic root)
- Salvia rosmarinus (Rosemary)
- Stachys officinalis (Wood betony)
- Tilia cordata (Lime tree, linden)
- Turnera diffusa (Damiana)
- Valeriana officinalis (Valerian, heliotrope, Mexican valerian (V. edulis))
- Verbena officinalis (Vervain)
- Ziziphus jujuba var. spinosa (Zizyphus, sour Chinese date, jujube, Da Zao, Suan Zao Ren)

Arrhythmia

- Angelica polymorpha (Dong quai, dang gui, Chinese angelica)
- Calendula officinalis (Calendula, marigold)
- Convallaria majalis (Lily of the valley)
- Coptis chinensis (Huanglian (China), makino (Japan))
- Corydalis ambigua (Corydalis)
- Harpagophytum procumbens (Devil's claw)
- Leonurus cardiaca (Motherwort)
- Panax ginseng (Ginseng, Ren Shen)
- Panax notoginseng (Tienchi ginseng (san qi, tian qi – Mandarin) Yunnan bayou)

Arteriosclerosis

- Allium sativum (Garlic)
- Astragalus membranaceus (Astragalus, milk vetch, huang qi (Chinese), ogi (Japanese))
- Crataegus monogyna (Hawthorn)
- Cynara scolymus (Globe artichoke)
- Ginkgo biloba (Maidenhair)
- Glycine max (Soy, soy germ, soy isoflavones (genistein), phyto-oestrogens, tofu (bean curd))
- Inula racemosa (Inula)

- Paeonia lactiflora (Peony, white peony, Bai Shao)
- Panax notoginseng (Tienchi ginseng (san qi, tian qi – Mandarin) Yunnan bayou)
- Tilia cordata (Lime tree, linden)
- Viscum album (Mistletoe)
- Zingiber officinale (Ginger, Sheng Jiang (fresh), Gan Jiang (dried))

Arthritis

- Actaea racemosa (Black cohosh, squawroot, snakeroot)
- Alpinia galanga (Greater galangal, Thai ginger)
- Apium graveolens (Celery seed, karafs)
- Arctium lappa (Burdock)
- Berberis vulgaris (Barberry)
- Betula pendula (Silver birch)
- Boswellia serrata (Boswellia, olibanum, frankincense)
- Capsicum spp. (Chilli, capsicum, pepper, paprika, cayenne)
- Centella asiatica (Gotu kola, brahmi, Indian pennywort)
- Curcuma longa (Turmeric)
- Elymus repens (Couch grass)
- Eupatorium perfoliatum (Boneset, feverwort)
- Guaiacum officinale (Guaiacum)
- Harpagophytum procumbens (Devil's claw)
- Rosa canina (Rosehip, dog rose)
- Rumex crispus (Yellow dock, curled dock)
- Salix spp. (Willow bark, white willow)
- Smilax ornata (Sarsaparilla)
- Symphytum officinale (Comfrey)
- Tanacetum parthenium (Feverfew)
- Thuja occidentalis (Thuja, white cedar, arbor-vitae)
- Uncaria tomentosa (Cat's claw)
- Urtica dioica folia (Nettle leaf, stinging nettle)
- Urtica dioica radix (Nettle root)
- Zingiber officinale (Ginger, Sheng Jiang (fresh), Gan Jiang (dried))

Asthma

- Albizia lebbeck (Albizia, sirisha)
- Alpinia galanga (Greater galangal, Thai ginger)
- Althaea officinalis (Marshmallow, white mallow)
- Asclepias tuberosa (Pleurisy root, butterfly weed)
- Boswellia serrata (olibanum, frankincense)
- Carica papaya (Paw paw, papaya)
- Cordyceps militaris (Cordyceps, orange catapillar fungus, dong chong xia cao (China), hyakurakusou (Japan))
- Crocus sativus (Saffron)
- Curcuma longa (Turmeric)
- Drosera spp. (Sundew)
- Ephedra sinensis (Ma-huang)

- Epimedium sagittatum (Horny goat weed, barrenwort, yin yang huo, Inyokaku)
- Euphorbia hirta (Euphorbia)
- Galium aparine (Clivers, cleavers)
- Glycyrrhiza spp. (Licorice, Liquorice, Gan Cao)
- Grindelia camporum (Gum weed)
- Houttuynia cordata (Yu Xing Cao, chameleon plant, fish mint)
- Inula helenium (Elecampane)
- Inula racemosa (Inula)
- Justicia adhatoda (Basak, vasaka, Malabar nut)
- Lobelia inflata (Indian tobacco)
- Lomatium dissectum (Fern-leaf biscuit root, tohza, desert parsley)
- Magnolia officinalis (Magnolia, Hou po)
- Matricaria chamomilla (Chamomile, German chamomile)
- Ocimum tenuiflorum (Tulsi, Holy basil)
- Panax ginseng (Ginseng, Ren Shen)
- Perilla frutescens (Perilla, su zi, shisu)
- Picrorhiza kurroa (Kutki)
- Pinus pinaster (Maritime bark)
- Plectranthus barbatus (Coleus, makandi)
- Pseudowintera colorata (Horopito)
- Scutellaria baicalensis (Baikal skullcap, baical skullcap, Chinese skullcap, Huang qin (Mandarin), ogon (Japanese))
- Thymus vulgaris (Thyme)
- Tussilago farfara (Coltsfoot)
- Uncaria tomentosa (Cat's claw)
- Viburnum prunifolium (Black haw, Sweet viburnum)

Asthma; bronchial

- Alpinia galanga (Greater galangal, Thai ginger)
- Asclepias tuberosa (Pleurisy root, butterfly weed)
- Ganoderma lucidum (Reishi, lingzhi)
- Hedera helix (Ivy leaf, English ivy)
- Ocimum tenuiflorum (Tulsi, Holy basil)
- Salvia rosmarinus (Rosemary)
- Tussilago farfara (Coltsfoot)

Atherosclerosis

- Allium sativum (Garlic)
- Astragalus membranaceus (Astragalus, milk vetch, huang qi (Chinese), ogi (Japanese))
- Camellia sinensis (Green tea (green, black or oolong according to processing))
- Coptis chinensis (Huanglian (China), makino (Japan))
- Curcuma longa (Turmeric)
- Cynara scolymus (Globe artichoke)
- Epimedium sagittatum (Horny goat weed, barrenwort, yin yang huo, Inyokaku)
- Ganoderma lucidum (Reishi, lingzhi)

- Ginkgo biloba (Maidenhair)
- Glycine max (Soy, soy germ, soy isoflavones (genistein), phyto-oestrogens, tofu (bean curd))
- Inula racemosa (Inula)
- Magnolia officinalis (Magnolia, Hou po)
- Panax notoginseng (Tienchi ginseng (san qi, tian qi – Mandarin) Yunnan bayou)
- Scutellaria baicalensis (Baikal skullcap, baical skullcap, Chinese skullcap, Huang qin (Mandarin), ogon (Japanese))
- Silybum marianum (St Mary's thistle, milk thistle, silymarin)

Autoimmune disease
- Astragalus membranaceus (Astragalus, milk vetch, huang qi (Chinese), ogi (Japanese))
- Bupleurum falcatum (Bupleurum, sickle-leaved hare's ear)
- Hemidesmus indicus (Anantamul, Indian sarsparilla)
- Nigella sativa (Black cumin)
- Picrorrhiza kurroa (Kutki)
- Rehmannia glutinosa (Rehmannia, sheng di huang (uncured), shu di huang (cured), Chinese foxglove)
- Salvia miltiorrhiza (Dan shen (Mandarin), red root sage)
- Scutellaria baicalensis (Baikal skullcap, baical skullcap, Chinese skullcap, Huang qin (Mandarin), ogon (Japanese))
- Uncaria tomentosa (Cat's claw)

Benign breast disease
- Calendula officinalis (Calendula, marigold)
- Ginkgo biloba (Maidenhair)
- Paeonia lactiflora (Peony, white peony, Bai Shao)
- Poria cocos (Hoelen, China root, sclerotium of tuckahoe, fu ling (Mandarin) and bukuryo (Japanese))
- Vitex agnus-castus (Chaste tree, Man Jing Zi)

Benign prostatic hyperplasia
- Crateva magna (Varuna)
- Elymus repens (Couch grass)
- Epilobium parviflorum (Willow herb)
- Epimedium sagittatum (Horny goat weed, barrenwort, yin yang huo, Inyokaku)
- Serenoa repens (Saw palmetto, cabbage palm, dwarf palmetto)
- Urtica dioica radix (Nettle root)

Bladder; atonic
- Crateva magna (Varuna)

Blood stasis
- Achillea millefolium (Yarrow)
- Corydalis ambigua (Corydalis)
- Panax notoginseng (Tienchi ginseng (san qi, tian qi – Mandarin) Yunnan bayou)

Boils
- Andrographis paniculata (Andrographis, kalmegh)
- Arctium lappa (Burdock)
- Berberis vulgaris (Barberry)
- Calendula officinalis (Calendula, marigold)
- Echinacea spp. (American coneflower)
- Houttuynia cordata (Yu Xing Cao, chameleon plant, fish mint)
- Macropiper excelsum (Kawakawa, New Zealand peppertree)
- Matricaria chamomilla (Chamomile, German chamomile)

Boils (poultice)
- Althaea officinalis (Marshmallow, white mallow)
- Calendula officinalis (Calendula, marigold)
- Ulmus fulva (Slippery elm, red elm)

Bronchitis
- Actaea racemosa (Black cohosh, squawroot, snakeroot)
- Alpinia galanga (Greater galangal, Thai ginger)
- Althaea officinalis (Marshmallow, white mallow)
- Andrographis paniculata (Andrographis, kalmegh)
- Angelica archangelica (European angelica, angelica)
- Armoracia rusticana (Horseradish)
- Asclepias tuberosa (Pleurisy root, butterfly weed)
- Bryonia dioica (Bryony)
- Codonopsis pilosula (Dang shen, codonopsis)
- Cordyceps militaris (Cordyceps, orange catapillar fungus, dong chong xia cao (China), hyakurakusou (Japan))
- Drosera spp. (Sundew)
- Echinacea spp. (Echinacea)
- Ephedra sinensis (Ma-huang)
- Eupatorium perfoliatum (Boneset, feverwort)
- Euphorbia hirta (Euphorbia)
- Glechoma hederacea (Ground ivy)
- Glycyrrhiza spp. (Licorice, Liquorice, Gan Cao)
- Grindelia camporum (Gum weed)
- Gynostemma pentaphyllum (Jiaogulan, xiancao)
- Hedera helix (Ivy leaf, English ivy)
- Hyssopus officinalis (Hyssop)
- Inula helenium (Elecampane)
- Inula racemosa (Inula)
- Justicia adhatoda (Basak, vasaka, Malabar nut)
- Lobelia inflata (Indian tobacco)
- Marrubium vulgare (White horehound)
- Ocimum tenuiflorum (Tulsi, Holy basil)
- Pelargonium sidoides (African geranium, umckaloabo (severe cough in Zulu))
- Pimpinella anisum (Aniseed)

- Plantago lanceolata (Ribwort, narrow-leaved plantain)
- Plectranthus barbatus (Coleus, makandi)
- Prunus serotina (Wild cherry, black cherry)
- Thuja occidentalis (Thuja, white cedar, arbor-vitae (American))
- Thymus vulgaris (Thyme)
- Trifolium pratense (Red clover, trifoil)
- Usnea spp. (Old man's beard, songluo)
- Verbascum thapsus (Mullein, candlewick plant, flannel-leaf, bunny's ears)
- Viola tricolor (Heartsease, wild pansy, viola)

Bruises (topically)

- Arnica montana (Arnica)
- Macropiper excelsum (Kawakawa, New Zealand peppertree)
- Symphytum officinale (Comfrey)

Buerger's disease

- Angelica polymorpha (Dong quai, dang gui, Chinese angelica)
- Salvia miltiorrhiza (Dan shen (Mandarin), red root sage)

Burns (topically)

- Aloe ferox (Aloe vera (gel), bitter aloes (resin))
- Calendula officinalis (Calendula, marigold)

Calculi; kidney and bladder

- Arctostaphylos uva-ursi (Bearberry)
- Asparagus racemosus (Shatavari (Sanskrit), satavari (Hindi), satmuli (Bengali))
- Bupleurum falcatum (Bupleurum, sickle-leaved hare's ear)
- Crateva magna (Varuna)
- Filipendula ulmaria (Meadowsweet)
- Hydrangea arborescens (Hydrangea)
- Quercus robur (Oak bark)
- Solidago virgaurea (Goldenrod)

Cancer; prevention/supportive treatment

- Annona muricata (Graviola, soursop, guanábana)
- Arctium lappa (Burdock)
- Artemisia annua (Sweet Annie, Chinese wormwood, qing hao)
- Asparagus racemosus (Shatavari (Sanskrit), satavari (Hindi), satmuli (Bengali))
- Astragalus membranaceus (Astragalus, milk vetch, huang qi (Chinese), ogi (Japanese))
- Atractylodes macrocephala (Atractylodes, bai zhu)
- Boswellia serrata (Boswellia, olibanum, frankincense)
- Bryonia dioica (Bryony)
- Bupleurum falcatum (Bupleurum, sickle-leaved hare's ear)
- Camellia sinensis (Green tea)

- Carica papaya (Paw paw, papaya)
- Codonopsis pilosula (Dang shen, codonopsis)
- Coptis chinensis (Huanglian (China), makino (Japan))
- Cordyceps militaris (Cordyceps, orange catapillar fungus, dong chong xia cao (China), hyakurakusou (Japan))
- Curcuma longa (Turmeric)
- Echinacea spp. (Echinacea)
- Eleutherococcus senticosus (Eleuthero, eleutherokokk, Siberian ginseng)
- Fucus vesiculosus (Bladderwrack)
- Ganoderma lucidum (Reishi, lingzhi)
- Glycine max (Soy, soy germ, soy isoflavones (genistein), phyto-oestrogens, tofu (bean curd))
- Handroanthus impetiginosus (Pau d'arco, lapacho (Spanish))
- Isatis tinctoria (Isatis, ban lan gen, woad, Chinese indigo)
- Isodon rubescens (Dong ling cao, Chinese sage bush, rabdosia)
- Ligustrum lucidum (Glossy privet, nu zhen zi, joteishi)
- Magnolia officinalis (Magnolia, Hou po)
- Nigella sativa (Black cumin)
- Panax ginseng (Ginseng, Ren Shen)
- Panax quinquefolium (American ginseng)
- Picrorhiza kurroa (Kutki)
- Poria cocos (Hoelen, China root, sclerotium of tuckahoe, fu ling (Mandarin) and bukuryo (Japanese))
- Punica granatum (Pomegranate)
- Rhodiola rosea (Golden root, rose root, arctic root)
- Salvia rosmarinus (Rosemary)
- Schisandra chinensis (Bei-Wuweizi, Schisandra, Chinese magnolia vine, Wu Wei Zi)
- Scutellaria baicalensis (Baikal skullcap, baical skullcap, Chinese skullcap, Huang qin (Mandarin), ogon (Japanese))
- Trametes versicolor (Turkey tail PSK, PSP)
- Uncaria tomentosa (Cat's claw)
- Viscum album (Mistletoe)
- Withania somnifera (Ashwaghanda, winter cherry)

Candidiasis

- Calendula officinalis (Calendula, marigold)
- Coptis chinensis (Huanglian (China), makino (Japan))
- Echinacea spp. (Echinacea)
- Handroanthus impetiginosus (Pau d'arco, lapacho (Spanish))
- Hydrastis canadensis (Goldenseal)
- Lomatium dissectum (Fern-leaf biscuit root, tohza, desert parsley)
- Pseudowintera colorata (Horopito)

- Ulmus fulva (Slippery elm, red elm)
- Usnea spp. (Old man's beard, songluo)

Capillary fragility

- Centella asiatica (Gotu kola, brahmi, Indian pennywort)
- Vaccinium myrtillus (Bilberry, blueberry)
- Viola tricolor (Heartsease, wild pansy, viola)
- Vitis vinifera (Grape vine, grapeseed extract)

Cardiac debility

- Asparagus racemosus (Shatavari (Sanskrit), satavari (Hindi), satmuli (Bengali))
- Inula racemosa (Inula)
- Leonurus cardiaca (Motherwort)
- Salvia miltiorrhiza (Dan shen (Mandarin), red root sage)
- Thuja occidentalis (Thuja, white cedar, arbor-vitae (American))

Cardiovascular disease prevention

- Andrographis paniculata (Andrographis, kalmegh)
- Astragalus membranaceus (Astragalus, milk vetch, huang qi (Chinese), ogi (Japanese))
- Coptis chinensis (Huanglian (China), makino (Japan))
- Crataegus monogyna (Hawthorn)
- Curcuma longa (Turmeric)
- Epimedium sagittatum (Horny goat weed, barrenwort, yin yang huo, Inyokaku)
- Harpagophytum procumbens (Devil's claw)
- Magnolia officinalis (Magnolia, Hou po)
- Panax ginseng (Ginseng, Ren Shen)
- Panax quinquefolium (American ginseng)
- Plectranthus barbatus (Coleus, makandi)
- Pueraria lobata (Kudzu)
- Salvia rosmarinus (Rosemary)
- Schisandra chinensis (Bei-Wuweizi, Schisandra, Chinese magnolia vine, Wu Wei Zi)
- Tribulus terrestris (Tribulus, calthrops, puncture vine, Bai Ji Li)

Carpal tunnel syndrome

- Aesculus hippocastanum (Horse chestnut)

Cataract and diabetic complications

- Ginkgo biloba (Maidenhair)
- Gymnema sylvestre (Gumar, meshashringi)
- Scutellaria baicalensis (Baikal skullcap, baical skullcap, Chinese skullcap, Huang qin (Mandarin), ogon (Japanese))
- Vaccinium myrtillus (Bilberry, blueberry)

Catarrh; naso-pharyngeal congestion

- Alpinia galanga (Greater galangal, Thai ginger)
- Armoracia rusticana (Horseradish)
- Bistorta officinalis (Bistort, common bistort, European bistort or meadow bistort)
- Echinacea spp. (Echinacea)
- Eupatorium perfoliatum (Boneset, feverwort)
- Euphrasia officinalis (Eyebright)
- Hydrastis canadensis (Goldenseal)
- Hyssopus officinalis (Hyssop)
- Isodon rubescens (Dong ling cao, Chinese sage bush, rabdosia)
- Plantago lanceolata (Ribwort, narrow-leaved plantain)
- Sambucus nigra (Elder, elderflower, elderberry, sambuco)
- Solidago virgaurea (Goldenrod)

Catarrhal deafness

- Capsella bursa-pastoris (Shepherd's purse)
- Ginkgo biloba (Maidenhair)
- Hydrastis canadensis (Goldenseal)
- Sambucus nigra (Elder, elderflower, elderberry, sambuco)

Cellulitis

- Centella asiatica (Gotu kola, brahmi, Indian pennywort)
- Vitis vinifera (Grape vine, grapeseed extract)

Cerebral ischaemia

- Angelica polymorpha (Dong quai, dang gui, Chinese angelica)
- Isodon rubescens (Dong ling cao, Chinese sage bush, rabdosia)

Cerebrovascular disease

- Angelica polymorpha (Dong quai, dang gui, Chinese angelica)
- Ginkgo biloba (Maidenhair)
- Plectranthus barbatus (Coleus, makandi)
- Salvia miltiorrhiza (Dan shen (Mandarin), red root sage)
- Vinca minor (Periwinkle, lesser periwinkle)

Chemotherapy; to minimise the side effects of

- Astragalus membranaceus (Astragalus, milk vetch, huang qi (Chinese), ogi (Japanese))
- Codonopsis pilosula (Dang shen, codonopsis)
- Echinacea spp. (Echinacea)
- Eleutherococcus senticosus (Eleuthero, eleutherokokk, Siberian ginseng)
- Panax ginseng (Ginseng, Ren Shen)
- Terminalia arjuna (Arjuna)
- Withania somnifera (Ashwaghanda, winter cherry)

Chilblains; unbroken (topically)

- Arnica montana (Arnica)
- Pseudowintera colorata (Horopito)
- Zanthoxylum clava-herculis (Prickly ash)

Childbirth recovery

- Aletris farinosa (True unicorn root, white colic root)
- Caulophyllum thalictroides (Blue cohosh)
- Mitchella repens (Partridgeberry)

Cholecystitis

- Berberis vulgaris (Barberry)
- Calendula officinalis (Calendula, marigold)
- Chelidonium majus (Greater celandine)
- Chionanthus virginicus (Fringe tree, old man's beard)
- Curcuma longa (Turmeric)
- Dioscorea spp. (Wild yam)
- Peumus boldus (Boldo)
- Rheum palmatum (Da Huang, Chinese rhubarb)
- Taraxacum officinale folia (Dandelion leaf, Pu Gong Ying)
- Taraxacum officinale radix (Dandelion root)
- Verbena officinalis (Vervain)

Chronic fatigue syndrome

- Andrographis paniculata (Andrographis, kalmegh)
- Astragalus membranaceus (Astragalus, milk vetch, huang qi (Chinese), ogi (Japanese))
- Atractylodes macrocephala (Atractylodes, bai zhu)
- Bacopa monnieri (Bacopa, brahmi)
- Bryonia dioica (Bryony)
- Centella asiatica (Gotu kola, brahmi, Indian pennywort)
- Codonopsis pilosula (Dang shen, codonopsis)
- Echinacea spp. (Echinacea)
- Eleutherococcus senticosus (Eleuthero, eleutherokokk, Siberian ginseng)
- Glycyrrhiza spp. (Licorice, Liquorice, Gan Cao)
- Gynostemma pentaphyllum (Jiaogulan, xiancao)
- Hypericum perforatum (St John's wort)
- Panax ginseng (Ginseng, Ren Shen)
- Rehmannia glutinosa (Rehmannia, sheng di huang (uncured), shu di huang (cured), Chinese foxglove)
- Schisandra chinensis (Bei-Wuweizi, Schisandra, Chinese magnolia vine, Wu Wei Zi)
- Uncaria tomentosa (Cat's claw)
- Withania somnifera (Ashwaghanda, winter cherry)

Circulation; peripheral; impaired

- Allium sativum (Garlic)
- Angelica archangelica (European angelica, angelica)
- Armoracia rusticana (Horseradish) Capsicum spp. (Chilli, capsicum, pepper, paprika, cayenne)
- Echinacea spp. (Echinacea)
- Ginkgo biloba (Maidenhair)
- Pseudowintera colorata (Horopito) Salvia miltiorrhiza (Dan shen (Mandarin), red root sage)
- Vaccinium myrtillus (Bilberry, blueberry)

- Zanthoxylum clava-herculis (Prickly ash)
- Zingiber officinale (Ginger)

Colic

- Cinnamomum verum (Cinnamon, cassia bark, rou gui)
- Dioscorea spp. (Wild yam)
- Lavandula angustifolia (Lavender)
- Nepeta cataria (Catnip, catmint, Jing Jie)
- Ulmus fulva (Slippery elm, red elm)

Colic; childhood

- Anethum graveolens (Dill)
- Foeniculum vulgare (Fennel)
- Matricaria chamomilla (Chamomile, German chamomile)
- Mentha x piperita (Peppermint, Bo He)
- Valeriana officinalis (Valerian, heliotrope, Mexican valerian (V. edulis))
- Zingiber officinale (Ginger, Sheng Jiang (fresh), Gan Jiang (dried))

Colic; flatulent

- Melissa officinalis (Lemon balm, Melissa)
- Mentha pulegium (Pennyroyal)
- Petroselinum crispum (Parsley root)
- Pimpinella anisum (Aniseed)

Colic; intestinal

- Alchemilla vulgaris (Lady's mantle)
- Alpinia galanga (Greater galangal, Thai ginger)
- Apium graveolens (Celery seed, karafs)
- Cinnamomum verum (Cinnamon, cassia bark, rou gui)
- Dioscorea spp. (Wild yam)
- Dulacia inopiflora (Muira puama)
- Foeniculum vulgare (Fennel)
- Matricaria chamomilla (Chamomile, German chamomile)
- Mentha pulegium (Pennyroyal)
- Mentha x piperita (Peppermint, Bo He)
- Momordica charantia (Bitter melon, bitter gourd, African or wild cucumber)
- Ruta graveolens (Rue)
- Valeriana officinalis (Valerian, heliotrope, Mexican valerian (V. edulis))
- Viburnum opulus (Cramp bark)
- Zingiber officinale (Ginger, Sheng Jiang (fresh), Gan Jiang (dried))

Colitis

- Agrimonia eupatoria (Agrimony)
- Althaea officinalis (Marshmallow, white mallow)
- Angelica archangelica (European angelica, angelica)
- Artemisia annua (Sweet Annie, Chinese wormwood, qing hao)

- Bistorta officinalis (Bistort, common bistort, European bistort or meadow bistort)
- Hamamelis virginiana (Witch hazel)
- Humulus lupulus (Hops)
- Hydrastis canadensis (Goldenseal)
- Matricaria chamomilla (Chamomile, German chamomile)
- Mitchella repens (Partridgeberry)
- Myrica cerifera (Bayberry, candleberry, wax myrtle)
- Symphytum officinale (Comfrey)
- Ulmus fulva (Slippery elm, red elm)

Common cold

- Achillea millefolium (Yarrow)
- Andrographis paniculata (Andrographis, kalmegh)
- Baptisia tinctoria (Wild indigo)
- Bidens tripartita (Burr marigold, water agrimony, gui zhen cao, longbacao)
- Cinnamomum verum (Cinnamon, cassia bark, rou gui)
- Coptis chinensis (Huanglian (China), makino (Japan))
- Echinacea spp. (Echinacea)
- Ephedra sinensis (Ma-huang)
- Euphrasia officinalis (Eyebright)
- Hedera helix (Ivy leaf, English ivy)
- Leptospermum scoparium (Manuka, tea tree)
- Lomatium dissectum (Fern-leaf biscuit root, tohza, desert parsley)
- Melissa officinalis (Lemon balm, Melissa)
- Mentha x piperita (Peppermint, Bo He)
- Myrica cerifera (Bayberry, candleberry, wax myrtle)
- Nepeta cataria (Catnip, catmint, Jing Jie)
- Ocimum tenuiflorum (Tulsi, Holy basil)
- Pelargonium sidoides (African geranium, umckaloabo (severe cough in Zulu))
- Pseudowintera colorata (Horopito)
- Rosa canina (Rosehip, dog rose)
- Sambucus nigra (Elder, elderflower, elderberry, sambuco)
- Thuja occidentalis (Thuja, white cedar, arbor-vitae (American))
- Tilia cordata (Lime tree, linden)

Congestive heart failure

- Astragalus membranaceus (Astragalus, milk vetch, huang qi (Chinese), ogi (Japanese))
- Convallaria majalis (Lily of the valley)
- Inula racemosa (Inula)
- Panax ginseng (Ginseng, Ren Shen)
- Panax notoginseng (Tienchi ginseng (san qi, tian qi – Mandarin) Yunnan bayou)
- Poria cocos (Hoelen, China root, sclerotium of tuckahoe, fu ling (Mandarin) and bukuryo (Japanese))

- Salvia miltiorrhiza (Dan shen (Mandarin), red root sage)
- Terminalia arjuna (Arjuna)

Conjunctivitis (locally as eye lotion)

- Euphrasia officinalis (Eyebright)
- Isatis tinctoria (Isatis, ban lan gen, woad, Chinese indigo)

Connective tissue disorders

- Centella asiatica (Gotu kola, brahmi, Indian pennywort)
- Echinacea spp. (Echinacea)
- Reynoutria multiflora (He Shou Wu, Fo-Ti)
- Vitis vinifera (Grape vine, grapeseed extract)
- Withania somnifera (Ashwaghanda, winter cherry)

Constipation

- Aloe ferox (Aloe vera (gel), bitter aloes (resin))
- Angelica polymorpha (Dong quai, dang gui, Chinese angelica)
- Cassia senna (Senna pod)
- Collinsonia canadensis (Stone root)
- Glycyrrhiza spp. (Licorice, Liquorice, Gan Cao)
- Iris versicolor (Blue flag)
- Juglans cinerea (Butternut bark, white walnut, lemon walnut)
- Magnolia officinalis (Magnolia, Hou po)
- Rhamnus frangula (Alder buckthorn)
- Rhamnus purshiana (Cascara sagrada (sacred bark), Californian buckthorn)
- Rheum palmatum (Da Huang, Chinese rhubarb)
- Rumex crispus (Yellow dock, curled dock)
- Taraxacum officinale folia (Dandelion leaf, Pu Gong Ying)
- Taraxacum officinale radix (Dandelion root)
- Turnera diffusa (Damiana)
- Ulmus fulva (Slippery elm, red elm)

Convalescence

- Andrographis paniculata (Andrographis, kalmegh)
- Astragalus membranaceus (Astragalus, milk vetch, huang qi (Chinese), ogi (Japanese))
- Atractylodes macrocephala (Atractylodes, bai zhu)
- Avena sativa (green) (Oats, green oats, oat straw)
- Avena sativa (seed) (Oats, groats, oatmeal)
- Bacopa monnieri (Bacopa, brahmi)
- Centella asiatica (Gotu kola, brahmi, Indian pennywort)
- Codonopsis pilosula (Dang shen, codonopsis)
- Eleutherococcus senticosus (Eleuthero, eleutherokokk, Siberian ginseng)
- Gentiana lutea (Gentian)
- Glycyrrhiza spp. (Licorice, Liquorice, Gan Cao)
- Panax ginseng (Ginseng, Ren Shen)
- Rehmannia glutinosa (Rehmannia, sheng di huang

(uncured), shu di huang (cured), Chinese foxglove)
- Schisandra chinensis (Bei-Wuweizi, Schisandra, Chinese magnolia vine, Wu Wei Zi)
- Trigonella foenum-graecum (Fenugreek)
- Uncaria tomentosa (Cat's claw)
- Withania somnifera (Ashwaghanda, winter cherry)

Cough
- Alpinia galanga (Greater galangal, Thai ginger)
- Althaea officinalis (Marshmallow, white mallow)
- Asclepias tuberosa (Pleurisy root, butterfly weed)
- Asparagus racemosus (Shatavari (Sanskrit), satavari (Hindi), satmuli (Bengali))
- Citrus reticulata (Chen pi, mandarin, tangerine)
- Crocus sativus (Saffron)
- Ephedra sinensis (Ma-huang)
- Euphorbia hirta (Euphorbia)
- Ganoderma lucidum (Reishi, lingzhi)
- Glycyrrhiza spp. (Licorice, Liquorice, Gan Cao)
- Inula helenium (Elecampane)
- Isodon rubescens (Dong ling cao, Chinese sage bush, rabdosia)
- Lobelia inflata (Indian tobacco)
- Lycopus spp. (Bugleweed, gypsy wort)
- Marrubium vulgare (White horehound)
- Nigella sativa (Black cumin)
- Ocimum tenuiflorum (Tulsi, Holy basil)
- Pimpinella anisum (Aniseed)
- Piscidia piscipula (Jamaican dogwood)
- Plantago lanceolata (Ribwort, narrow-leaved plantain)
- Prunus serotina (Wild cherry, black cherry)
- Pseudowintera colorata (Horopito)
- Ruta graveolens (Rue)
- Sambucus nigra (Elder, elderflower, elderberry, sambuco)
- Syzygium aromaticum (Cloves)
- Thymus vulgaris (Thyme)
- Trifolium pratense (Red clover, trifoil)
- Tussilago farfara (Coltsfoot)
- Ulmus fulva (Slippery elm, red elm)
- Usnea spp. (Old man's beard, songluo)
- Verbascum thapsus (Mullein, candlewick plant, flannel-leaf, bunny's ears)

Cramps; muscular spasm; muscular tension
- Paeonia lactiflora (Peony, white peony, Bai Shao)
- Piper methysticum (Kava)
- Valeriana officinalis (Valerian, heliotrope, Mexican valerian (V. edulis))
- Viburnum opulus (Cramp bark)
- Zanthoxylum clava-herculis (Prickly ash)

Crohn's disease
- Boswellia serrata (Boswellia, olibanum, frankincense)
- Glycine max (Soy, soy germ, soy isoflavones (genistein), phyto-oestrogens, tofu (bean curd))
- Mentha x piperita (Peppermint, Bo He)
- Ulmus fulva (Slippery elm, red elm)
- Uncaria tomentosa (Cat's claw)

Cystic hyperplasia
- Aletris farinosa (True unicorn root, white colic root)
- Chamaelirium luteum (False unicorn root, helonias)
- Dioscorea spp. (Wild yam)
- Trillium erectum (Beth root, birth root)
- Vitex agnus-castus (Chaste tree, chasteberry, Man Jing Zi)

Cystitis
- Agathosma betulina (Buchu)
- Agrimonia eupatoria (Agrimony)
- Althaea officinalis (Marshmallow, white mallow)
- Apium graveolens (Celery seed, karafs)
- Arctostaphylos uva-ursi (Bearberry)
- Capsella bursa-pastoris (Shepherd's purse)
- Crateva magna (Varuna)
- Dioscorea spp. (Wild yam)
- Echinacea spp. (Echinacea)
- Elymus repens (Couch grass)
- Eutrochium purpureum (Gravel root, Joe Pye weed)
- Filipendula ulmaria (Meadowsweet)
- Glechoma hederacea (Ground ivy)
- Hydrangea arborescens (Hydrangea)
- Juniperus communis (Juniper)
- Macropiper excelsum (Kawakawa, New Zealand peppertree)
- Petroselinum crispum (Parsley root)
- Peumus boldus (Boldo)
- Plantago major (Plantain, broad-leaved plantain, Che Qian Zi)
- Serenoa repens (Saw palmetto, cabbage palm, dwarf palmetto)
- Solidago virgaurea (Goldenrod)
- Thuja occidentalis (Thuja, white cedar, arbor-vitae (American))
- Ulmus fulva (Slippery elm, red elm)
- Viola tricolor (Heartsease, wild pansy, viola)
- Zea mays (Corn silk, maize)

Cystitis with haematuria
- Equisetum arvense (Horsetail)
- Plantago major (Plantain, broad-leaved plantain, Che Qian Zi)

DVT prophylaxis
- Ginkgo biloba (Maidenhair)

Debility
- Andrographis paniculata (Andrographis, kalmegh)
- Astragalus membranaceus (Astragalus, milk vetch, huang qi (Chinese), ogi (Japanese))
- Bacopa monnieri (Bacopa, brahmi)
- Eleutherococcus senticosus (Eleuthero, eleutherokokk, Siberian ginseng)
- Ganoderma lucidum (Reishi, lingzhi)
- Ligustrum lucidum (Glossy privet, nu zhen zi, joteishi)
- Panax ginseng (Ginseng, Ren Shen)
- Salvia rosmarinus (Rosemary)
- Uncaria tomentosa (Cat's claw)
- Verbena officinalis (Vervain)
- Withania somnifera (Ashwaghanda, winter cherry)

Dementia
- Bacopa monnieri (Bacopa, brahmi)
- Curcuma longa (Turmeric)
- Epimedium sagittatum (Horny goat weed, barrenwort, yin yang huo, Inyokaku)
- Ginkgo biloba (Maidenhair)
- Isodon rubescens (Dong ling cao, Chinese sage bush, rabdosia)
- Magnolia officinalis (Magnolia, Hou po)
- Panax quinquefolium (American ginseng)
- Salvia officinalis (Sage)

Depression
- Actaea racemosa (Black cohosh, squawroot, snakeroot)
- Annona muricata (Graviola, soursop, guanábana)
- Avena sativa (green) (Oats, green oats, oat straw)
- Avena sativa (seed) (Oats, groats, oatmeal)
- Cola spp. (Kola nut, cola nut)
- Crocus sativus (Saffron)
- Dulacia inopiflora (Muira puama)
- Epimedium sagittatum (Horny goat weed, barrenwort, yin yang huo, Inyokaku)
- Ginkgo biloba (Maidenhair)
- Hypericum perforatum (St John's wort)
- Lavandula angustifolia (Lavender)
- Magnolia officinalis (Magnolia, Hou po)
- Melissa officinalis (Lemon balm, Melissa)
- Panax ginseng (Ginseng, Ren Shen)
- Rhodiola rosea (Golden root, rose root, arctic root)
- Salvia rosmarinus (Rosemary)
- Scutellaria lateriflora (Blue skulcap)
- Tribulus terrestris (Tribulus, calthrops, puncture vine, Bai Ji Li)
- Trillium erectum (Beth root, birth root)
- Turnera diffusa (Damiana)
- Uncaria tomentosa (Cat's claw)
- Verbena officinalis (Vervain)
- Vinca minor (Periwinkle, lesser or common periwinkle)
- Vitex agnus-castus (Chaste tree, chasteberry, Man Jing Zi)
- Withania somnifera (Ashwaghanda, winter cherry)
- Ziziphus jujuba var. spinosa (Zizyphus, sour Chinese date, jujube, Da Zao, Suan Zao Ren)

Depression; postnatal
- Hypericum perforatum (St John's wort)
- Lavandula angustifolia (Lavender)
- Piper methysticum (Kava)
- Vitex agnus-castus (Chaste tree, chasteberry, Man Jing Zi)

Dermatitis
- Althaea officinalis (Marshmallow, white mallow)
- Berberis aquifolium (Oregon grape, mountain grape)
- Houttuynia cordata (Yu Xing Cao, chameleon plant, fish mint)

Diabetes
- Alpinia galanga (Greater galangal, Thai ginger)
- Anethum graveolens (Dill)
- Annona muricata (Graviola, soursop, guanábana)
- Berberis aristata (Daruharidra, Daruhaldi, Darvi, Chitra, Indian barberry)
- Carica papaya (Paw paw, papaya)
- Centaurium erythraea (Centaury)
- Cinnamomum verum (Cinnamon, cassia bark, rou gui)
- Cnicus benedictus (Blessed or holy thistle)
- Codonopsis pilosula (Dang shen, codonopsis)
- Coptis chinensis (Huanglian (China), makino (Japan))
- Cryptolepis sanguinolenta (Yellow dye root, delboi)
- Cynara scolymus (Globe artichoke)
- Dipsacus asper (Teasel root)
- Fucus vesiculosus (Bladderwrack)
- Galega officinalis (Goat's rue)
- Ganoderma lucidum (Reishi, lingzhi)
- Ginkgo biloba (Maidenhair)
- Gynostemma pentaphyllum (Jiaogulan, xiancao)
- Houttuynia cordata (Yu Xing Cao, chameleon plant, fish mint)
- Humulus lupulus (Hops)
- Ligustrum lucidum (Glossy privet, nu zhen zi, joteishi)
- Nigella sativa (Black cumin)
- Ocimum tenuiflorum (Tulsi, Holy basil)
- Perilla frutescens (Perilla, su zi, shisu)

- Phyllanthus spp. (Phyllanthus)
- Pinus pinaster (Maritime bark)
- Pueraria lobata (Kudzu)
- Punica granatum (Pomegranate)
- Salvia miltiorrhiza (Dan shen (Mandarin), red root sage)
- Stevia rebaudiana (Stevia)
- Syzygium aromaticum (Cloves)
- Terminalia arjuna (Arjuna)
- Trigonella foenum-graecum (Fenugreek)

Diabetes; gestational

- Cinnamomum verum (Cinnamon, cassia bark, rou gui)
- Codonopsis pilosula (Dang shen, codonopsis)
- Cynara scolymus (Globe artichoke)

Diabetic foot pain

- Capsicum spp. (Chilli, capsicum, pepper, paprika, cayenne)

Diabetic neuropathy

- Coptis chinensis (Huanglian (China), makino (Japan))
- Ginkgo biloba (Maidenhair)
- Gymnema sylvestre (Gumar, meshashringi)
- Perilla frutescens (Perilla, su zi, shisu)
- Pueraria lobata (Kudzu)
- Salvia miltiorrhiza (Dan shen, red root sage)
- Vaccinium myrtillus (Bilberry, blueberry)
- Vitis vinifera (Grape vine, grapeseed extract)

Diabetic retinopathy

- Ginkgo biloba (Maidenhair)
- Gymnema sylvestre (Gumar, meshashringi)
- Pinus pinaster (Maritime bark)
- Pueraria lobata (Kudzu)
- Vaccinium myrtillus (Bilberry, blueberry)
- Vitis vinifera (Grape vine, grapeseed extract)

Diarrhoea

- Agrimonia eupatoria (Agrimony)
- Alchemilla vulgaris (Lady's mantle)
- Alpinia galanga (Greater galangal, Thai ginger)
- Andrographis paniculata (Andrographis, kalmegh)
- Asparagus racemosus (Shatavari (Sanskrit), satavari (Hindi), satmuli (Bengali))
- Atractylodes macrocephala (Atractylodes, bai zhu)
- Berberis aquifolium (Oregon grape, mountain grape)
- Berberis aristata (Daruharidra, Daruhaldi, Darvi, Chitra, Indian barberry)
- Bistorta officinalis (Bistort, common bistort, European bistort or meadow bistort)
- Cinnamomum verum (Cinnamon, cassia bark, rou gui)

- Cryptolepis sanguinolenta (Yellow dye root, delboi)
- Echinacea spp. (Echinacea)
- Filipendula ulmaria (Meadowsweet)
- Geranium maculatum (Cranesbill)
- Glechoma hederacea (Ground ivy)
- Glycine max (Soy, soy germ, soy isoflavones (genistein), phyto-oestrogens, tofu (bean curd))
- Hamamelis virginiana (Witch hazel)
- Harpagophytum procumbens (Devil's claw)
- Juglans nigra (Black walnut)
- Matricaria chamomilla (Chamomile, German chamomile)
- Myrica cerifera (Bayberry, candleberry, wax myrtle)
- Poria cocos (Hoelen, China root, sclerotium of tuckahoe, fu ling (Mandarin) and bukuryo (Japanese))
- Punica granatum (Pomegranate)
- Quercus robur (Oak bark)
- Rheum palmatum (Da Huang, Chinese rhubarb)
- Rosa canina (Rosehip, dog rose)
- Rubus idaeus (Raspberry leaf)
- Thymus vulgaris (Thyme)
- Ulmus fulva (Slippery elm, red elm)

Digestive complaints

- Achillea millefolium (Yarrow)
- Aletris farinosa (True unicorn root, white colic root)
- Alpinia galanga (Greater galangal, Thai ginger)
- Andrographis paniculata (Andrographis, kalmegh)
- Angelica archangelica (European angelica, angelica)
- Angelica polymorpha (Dong quai, dang gui, Chinese angelica)
- Annona muricata (Graviola, soursop, guanábana)
- Capsicum spp. (Chilli, capsicum, pepper, paprika, cayenne)
- Centaurium erythraea (Centaury)
- Chamaelirium luteum (False unicorn root, helonias)
- Citrus reticulata (Chen pi, mandarin, tangerine)
- Codonopsis pilosula (Dang shen, codonopsis)
- Curcuma longa (Turmeric)
- Cynara scolymus (Globe artichoke)
- Fumaria officinalis (Fumitory)
- Gentiana lutea (Gentian)
- Glycine max (Soy, soy germ, soy isoflavones (genistein), phyto-oestrogens, tofu (bean curd))
- Lavandula angustifolia (Lavender)
- Plectranthus barbatus (Coleus, makandi)
- Silybum marianum (St Mary's thistle, milk thistle, silymarin)
- Taraxacum officinale folia (Dandelion leaf, Pu Gong Ying)
- Taraxacum officinale radix (Dandelion root)

- Ulmus fulva (Slippery elm, red elm)
- Zingiber officinale (Ginger, Sheng Jiang (fresh), Gan Jiang (dried))

Digestive weakness

- Aletris farinosa (True unicorn root, white colic root)
- Andrographis paniculata (Andrographis, kalmegh)
- Angelica archangelica (European angelica, angelica)
- Capsicum spp. (Chilli, capsicum, pepper, paprika, cayenne)
- Chamaelirium luteum (False unicorn root, helonias)
- Citrus reticulata (Chen pi, mandarin, tangerine)
- Codonopsis pilosula (Dang shen, codonopsis)
- Curcuma longa (Turmeric)
- Cynara scolymus (Globe artichoke)
- Fumaria officinalis (Fumitory)
- Harpagophytum procumbens (Devil's claw)
- Lavandula angustifolia (Lavender)
- Plectranthus barbatus (Coleus, makandi)

Diverticulitis

- Dioscorea spp. (Wild yam)
- Ulmus fulva (Slippery elm, red elm)
- Uncaria tomentosa (Cat's claw)

Dysentery

- Alchemilla vulgaris (Lady's mantle)
- Andrographis paniculata (Andrographis, kalmegh)
- Asparagus racemosus (Shatavari (Sanskrit), satavari (Hindi), satmuli (Bengali))
- Bidens tripartita (Burr marigold, water agrimony, gui zhen cao, longbacao)
- Bistorta officinalis (Bistort, common bistort, European bistort or meadow bistort)
- Collinsonia canadensis (Stone root)
- Coptis chinensis (Huanglian (China), makino (Japan))
- Echinacea spp. (Echinacea)
- Euphorbia hirta (Euphorbia)
- Geranium maculatum (Cranesbill)
- Nigella sativa (Black cumin)

Dyslipidaemia

- Agrimonia eupatoria (Agrimony)
- Allium sativum (Garlic)
- Anethum graveolens (Dill)
- Asparagus racemosus (Shatavari (Sanskrit), satavari (Hindi), satmuli (Bengali))
- Avena sativa (seed) (Oats, groats, oatmeal)
- Coptis chinensis (Huanglian (China), makino (Japan))
- Cordyceps militaris (Cordyceps, orange catapilar fungus, dong chong xia cao (China), hyakurakusou (Japan))
- Crocus sativus (Saffron)
- Ganoderma lucidum (Reishi, lingzhi)
- Gynostemma pentaphyllum (Jiaogulan, xiancao)
- Momordica charantia (Bitter melon, bitter gourd, African or wild cucumber)
- Nigella sativa (Black cumin)
- Olea europaea (Olive tree)
- Pinus pinaster (Maritime bark)
- Pueraria lobata (Kudzu)
- Punica granatum (Pomegranate)
- Salvia rosmarinus (Rosemary)
- Schisandra chinensis (Bei-Wuweizi, Schisandra, Chinese magnolia vine, Wu Wei Zi)
- Silybum marianum (St Mary's thistle, milk thistle, silymarin)
- Terminalia arjuna (Arjuna)
- Tribulus terrestris (Tribulus, calthrops, puncture vine, Bai Ji Li)
- Trigonella foenum-graecum (Fenugreek)
- Ulmus fulva (Slippery elm, red elm)

Dysmenorrhoea

- Actaea racemosa (Black cohosh, squawroot, snakeroot)
- Alchemilla vulgaris (Lady's mantle)
- Anemone pulsatilla (Pulsatilla)
- Angelica polymorpha (Dong quai, dang gui, Chinese angelica)
- Capsella bursa-pastoris (Shepherd's purse)
- Caulophyllum thalictroides (Blue cohosh)
- Chamaelirium luteum (False unicorn root, helonias)
- Corydalis ambigua (Corydalis)
- Crocus sativus (Saffron)
- Dioscorea spp. (Wild yam)
- Dulacia inopiflora (Muira puama)
- Ginkgo biloba (Maidenhair)
- Humulus lupulus (Hops)
- Hydrastis canadensis (Goldenseal)
- Lamium album (White dead nettle)
- Mentha x piperita (Peppermint, Bo He)
- Mitchella repens (Partridgeberry)
- Nigella sativa (Black cumin)
- Paeonia lactiflora (Peony, white peony, Bai Shao)
- Piscidia piscipula (Jamaican dogwood)
- Poria cocos (Hoelen, China root, sclerotium of tuckahoe, fu ling (Mandarin) and bukuryo (Japanese))
- Valeriana officinalis (Valerian, heliotrope, Mexican valerian (V. edulis))
- Verbena officinalis (Vervain)
- Viburnum opulus (Cramp bark)
- Viburnum prunifolium (Black haw, Sweet viburnum)
- Vitex agnus-castus (Chaste tree, chasteberry, Man Jing Zi)

- Zingiber officinale (Ginger, Sheng Jiang (fresh), Gan Jiang (dried))

Dysmenorrhoea; congestive

- Angelica polymorpha (Dong quai, dang gui, Chinese angelica)
- Ginkgo biloba (Maidenhair)
- Vitis vinifera (Grape vine, grapeseed extract)

Dysmenorrhoea; spasmodic

- Calendula officinalis (Calendula, marigold)
- Dioscorea spp. (Wild yam)
- Paeonia lactiflora (Peony, white peony, Bai Shao)
- Viburnum opulus (Cramp bark)

Dyspepsia

- Achillea millefolium (Yarrow)
- Aletris farinosa (True unicorn root, white colic root)
- Alpinia galanga (Greater galangal, Thai ginger)
- Althaea officinalis (Marshmallow, white mallow)
- Andrographis paniculata (Andrographis, kalmegh)
- Angelica archangelica (European angelica, angelica)
- Artemisia absinthium (Wormwood, absinthe)
- Asparagus racemosus (Shatavari (Sanskrit), satavari (Hindi), satmuli (Bengali))
- Berberis aquifolium (Oregon grape, mountain grape)
- Centaurium erythraea (Centaury)
- Cinnamomum verum (Cinnamon, cassia bark, rou gui)
- Dulacia inopiflora (Muira puama)
- Filipendula ulmaria (Meadowsweet)
- Ganoderma lucidum (Reishi, lingzhi)
- Gentiana lutea (Gentian)
- Magnolia officinalis (Magnolia, Hou po)
- Marrubium vulgare (White horehound)
- Matricaria chamomilla (Chamomile, German chamomile)
- Mentha pulegium (Pennyroyal)
- Momordica charantia (Bitter melon, bitter gourd, African or wild cucumber)
- Nigella sativa (Black cumin)
- Panax quinquefolium (American ginseng)
- Peumus boldus (Boldo)
- Rheum palmatum (Da Huang, Chinese rhubarb)
- Taraxacum officinale folia (Dandelion leaf, Pu Gong Ying)
- Taraxacum officinale radix (Dandelion root)
- Thymus vulgaris (Thyme)
- Trigonella foenum-graecum (Fenugreek)

Dyspepsia; flatulent

- Anethum graveolens (Dill)
- Angelica archangelica (European angelica, angelica)

- Artemisia absinthium (Wormwood, absinthe)
- Cinnamomum verum (Cinnamon, cassia bark, rou gui)
- Cnicus benedictus (Blessed or holy thistle)
- Foeniculum vulgare (Fennel)
- Lavandula angustifolia (Lavender)
- Matricaria chamomilla (Chamomile, German chamomile)
- Melissa officinalis (Lemon balm, Melissa)
- Mentha x piperita (Peppermint, Bo He)
- Petroselinum crispum (Parsley root)
- Salvia officinalis (Sage)
- Salvia rosmarinus (Rosemary)
- Zingiber officinale (Ginger, Sheng Jiang (fresh), Gan Jiang (dried))

Dyspepsia; nervous

- Althaea officinalis (Marshmallow, white mallow)
- Artemisia vulgaris (Mugwort)
- Ballota nigra (Black horehound)
- Eschscholzia californica (Californian poppy)
- Filipendula ulmaria (Meadowsweet)
- Humulus lupulus (Hops)
- Matricaria chamomilla (Chamomile, German chamomile)
- Melissa officinalis (Lemon balm, Melissa)
- Nepeta cataria (Catnip, catmint, Jing Jie)
- Prunus serotina (Wild cherry, black cherry)
- Turnera diffusa (Damiana)

Dysuria

- Agathosma betulina (Buchu)
- Arctostaphylos uva-ursi (Bearberry)
- Eutrochium purpureum (Gravel root, Joe Pye weed)
- Solidago virgaurea (Goldenrod)
- Terminalia arjuna (Arjuna)
- Viola tricolor (Heartsease, wild pansy, viola)

Eczema

- Albizia lebbeck (Albizia, sirisha)
- Althaea officinalis (Marshmallow, white mallow)
- Arctium lappa (Burdock)
- Berberis aquifolium (Oregon grape, mountain grape)
- Berberis vulgaris (Barberry)
- Calendula officinalis (Calendula, marigold)
- Carica papaya (Paw paw, papaya)
- Curcuma longa (Turmeric)
- Echinacea spp. (Echinacea)
- Fumaria officinalis (Fumitory)
- Galium aparine (Clivers, cleavers)
- Glycyrrhiza spp. (Licorice, Liquorice, Gan Cao)
- Hemidesmus indicus (Anantamul, Indian sarsparilla)

- Hydrastis canadensis (Goldenseal)
- Iris versicolor (Blue flag)
- Isatis tinctoria (Isatis, ban lan gen, woad, Chinese indigo)
- Juglans nigra (Black walnut)
- Macropiper excelsum (Kawakawa, New Zealand peppertree)
- Plantago lanceolata (Ribwort, narrow-leaved plantain)
- Quercus robur (Oak bark)
- Rumex crispus (Yellow dock, curled dock)
- Scrophularia nodosa (Figwort)
- Scutellaria baicalensis (Baikal skullcap, baical skullcap, Chinese skullcap, Huang qin (Mandarin), ogon (Japanese))
- Smilax ornata (Sarsaparilla)
- Stellaria media (Chickweed, starweed)
- Trifolium pratense (Red clover, trifoil)
- Urtica dioica folia (Nettle leaf, stinging nettle)
- Viola tricolor (Heartsease, wild pansy, viola)

Eczema (topically)

- Avena sativa (green) (Oats, green oats, oat straw)
- Avena sativa (seed) (Oats, groats, oatmeal)
- Calendula officinalis (Calendula, marigold)
- Hypericum perforatum (St John's wort)
- Matricaria chamomilla (Chamomile, German chamomile)
- Quercus robur (Oak bark)
- Stellaria media (Chickweed, starweed)

Emaciation

- Withania somnifera (Ashwaghanda, winter cherry)

Emphysema

- Asclepias tuberosa (Pleurisy root, butterfly weed)
- Euphorbia hirta (Euphorbia)
- Glycyrrhiza spp. (Licorice, Liquorice, Gan Cao)
- Hedera helix (Ivy leaf, English ivy)
- Inula helenium (Elecampane)
- Lobelia inflata (Indian tobacco)
- Panax ginseng (Ginseng, Ren Shen)
- Tussilago farfara (Coltsfoot)

Endometriosis

- Actaea racemosa (Black cohosh, squawroot, snakeroot)
- Anemone pulsatilla (Pulsatilla)
- Angelica polymorpha (Dong quai, dang gui, Chinese angelica)
- Caulophyllum thalictroides (Blue cohosh)
- Centella asiatica (Gotu kola, brahmi, Indian pennywort)
- Chamaelirium luteum (False unicorn root, helonias)
- Corydalis ambigua (Corydalis)

- Curcuma longa (Turmeric)
- Dioscorea spp. (Wild yam)
- Glycyrrhiza spp. (Licorice, Liquorice, Gan Cao)
- Paeonia lactiflora (Peony, white peony, Bai Shao)
- Salvia miltiorrhiza (Dan shen (Mandarin), red root sage)
- Viburnum opulus (Cramp bark)
- Vitex agnus-castus (Chaste tree, chasteberry, Man Jing Zi)
- Zingiber officinale (Ginger, Sheng Jiang (fresh), Gan Jiang (dried))

Enuresis

- Ephedra sinensis (Ma-huang)
- Equisetum arvense (Horsetail)
- Leptospermum scoparium (Manuka, tea tree)
- Thuja occidentalis (Thuja, white cedar, arbor-vitae (American))
- Thymus vulgaris (Thyme)
- Viburnum opulus (Cramp bark)
- Zea mays (Corn silk, maize)

Epilepsy

- Bacopa monnieri (Bacopa, brahmi)
- Paeonia lactiflora (Peony, white peony, Bai Shao)
- Reynoutria multiflora (He Shou Wu, Fo-Ti)
- Scutellaria lateriflora (Blue skulcap)
- Tilia cordata (Lime tree, linden)

Erectile dysfunction

- Crocus sativus (Saffron)
- Epimedium sagittatum (Horny goat weed, barrenwort, yin yang huo, Inyokaku)
- Panax ginseng (Ginseng, Ren Shen)
- Tribulus terrestris (calthrops, puncture vine, Bai Ji Li)

Excitability

- Humulus lupulus (Hops)
- Valeriana officinalis (Valerian, heliotrope, Mexican valerian (V. edulis))

Exhaustion

- Astragalus membranaceus (Astragalus, milk vetch, huang qi (Chinese), ogi (Japanese))
- Atractylodes macrocephala (Atractylodes, bai zhu)
- Avena sativa (green) (Oats, green oats, oat straw)
- Avena sativa (seed) (Oats, groats, oatmeal)
- Codonopsis pilosula (Dang shen, codonopsis)
- Cola spp. (Kola nut, cola nut)
- Eleutherococcus senticosus (Eleuthero, eleutherokokk, Siberian ginseng)
- Panax ginseng (Ginseng, Ren Shen)
- Panax quinquefolium (American ginseng)
- Rehmannia glutinosa (Rehmannia, sheng di huang (uncured), shu di huang (cured), Chinese foxglove)

- Rhodiola rosea (Golden root, rose root, arctic root)
- Withania somnifera (Ashwaghanda, winter cherry)

Fatigue

- Asparagus racemosus (Shatavari (Sanskrit), satavari (Hindi), satmuli (Bengali))
- Astragalus membranaceus (Astragalus, milk vetch, huang qi (Chinese), ogi (Japanese))
- Bryonia dioica (Bryony)
- Eleutherococcus senticosus (Eleuthero)
- Epimedium sagittatum (Horny goat weed, barrenwort, yin yang huo, Inyokaku)
- Ganoderma lucidum (Reishi, lingzhi)
- Gynostemma pentaphyllum (Jiaogulan, xiancao)
- Ligustrum lucidum (Glossy privet, nu zhen zi, joteishi)
- Panax ginseng (Ginseng, Ren Shen)
- Panax quinquefolium (American ginseng)
- Quercus robur (Oak bark)

Fever

- Achillea millefolium (Yarrow)
- Alpinia galanga (Greater galangal, Thai ginger)
- Annona muricata (Graviola, soursop, guanábana)
- Baptisia tinctoria (Wild indigo)
- Carica papaya (Paw paw, papaya)
- Centaurium erythraea (Centaury)
- Crocus sativus (Saffron)
- Cryptolepis sanguinolenta (Yellow dye root, delboi)
- Echinacea spp. (Echinacea)
- Ephedra sinensis (Ma-huang)
- Isatis tinctoria (Isatis, ban lan gen, woad, Chinese indigo)
- Lobelia inflata (Indian tobacco)
- Lomatium dissectum (Fern-leaf biscuit root, tohza, desert parsley)
- Melissa officinalis (Lemon balm, Melissa)
- Mentha x piperita (Peppermint, Bo He)
- Myrica cerifera (Bayberry, candleberry, wax myrtle)
- Nigella sativa (Black cumin)
- Ocimum tenuiflorum (Tulsi, Holy basil)
- Phyllanthus spp. (Phyllanthus)
- Sambucus nigra (Elder, elderflower, elderberry, sambuco)
- Tilia cordata (Lime tree, linden)
- Usnea spp. (Old man's beard, songluo)
- Verbena officinalis (Vervain)
- Zingiber officinale (Ginger, Sheng Jiang (fresh), Gan Jiang (dried))

Fever; childhood

- Hyssopus officinalis (Hyssop)
- Melissa officinalis (Lemon balm, Melissa)
- Mentha x piperita (Peppermint, Bo He)

Fibroids

- Actaea racemosa (Black cohosh, squawroot, snakeroot)
- Chamaelirium luteum (False unicorn root, helonias)
- Paeonia lactiflora (Peony, white peony, Bai Shao)
- Panax notoginseng (Tienchi ginseng (san qi, tian qi – Mandarin) Yunnan bayou)
- Poria cocos (Hoelen, China root, sclerotium of tuckahoe, fu ling (Mandarin) and bukuryo (Japanese))
- Ruta graveolens (Rue)
- Turnera diffusa (Damiana)
- Vitex agnus-castus (Chaste tree, chasteberry, Man Jing Zi)

Flatulence

- Aletris farinosa (True unicorn root, white colic root)
- Andrographis paniculata (Andrographis, kalmegh)
- Angelica archangelica (European angelica, angelica)
- Apium graveolens (Celery seed, karafs)
- Cinnamomum verum (Cinnamon, cassia bark, rou gui)
- Dioscorea spp. (Wild yam)
- Filipendula ulmaria (Meadowsweet)
- Gentiana lutea (Gentian)
- Juniperus communis (Juniper)
- Lamium album (White dead nettle)
- Matricaria chamomilla (Chamomile, German chamomile)
- Melissa officinalis (Lemon balm, Melissa)
- Mentha pulegium (Pennyroyal)
- Mentha x piperita (Peppermint, Bo He)
- Pimpinella anisum (Aniseed)
- Ulmus fulva (Slippery elm, red elm)

Flavouring

- Anethum graveolens (Dill)
- Glycyrrhiza spp. (Licorice, Liquorice, Gan Cao)
- Mentha x piperita (Peppermint, Bo He)

Fluid retention

- Aesculus hippocastanum (Horse chestnut)
- Apium graveolens (Celery seed, karafs)
- Asparagus racemosus (Shatavari (Sanskrit), satavari (Hindi), satmuli (Bengali))
- Galega officinalis (Goat's rue)
- Pinus pinaster (Maritime bark)
- Poria cocos (Hoelen, China root, sclerotium of tuckahoe, fu ling (Mandarin) and bukuryo (Japanese))
- Taraxacum officinale folia (Dandelion leaf, pu gong ying)

Fluid retention; premenstrual

- Aesculus hippocastanum (Horse chestnut)

- Taraxacum officinale folia (Dandelion leaf, Pu Gong Ying)

Follicular cyst

- Vitex agnus-castus (Chaste tree, chasteberry, man jing zi)

Furunculosis

- Baptisia tinctoria (Wild indigo)
- Echinacea spp. (Echinacea)

Galactorrhoea

- Salvia officinalis (Sage)

Gall stones (cholelithiasis)

- Asparagus racemosus (Shatavari (Sanskrit), satavari (Hindi), satmuli (Bengali))
- Berberis aquifolium (Oregon grape, mountain grape)
- Berberis vulgaris (Barberry)
- Chelidonium majus (Greater celandine)
- Chionanthus virginicus (Fringe tree, old man's beard)
- Cynara scolymus (Globe artichoke)
- Hedera helix (Ivy leaf, English ivy)
- Peumus boldus (Boldo)

Gallbladder disorders

- Berberis aquifolium (Oregon grape, mountain grape)
- Berberis vulgaris (Barberry)
- Cynara scolymus (Globe artichoke)
- Dioscorea spp. (Wild yam)
- Fumaria officinalis (Fumitory)
- Juglans cinerea (Butternut bark, white walnut, lemon walnut)
- Peumus boldus (Boldo)
- Silybum marianum (St Mary's thistle, milk thistle, silymarin)
- Taraxacum officinale folia (Dandelion leaf, Pu Gong Ying)
- Taraxacum officinale radix (Dandelion root)

Gastric reflux

- Filipendula ulmaria (Meadowsweet)
- Mentha x piperita (Peppermint, Bo He)
- Ulmus fulva (Slippery elm, red elm)

Gastritis

- Alpinia galanga (Greater galangal, Thai ginger)
- Althaea officinalis (Marshmallow, white mallow)
- Bidens tripartita (Burr marigold, water agrimony, gui zhen cao, longbacao)
- Calendula officinalis (Calendula, marigold)
- Collinsonia canadensis (Stone root)
- Filipendula ulmaria (Meadowsweet)
- Glechoma hederacea (Ground ivy)
- Glycyrrhiza spp. (Licorice, Liquorice, Gan Cao)

- Hydrastis canadensis (Goldenseal)
- Lamium album (White dead nettle)
- Macropiper excelsum (Kawakawa, New Zealand peppertree)
- Matricaria chamomilla (Chamomile, German chamomile)
- Poria cocos (Hoelen, China root, sclerotium of tuckahoe, fu ling (Mandarin) and bukuryo (Japanese))
- Rosa canina (Rosehip, dog rose)
- Thymus vulgaris (Thyme)
- Trigonella foenum-graecum (Fenugreek)
- Ulmus fulva (Slippery elm, red elm)
- Uncaria tomentosa (Cat's claw)

Gastroenteritis

- Althaea officinalis (Marshmallow, white mallow)
- Cryptolepis sanguinolenta (Yellow dye root, delboi)
- Isatis tinctoria (Isatis, ban lan gen, woad, Chinese indigo)
- Phyllanthus spp. (Phyllanthus)

Gastrointestinal amoebiasis

- Cryptolepis sanguinolenta (Yellow dye root, delboi)
- Euphorbia hirta (Euphorbia)

Gastrointestinal catarrh

- Angelica archangelica (European angelica, angelica)
- Berberis aquifolium (Oregon grape, mountain grape)
- Berberis vulgaris (Barberry)
- Citrus reticulata (Chen pi, mandarin, tangerine)
- Filipendula ulmaria (Meadowsweet)
- Hydrastis canadensis (Goldenseal)
- Lamium album (White dead nettle)
- Matricaria chamomilla (Chamomile, German chamomile)
- Mitchella repens (Partridgeberry)
- Ulmus fulva (Slippery elm, red elm)

Gastrointestinal tract dysbiosis

- Coptis chinensis (Huanglian (China), makino (Japan))
- Euphorbia hirta (Euphorbia)
- Handroanthus impetiginosus (Pau d'arco, lapacho (Spanish))
- Hydrastis canadensis (Goldenseal)
- Matricaria chamomilla (Chamomile, German chamomile)
- Propolis (Propolis)
- Ulmus fulva (Slippery elm, red elm)

Gastrointestinal tract infestation

- Andrographis paniculata (Andrographis, kalmegh)
- Artemisia vulgaris (Mugwort)
- Atractylodes macrocephala (Atractylodes, bai zhu)

- Euphorbia hirta (Euphorbia)
- Hydrastis canadensis (Goldenseal)

Gingivitis

- Baptisia tinctoria (Wild indigo)
- Bistorta officinalis (Bistort, common bistort, European bistort or meadow bistort)
- Carica papaya (Paw paw, papaya)
- Commiphora myrrha (Myrrh)
- Echinacea spp. (Echinacea)
- Isodon rubescens (Dong ling cao, Chinese sage bush, rabdosia)
- Justicia adhatoda (Basak, vasaka, Malabar nut)
- Leptospermum scoparium (Manuka, tea tree)
- Lomatium dissectum (Fern-leaf biscuit root, tohza, desert parsley)
- Matricaria chamomilla (Chamomile, German chamomile)
- Pinus pinaster (Maritime bark)
- Propolis (Propolis)
- Verbena officinalis (Vervain)

Glands; swollen

- Calendula officinalis (Calendula, marigold)
- Echinacea spp. (Echinacea)
- Galium aparine (Clivers, cleavers)
- Phytolacca americana (Poke root, pokeweed)

Gout

- Agathosma betulina (Buchu)
- Apium graveolens (Celery seed, karafs)
- Arctium lappa (Burdock)
- Berberis aquifolium (Oregon grape, mountain grape)
- Berberis vulgaris (Barberry)
- Betula pendula (Silver birch)
- Bidens tripartita (Burr marigold, water agrimony, gui zhen cao, longbacao)
- Elymus repens (Couch grass)
- Eupatorium perfoliatum (Boneset, feverwort)
- Eutrochium purpureum (Gravel root, Joe Pye weed)
- Filipendula ulmaria (Meadowsweet)
- Galium aparine (Clivers, cleavers)
- Glycyrrhiza spp. (Licorice, Liquorice, Gan Cao)
- Guaiacum officinale (Guaiacum)
- Harpagophytum procumbens (Devil's claw)
- Matricaria chamomilla (Chamomile, German chamomile)
- Olea europaea (Olive tree)
- Rumex crispus (Yellow dock, curled dock)
- Salix spp. (Willow bark, white willow)
- Smilax ornata (Sarsaparilla)
- Urtica dioica folia (Nettle leaf, stinging nettle)

Graves' disease

- Leonurus cardiaca (Motherwort)
- Lycopus spp. (Bugleweed, gypsy wort)

Gums; bleeding

- Vaccinium myrtillus (Bilberry, blueberry)
- Vitis vinifera (Grape vine, grapeseed extract)

Haematemesis

- Geranium maculatum (Cranesbill)
- Panax notoginseng (Tienchi ginseng (san qi, tian qi – Mandarin) Yunnan bayou)

Haematuria

- Agathosma betulina (Buchu)
- Panax notoginseng (Tienchi ginseng (san qi, tian qi – Mandarin) Yunnan bayou)
- Plantago major (Plantain, broad-leaved plantain, Che Qian Zi)
- Rehmannia glutinosa (Rehmannia, sheng di huang (uncured), shu di huang (cured), Chinese foxglove)
- Trillium erectum (Beth root, birth root)

Haemorrhage; postpartum

- Alchemilla vulgaris (Lady's mantle)
- Justicia adhatoda (Basak, vasaka, Malabar nut)
- Mitchella repens (Partridgeberry)
- Panax notoginseng (Tienchi ginseng (san qi, tian qi – Mandarin) Yunnan bayou)
- Trillium erectum (Beth root, birth root)

Haemorrhoids

- Aesculus hippocastanum (Horse chestnut)
- Berberis aristata (Daruharidra, Daruhaldi, Darvi, Chitra, Indian barberry)
- Bidens tripartita (Burr marigold, water agrimony, gui zhen cao, longbacao)
- Geranium maculatum (Cranesbill)
- Glechoma hederacea (Ground ivy)
- Hamamelis virginiana (Witch hazel)
- Isatis tinctoria (Isatis, ban lan gen, woad, Chinese indigo)
- Nigella sativa (Black cumin)
- Plantago lanceolata (Ribwort, narrow-leaved plantain)
- Plantago major (Plantain, broad-leaved plantain, Che Qian Zi)
- Quercus robur (Oak bark)
- Ruscus aculeatus (Butcher's broom, box holly)

Haemorrhoids (topically)

- Aesculus hippocastanum (Horse chestnut)
- Bistorta officinalis (Bistort, common bistort, European bistort or meadow bistort)
- Calendula officinalis (Calendula, marigold)
- Collinsonia canadensis (Stone root)
- Commiphora myrrha (Myrrh)

- Hamamelis virginiana (Witch hazel)
- Matricaria chamomilla (Chamomile, German chamomile)
- Punica granatum (Pomegranate)
- Quercus robur (Oak bark)
- Uncaria tomentosa (Cat's claw)

Halitosis
- Gentiana lutea (Gentian)
- Mentha x piperita (Peppermint, Bo He)
- Zingiber officinale (Ginger, Sheng Jiang (fresh), Gan Jiang (dried))

Hayfever
- Albizia lebbeck (Albizia, sirisha)
- Armoracia rusticana (Horseradish)
- Echinacea spp. (Echinacea)
- Ephedra sinensis (Ma-huang) Euphrasia officinalis (Eyebright)
- Matricaria chamomilla (Chamomile, German chamomile)
- Perilla frutescens (Perilla, su zi, shisu)
- Plectranthus barbatus (Coleus, makandi)
- Scutellaria baicalensis (Baikal skullcap, baical skullcap, Chinese skullcap, Huang qin (Mandarin), ogon (Japanese))
- Uncaria tomentosa (Cat's claw)

Headache
- Anemone pulsatilla (Pulsatilla)
- Corydalis ambigua (Corydalis)
- Isodon rubescens (Dong ling cao, Chinese sage bush, rabdosia)
- Lavandula angustifolia (Lavender)
- Nepeta cataria (Catnip, catmint, Jing Jie)
- Nigella sativa (Black cumin)
- Piper methysticum (Kava)
- Salvia rosmarinus (Rosemary)
- Syzygium aromaticum (Cloves)
- Usnea spp. (Old man's beard, songluo)
- Vinca minor (Periwinkle, lesser or common periwinkle)
- Viscum album (Mistletoe)

Hepatic steatosis
- Dipsacus asper (Teasel root)
- Ligustrum lucidum (Glossy privet, nu zhen zi, joteishi)

Hepatitis
- Andrographis paniculata (Andrographis, kalmegh)
- Astragalus membranaceus (Astragalus, milk vetch, huang qi (Chinese), ogi (Japanese))
- Berberis aristata (Daruharidra, Daruhaldi, Darvi, Chitra, Indian barberry)
- Codonopsis pilosula (Dang shen, codonopsis)
- Cordyceps militaris (Cordyceps, orange

catapillar fungus, dong chong xia cao (China), hyakurakusou (Japan))
- Cryptolepis sanguinolenta (Yellow dye root, delboi)
- Cynara scolymus (Globe artichoke)
- Ganoderma lucidum (Reishi, lingzhi)
- Glycyrrhiza spp. (Licorice, Liquorice, Gan Cao)
- Isodon rubescens (Dong ling cao, Chinese sage bush, rabdosia)
- Nigella sativa (Black cumin)
- Phyllanthus spp. (Phyllanthus)
- Picrorhiza kurroa (Kutki)
- Punica granatum (Pomegranate)
- Salvia rosmarinus (Rosemary)
- Schisandra chinensis (Bei-Wuweizi, Schisandra, Chinese magnolia vine, Wu Wei Zi)
- Scutellaria baicalensis (Baikal skullcap, baical skullcap, Chinese skullcap, Huang qin (Mandarin), ogon (Japanese))
- Silybum marianum (St Mary's thistle, milk thistle, silymarin)
- Trametes versicolor (Turkey tail PSK, PSP)

Herpes (topically)
- Avena sativa (green) (Oats, green oats, oat straw)
- Glycyrrhiza spp. (Licorice, Liquorice, Gan Cao)
- Melissa officinalis (Lemon balm, Melissa)
- Uncaria tomentosa (Cat's claw)

Herpes simplex
- Avena sativa (green) (Oats, green oats, oat straw)
- Calendula officinalis (Calendula, marigold)
- Echinacea spp. (Echinacea)
- Hypericum perforatum (St John's wort)
- Matricaria chamomilla (Chamomile, German chamomile)
- Melissa officinalis (Lemon balm, Melissa)

Hyperactivity
- Anemone pulsatilla (Pulsatilla)
- Eschscholzia californica (Californian poppy)
- Ulmus fulva (Slippery elm, red elm)
- Valeriana officinalis (Valerian, heliotrope, Mexican valerian (V. edulis))

Hyperchlorhydria
- Filipendula ulmaria (Meadowsweet)
- Hyperhydrosis including sweating with menopause
- Salvia officinalis (Sage)

Hypertension
- Achillea millefolium (Yarrow)
- Actaea racemosa (Black cohosh, squawroot, snakeroot)
- Alchemilla vulgaris (Lady's mantle)
- Allium sativum (Garlic)

- Alpinia galanga (Greater galangal, Thai ginger)
- Angelica polymorpha (Dong quai, dang gui, Chinese angelica)
- Annona muricata (Graviola, soursop, guanábana)
- Astragalus membranaceus (Astragalus, milk vetch, huang qi (Chinese), ogi (Japanese))
- Avena sativa (seed) (Oats, groats, oatmeal)
- Calendula officinalis (Calendula, marigold)
- Carica papaya (Paw paw, papaya)
- Centaurium erythraea (Centaury)
- Coptis chinensis (Huanglian (China), makino (Japan))
- Crataegus monogyna (Hawthorn)
- Cryptolepis sanguinolenta (Yellow dye root, delboi)
- Glycine max (Soy, soy germ, soy isoflavones (genistein), phyto-oestrogens, tofu (bean curd))
- Gynostemma pentaphyllum (Jiaogulan, xiancao)
- Handroanthus impetiginosus (Pau d'arco, lapacho (Spanish))
- Harpagophytum procumbens (Devil's claw)
- Hedera helix (Ivy leaf, English ivy)
- Nigella sativa (Black cumin)
- Olea europaea (Olive tree)
- Pinus pinaster (Maritime bark)
- Piper methysticum (Kava)
- Plectranthus barbatus (Coleus, makandi)
- Pueraria lobata (Kudzu)
- Ruta graveolens (Rue)
- Salvia miltiorrhiza (Dan shen (Mandarin), red root sage)
- Scutellaria baicalensis (Baikal skullcap, baical skullcap, Chinese skullcap, Huang qin (Mandarin), ogon (Japanese))
- Stachys officinalis (Wood betony)
- Stevia rebaudiana (Stevia)
- Terminalia arjuna (Arjuna)
- Tilia cordata (Lime tree, linden)
- Valeriana officinalis (Valerian, heliotrope, Mexican valerian (V. edulis))
- Vinca minor (Periwinkle, lesser periwinkle)
- Viscum album (Mistletoe)
- Withania somnifera (Ashwaghanda, winter cherry)
- Ziziphus jujuba var. spinosa (Zizyphus, sour Chinese date, jujube, Da Zao, Suan Zao Ren)

Hyperthyroidism

- Leonurus cardiaca (Motherwort)
- Lycopus spp. (Bugleweed, gypsy wort)

Hypochlorhydria

- Agrimonia eupatoria (Agrimony)
- Andrographis paniculata (Andrographis, kalmegh)
- Angelica archangelica (European angelica, angelica)

- Capsicum spp. (Chilli, capsicum, pepper, paprika, cayenne)
- Gentiana lutea (Gentian)
- Hydrastis canadensis (Goldenseal)
- Zingiber officinale (Ginger)

Hypoglycaemia

- Avena sativa (seed) (Oats, groats, oatmeal)
- Bupleurum falcatum (Bupleurum, sickle-leaved hare's ear)
- Codonopsis pilosula (Dang shen, codonopsis)
- Gymnema sylvestre (Gumar, meshashringi)

Hysterectomy recovery

- Aletris farinosa (True unicorn root, white colic root)

Immune deficiency

- Andrographis paniculata (Andrographis, kalmegh)
- Astragalus membranaceus (Astragalus, milk vetch, huang qi (Chinese), ogi (Japanese))
- Cordyceps militaris (Cordyceps, orange catapillar fungus, dong chong xia cao (China), hyakurakusou (Japan))
- Echinacea spp. (Echinacea)
- Eleutherococcus senticosus (Eleuthero, eleutherokokk, Siberian ginseng)
- Ganoderma lucidum (Reishi, lingzhi)
- Handroanthus impetiginosus (Pau d'arco, lapacho)
- Panax ginseng (Ginseng, Ren Shen)
- Picrorhiza kurroa (Kutki)
- Trametes versicolor (Turkey tail PSK, PSP)
- Uncaria tomentosa (Cat's claw)
- Withania somnifera (Ashwaghanda, winter cherry)

Impotence

- Panax ginseng (Ginseng, Ren Shen)
- Tribulus terrestris (Tribulus, calthrops, puncture vine, Bai Ji Li)
- Withania somnifera (Ashwaghanda, winter cherry)

Incontinence

- Collinsonia canadensis (Stone root)
- Crateva magna (Varuna)
- Leptospermum scoparium (Manuka, tea tree)

Indigestion

- Annona muricata (Graviola, soursop, guanábana)
- Apium graveolens (Celery seed, karafs)
- Artemisia absinthium (Wormwood, absinthe)
- Atractylodes macrocephala (Atractylodes, bai zhu)
- Carica papaya (Paw paw, papaya)
- Codonopsis pilosula (Dang shen, codonopsis)
- Filipendula ulmaria (Meadowsweet)
- Foeniculum vulgare (Fennel)
- Gynostemma pentaphyllum (Jiaogulan, xiancao)
- Matricaria chamomilla (Chamomile, German chamomile)

- Mentha x piperita (Peppermint, Bo He)
- Rumex crispus (Yellow dock, curled dock)
- Stachys officinalis (Wood betony)
- Syzygium aromaticum (Cloves)
- Ulmus fulva (Slippery elm, red elm)

Infection; bacterial

- Alpinia galanga (Greater galangal, Thai ginger)
- Annona muricata (Graviola, soursop, guanábana)
- Astragalus membranaceus (Astragalus, milk vetch, huang qi (Chinese), ogi (Japanese))
- Houttuynia cordata (Yu Xing Cao, chameleon plant, fish mint)
- Isodon rubescens (Dong ling cao, Chinese sage bush, rabdosia)
- Pseudowintera colorata (Horopito)
- Syzygium aromaticum (Cloves)

Infection; fungal

- Alpinia galanga (Greater galangal, Thai ginger)
- Berberis aristata (Daruharidra, Daruhaldi, Darvi, Chitra, Indian barberry)
- Echinacea spp. (Echinacea)
- Houttuynia cordata (Yu Xing Cao, chameleon plant, fish mint)
- Propolis (Propolis)
- Pseudowintera colorata (Horopito)
- Syzygium aromaticum (Cloves)
- Uncaria tomentosa (Cat's claw)
- Usnea spp. (Old man's beard, songluo)

Infection; gastrointestinal system

- Allium sativum (Garlic)
- Alpinia galanga (Greater galangal, Thai ginger)
- Astragalus membranaceus (Astragalus, milk vetch, huang qi (Chinese), ogi (Japanese))
- Berberis aristata (Daruharidra, Daruhaldi, Darvi, Chitra, Indian barberry)
- Bidens tripartita (Burr marigold, water agrimony, gui zhen cao, longbacao)
- Bupleurum falcatum (Bupleurum, sickle-leaved hare's ear)
- Calendula officinalis (Calendula, marigold)
- Carica papaya (Paw paw, papaya)
- Echinacea spp. (Echinacea)
- Ganoderma lucidum (Reishi, lingzhi)
- Hydrastis canadensis (Goldenseal)
- Olea europaea (Olive tree)
- Propolis (Propolis)
- Scutellaria baicalensis (Baikal skullcap, baical skullcap, Chinese skullcap, Huang qin (Mandarin), ogon (Japanese))
- Stellaria media (Chickweed, starweed)
- Trametes versicolor (Turkey tail PSK, PSP)
- Ulmus fulva (Slippery elm, red elm)

Infection; genitourinary tract

- Berberis aristata (Daruharidra, Daruhaldi, Darvi, Chitra, Indian barberry)
- Cryptolepis sanguinolenta (Yellow dye root, delboi)
- Usnea spp. (Old man's beard, songluo)

Infection; protozoal

- Berberis aristata (Daruharidra, Daruhaldi, Darvi, Chitra, Indian barberry)
- Echinacea spp. (Echinacea)
- Propolis (Propolis)

Infection; respiratory tract

- Allium sativum (Garlic)
- Alpinia galanga (Greater galangal, Thai ginger)
- Andrographis paniculata (Andrographis, kalmegh)
- Angelica archangelica (European angelica, angelica)
- Annona muricata (Graviola, soursop, guanábana)
- Berberis aristata (Daruharidra, Daruhaldi, Darvi, Chitra, Indian barberry)
- Bidens tripartita (Burr marigold, water agrimony, gui zhen cao, longbacao)
- Cryptolepis sanguinolenta (Yellow dye root, delboi)
- Echinacea spp. (Echinacea)
- Ephedra sinensis (Ma-huang)
- Hedera helix (Ivy leaf, English ivy)
- Houttuynia cordata (Yu Xing Cao, chameleon plant, fish mint)
- Inula helenium (Elecampane)
- Isatis tinctoria (Isatis, ban lan gen, woad, Chinese indigo)
- Lomatium dissectum (Fern-leaf biscuit root, tohza, desert parsley)
- Propolis (Propolis)
- Scutellaria baicalensis (Baikal skullcap, baical skullcap, Chinese skullcap, Huang qin (Mandarin), ogon (Japanese))
- Thymus vulgaris (Thyme)
- Trametes versicolor (Turkey tail PSK, PSP)
- Usnea spp. (Old man's beard, songluo)

Infection; skin

- Andrographis paniculata (Andrographis, kalmegh)
- Berberis aquifolium (Oregon grape, mountain grape)
- Berberis aristata (Daruharidra, Daruhaldi, Darvi, Chitra, Indian barberry)
- Bidens tripartita (Burr marigold, water agrimony, gui zhen cao, longbacao)
- Calendula officinalis (Calendula, marigold)
- Carica papaya (Paw paw, papaya)
- Echinacea spp. (Echinacea)
- Leptospermum scoparium (Manuka, tea tree)

Infection; systemic

- Andrographis paniculata (Andrographis, kalmegh)
- Astragalus membranaceus (Astragalus, milk vetch, huang qi (Chinese), ogi (Japanese))
- Echinacea spp. (Echinacea)
- Eleutherococcus senticosus (Eleuthero, eleutherokokk, Siberian ginseng)
- Picrorhiza kurroa (Kutki)
- Uncaria tomentosa (Cat's claw)

Infection; throat

- Baptisia tinctoria (Wild indigo)
- Bidens tripartita (Burr marigold, water agrimony, gui zhen cao, longbacao)
- Echinacea spp. (Echinacea)
- Solidago virgaurea (Goldenrod)
- Thuja occidentalis (Thuja, white cedar, arbor-vitae (American))
- Thymus vulgaris (Thyme)

Infection; to improve resistance to

- Andrographis paniculata (Andrographis, kalmegh)
- Astragalus membranaceus (Astragalus, milk vetch, huang qi (Chinese), ogi (Japanese))
- Echinacea spp. (Echinacea)
- Eleutherococcus senticosus (Eleuthero, eleutherokokk, Siberian ginseng)
- Panax ginseng (Ginseng, Ren Shen)

Infection; urinary tract

- Althaea officinalis (Marshmallow, white mallow)
- Andrographis paniculata (Andrographis, kalmegh)
- Armoracia rusticana (Horseradish)
- Bidens tripartita (Burr marigold, water agrimony, gui zhen cao, longbacao)
- Elymus repens (Couch grass)
- Houttuynia cordata (Yu Xing Cao, chameleon plant, fish mint)
- Lomatium dissectum (Fern-leaf biscuit root, tohza, desert parsley)
- Nigella sativa (Black cumin)

Infection; viral

- Andrographis paniculata (Andrographis, kalmegh)
- Astragalus membranaceus (Astragalus, milk vetch, huang qi (Chinese), ogi (Japanese))
- Echinacea spp. (Echinacea)
- Houttuynia cordata (Yu Xing Cao, chameleon plant, fish mint)
- Hypericum perforatum (St John's wort)
- Isatis tinctoria (Isatis, ban lan gen, woad, Chinese indigo)
- Lomatium dissectum (Fern-leaf biscuit root, tohza, desert parsley)
- Phyllanthus spp. (Phyllanthus)
- Propolis (Propolis)

- Punica granatum (Pomegranate)

Infertility

- Aletris farinosa (True unicorn root, white colic root)
- Angelica polymorpha (Dong quai, dang gui, Chinese angelica)
- Asparagus racemosus (Shatavari (Sanskrit), satavari (Hindi), satmuli (Bengali))
- Chamaelirium luteum (False unicorn root, helonias)
- Crocus sativus (Saffron)
- Epimedium sagittatum (Horny goat weed, barrenwort, yin yang huo, Inyokaku)
- Glycyrrhiza spp. (Licorice, Liquorice, Gan Cao)
- Paeonia lactiflora (Peony, white peony, Bai Shao)
- Poria cocos (Hoelen, China root, sclerotium of tuckahoe, fu ling (Mandarin) and bukuryo (Japanese))
- Tribulus terrestris (Tribulus, calthrops, puncture vine, Bai Ji Li)
- Vitex agnus-castus (Chaste tree, chasteberry, Man Jing Zi)

Inflammation

- Cnicus benedictus (Blessed or holy thistle)
- Poria cocos (Hoelen, China root, sclerotium of tuckahoe, fu ling (Mandarin) and bukuryo (Japanese))
- Pseudowintera colorata (Horopito)
- Withania somnifera (Ashwaghanda, winter cherry)

Inflammation; gastrointestinal tract

- Aloe ferox (Aloe vera (gel), bitter aloes (resin))
- Alpinia galanga (Greater galangal, Thai ginger)
- Althaea officinalis (Marshmallow, white mallow)
- Angelica archangelica (European angelica, angelica)
- Arctium lappa (Burdock)
- Asparagus racemosus (Shatavari (Sanskrit), satavari (Hindi), satmuli (Bengali))
- Calendula officinalis (Calendula, marigold)
- Filipendula ulmaria (Meadowsweet)
- Matricaria chamomilla (Chamomile, German chamomile)
- Ulmus fulva (Slippery elm, red elm)

Inflammation; kidney and bladder

- Cordyceps militaris (Cordyceps, orange cataplillar fungus, dong chong xia cao (China), hyakurakusou (Japan))
- Elymus repens (Couch grass)
- Epilobium parviflorum (Willow herb)

Inflammation; oral cavity

- Althaea officinalis (Marshmallow, white mallow)
- Echinacea spp. (Echinacea)
- Matricaria chamomilla (Chamomile, German chamomile)

- Propolis (Propolis)
- Rubus idaeus (Raspberry leaf)
- Salvia officinalis (Sage)
- Thymus vulgaris (Thyme)

Inflammation; ovaries/testes
- Anemone pulsatilla (Pulsatilla)

Inflammation; pelvic
- Chamaelirium luteum (False unicorn root, helonias)

Inflammation; respiratory tract
- Alpinia galanga (Greater galangal, Thai ginger)
- Althaea officinalis (Marshmallow, white mallow)
- Ephedra sinensis (Ma-huang)
- Glycyrrhiza spp. (Licorice, Liquorice, Gan Cao)
- Phytolacca americana (Poke root, pokeweed)

Inflammation; skin (topically)
- Achillea millefolium (Yarrow)
- Aloe ferox (Aloe vera (gel), bitter aloes (resin))
- Macropiper excelsum (Kawakawa, New Zealand peppertree)
- Pseudowintera colorata (Horopito)

Inflammatory bowel disease
- Angelica archangelica (European angelica, angelica)
- Cinnamomum verum (Cinnamon, cassia bark, rou gui)
- Filipendula ulmaria (Meadowsweet)
- Foeniculum vulgare (Fennel)
- Matricaria chamomilla (Chamomile, German chamomile)
- Melissa officinalis (Lemon balm, Melissa)
- Mentha x piperita (Peppermint, Bo He)
- Nepeta cataria (Catnip, catmint, Jing Jie)
- Pimpinella anisum (Aniseed)
- Ulmus fulva (Slippery elm, red elm)

Influenza
- Andrographis paniculata (Andrographis, kalmegh)
- Asclepias tuberosa (Pleurisy root, butterfly weed)
- Bidens tripartita (Burr marigold, water agrimony, gui zhen cao, longbacao)
- Cinnamomum verum (Cinnamon, cassia bark, rou gui)
- Coptis chinensis (Huanglian (China), makino (Japan))
- Echinacea spp. (Echinacea)
- Ephedra sinensis (Ma-huang)
- Eupatorium perfoliatum (Boneset, feverwort)
- Eutrochium purpureum (Gravel root, Joe Pye weed)
- Isatis tinctoria (Isatis, ban lan gen, woad, Chinese indigo)
- Leptospermum scoparium (Manuka, tea tree)

- Lomatium dissectum (Fern-leaf biscuit root, tohza, desert parsley)
- Melissa officinalis (Lemon balm, Melissa)
- Ocimum tenuiflorum (Tulsi, Holy basil)
- Pelargonium sidoides (African geranium, umckaloabo (severe cough in Zulu))
- Salix spp. (Willow bark, white willow)
- Sambucus nigra (Elder, elderflower, elderberry)
- Solidago virgaurea (Goldenrod)
- Verbascum thapsus (Mullein, candlewick plant, flannel-leaf, bunny's ears)

Insomnia
- Alchemilla vulgaris (Lady's mantle)
- Anemone pulsatilla (Pulsatilla)
- Angelica archangelica (European angelica, angelica)
- Avena sativa (green) (Oats, green oats, oat straw)
- Avena sativa (seed) (Oats, groats, oatmeal)
- Ballota nigra (Black horehound)
- Corydalis ambigua (Corydalis)
- Cryptolepis sanguinolenta (Yellow dye root, delboi)
- Eschscholzia californica (Californian poppy)
- Humulus lupulus (Hops)
- Hypericum perforatum (St John's wort)
- Leptospermum scoparium (Manuka, tea tree)
- Magnolia officinalis (Magnolia, Hou po)
- Matricaria chamomilla (Chamomile, German chamomile)
- Melissa officinalis (Lemon balm, Melissa)
- Nepeta cataria (Catnip, catmint, Jing Jie)
- Passiflora incarnata (Passion flower)
- Piper methysticum (Kava)
- Piscidia piscipula (Jamaican dogwood)
- Poria cocos (Hoelen, China root, sclerotium of tuckahoe, fu ling (Mandarin) and bukuryo (Japanese))
- Reynoutria multiflora (He Shou Wu, Fo-Ti)
- Scutellaria lateriflora (Blue skulcap)
- Tribulus terrestris (Tribulus, calthrops, puncture vine, Bai Ji Li)
- Valeriana officinalis (Valerian, heliotrope, Mexican valerian (V. edulis))
- Vitex agnus-castus (Chaste tree, chasteberry, Man Jing Zi)
- Ziziphus jujuba var. spinosa (Zizyphus, sour Chinese date, jujube, Da Zao, Suan Zao Ren)

Intermittent claudication
- Capsicum spp. (Chilli, capsicum, pepper, paprika, cayenne)
- Dioscorea spp. (Wild yam)
- Ginkgo biloba (Maidenhair)
- Pseudowintera colorata (Horopito)

- Salvia miltiorrhiza (Dan shen (Mandarin), red root sage)
- Zanthoxylum clava-herculis (Prickly ash)

Intestinal worms
- Annona muricata (Graviola, soursop, guanábana)
- Artemisia absinthium (Wormwood, absinthe)
- Artemisia annua (Sweet Annie, Chinese wormwood, qing hao)
- Artemisia vulgaris (Mugwort)
- Echinacea spp. (Echinacea)
- Juglans nigra (Black walnut)
- Nigella sativa (Black cumin)
- Ruta graveolens (Rue)
- Syzygium aromaticum (Cloves)
- Vitis vinifera (Grape vine, grapeseed extract)

Irritability
- Hypericum perforatum (St John's wort)
- Matricaria chamomilla (Chamomile, German chamomile)
- Ziziphus jujuba var. spinosa (Zizyphus, sour Chinese date, jujube, Da Zao, Suan Zao Ren)

Irritable bowel syndrome
- Aloe ferox (Aloe vera (gel), bitter aloes (resin))
- Commiphora myrrha (Myrrh)
- Coptis chinensis (Huanglian (China), makino (Japan))
- Echinacea spp. (Echinacea)
- Filipendula ulmaria (Meadowsweet)
- Glycyrrhiza spp. (Licorice, Liquorice, Gan Cao)
- Magnolia officinalis (Magnolia, Hou po)
- Matricaria chamomilla (Chamomile, German chamomile)
- Melissa officinalis (Lemon balm, Melissa)
- Mentha x piperita (Peppermint, Bo He)
- Paeonia lactiflora (Peony, white peony, Bai Shao)
- Syzygium aromaticum (Cloves)

Jaundice
- Berberis aristata (Daruharidra, Daruhaldi, Darvi, Chitra, Indian barberry)
- Berberis vulgaris (Barberry)
- Chionanthus virginicus (Fringe tree, old man's beard)
- Nigella sativa (Black cumin)
- Rumex crispus (Yellow dock, curled dock)
- Silybum marianum (St Mary's thistle, milk thistle, silymarin)
- Taraxacum officinale radix (Dandelion root)
- Verbascum thapsus (Mullein, candlewick plant, flannel-leaf, bunny's ears)
- Verbena officinalis (Vervain)

Lactation; poor
- Asparagus racemosus (Shatavari (Sanskrit), satavari (Hindi), satmuli (Bengali))
- Foeniculum vulgare (Fennel)
- Galega officinalis (Goat's rue)
- Trigonella foenum-graecum (Fenugreek)
- Vitex agnus-castus (Chaste tree, chasteberry, Man Jing Zi)

Laryngitis
- Baptisia tinctoria (Wild indigo)
- Collinsonia canadensis (Stone root)
- Hedera helix (Ivy leaf, English ivy)
- Isatis tinctoria (Isatis, ban lan gen, woad, Chinese indigo)
- Phytolacca americana (Poke root, pokeweed)
- Plantago lanceolata (Ribwort, narrow-leaved plantain)
- Syzygium aromaticum (Cloves)
- Thymus vulgaris (Thyme)

Latent hyperprolactinaemia
- Vitex agnus-castus (Chaste tree, chasteberry, Man Jing Zi)

Leucorrhoea
- Alchemilla vulgaris (Lady's mantle)
- Chamaelirium luteum (False unicorn root, helonias)
- Houttuynia cordata (Yu Xing Cao, chameleon plant, fish mint)
- Lamium album (White dead nettle)
- Paeonia lactiflora (Peony, white peony, Bai Shao)
- Poria cocos (Hoelen, sclerotium of tuckahoe, fu ling (Mandarin) and bukuryo (Japanese))
- Trillium erectum (Beth root, birth root)
- Usnea spp. (Old man's beard, songluo)
- Vinca minor (Periwinkle, lesser or common periwinkle)

Leucorrhoea and vaginitis (douche)
- Baptisia tinctoria (Wild indigo)
- Bidens tripartita (Burr marigold, water agrimony, gui zhen cao, longbacao)
- Bistorta officinalis (Bistort, common bistort, European bistort or meadow bistort)
- Lamium album (White dead nettle)
- Myrica cerifera (Bayberry, candleberry, wax myrtle)
- Paeonia lactiflora (Peony, white peony, Bai Shao)
- Trillium erectum (Beth root, birth root)

Leukopenia
- Gynostemma pentaphyllum (Jiaogulan, xiancao)

Libido; low
- Crocus sativus (Saffron)
- Panax ginseng (Ginseng, Ren Shen)
- Trigonella foenum-graecum (Fenugreek)

Lithuria
- Arctostaphylos uva-ursi (Bearberry)
- Elymus repens (Couch grass)

Liver cirrhosis
- Angelica polymorpha (Dong quai, dang gui, Chinese angelica)
- Cordyceps militaris (Cordyceps, orange catapillar fungus, dong chong xia cao (China), hyakurakusou (Japan))
- Silybum marianum (St Mary's thistle, milk thistle, silymarin)

Liver congestion
- Crocus sativus (Saffron)
- Rheum palmatum (Da Huang, Chinese rhubarb)
- Rumex crispus (Yellow dock, curled dock)
- Schisandra chinensis (Bei-Wuweizi, Schisandra, Chinese magnolia vine, Wu Wei Zi)

Liver insufficiency
- Andrographis paniculata (Andrographis, kalmegh)
- Chionanthus virginicus (Fringe tree, old man's beard)
- Curcuma longa (Turmeric)
- Cynara scolymus (Globe artichoke)
- Fumaria officinalis (Fumitory)
- Juglans cinerea (Butternut bark, white walnut, lemon walnut)
- Rumex crispus (Yellow dock, curled dock)
- Schisandra chinensis (Bei-Wuweizi, Schisandra, Chinese magnolia vine, Wu Wei Zi)
- Silybum marianum (St Mary's thistle, milk thistle, silymarin)
- Taraxacum officinale radix (Dandelion root)
- Tribulus terrestris (Tribulus, calthrops)

Liver toxicity
- Agrimonia eupatoria (Agrimony)
- Andrographis paniculata (Andrographis, kalmegh)
- Rumex crispus (Yellow dock, curled dock)
- Schisandra chinensis (Bei-Wuweizi, Schisandra, Chinese magnolia vine, Wu Wei Zi)
- Silybum marianum (St Mary's thistle, milk thistle, silymarin)
- Taraxacum officinale radix (Dandelion root)

Longevity
- Astragalus membranaceus (Astragalus, milk vetch, huang qi (Chinese), ogi (Japanese))
- Panax ginseng (Ginseng, Ren Shen)
- Poria cocos (Hoelen, China root, sclerotium of tuckahoe, fu ling (Mandarin) and bukuryo (Japanese))
- Reynoutria multiflora (He Shou Wu, Fo-Ti)
- Schisandra chinensis (Bei-Wuweizi, Schisandra, Chinese magnolia vine, Wu Wei Zi)

Luteal phase complaints
- Paeonia lactiflora (Peony, white peony, Bai Shao)
- Vitex agnus-castus (Chaste tree, chasteberry, Man Jing Zi)

Lymphadenitis
- Baptisia tinctoria (Wild indigo)
- Phytolacca americana (Poke root, pokeweed)

Lymphadenopathy
- Galium aparine (Clivers, cleavers)
- Iris versicolor (Blue flag)
- Phytolacca americana (Poke root, pokeweed)

Lymphoma treatment; as an adjunct to
- Albizia lebbeck (Albizia, sirisha)
- Quercus robur (Oak bark)
- Salvia miltiorrhiza (Dan shen (Mandarin), red root sage)

Malaria
- Artemisia absinthium (Wormwood, absinthe)
- Artemisia annua (Sweet Annie, Chinese wormwood, qing hao)
- Berberis aristata (Daruharidra, Daruhaldi, Darvi, Chitra, Indian barberry)
- Carica papaya (Paw paw, papaya)
- Cryptolepis sanguinolenta (Yellow dye root, delboi)

Mammary abscess (poultice)
- Phytolacca americana (Poke root, pokeweed)
- Zingiber officinale (Ginger, Sheng Jiang (fresh), Gan Jiang (dried))

Mastalgia
- Ginkgo biloba (Maidenhair)
- Paeonia lactiflora (Peony, white peony, Bai Shao)
- Symphytum officinale (Comfrey)
- Vitex agnus-castus (Chaste tree, chasteberry, Man Jing Zi)

Mastitis
- Phytolacca americana (Poke root, pokeweed)
- Zingiber officinale (Ginger, Sheng Jiang (fresh), Gan Jiang (dried))

Memory and concentration; poor
- Asparagus racemosus (Shatavari (Sanskrit), satavari (Hindi), satmuli (Bengali))
- Bacopa monnieri (Bacopa, brahmi)
- Centella asiatica (Gotu kola, brahmi, Indian pennywort)
- Crocus sativus (Saffron)
- Ginkgo biloba (Maidenhair)
- Magnolia officinalis (Magnolia, Hou po)
- Paeonia lactiflora (Peony, white peony, Bai Shao)
- Panax ginseng (Ginseng, Ren Shen)
- Panax quinquefolium (American ginseng)

- Poria cocos (Hoelen, China root, sclerotium of tuckahoe, fu ling (Mandarin) and bukuryo (Japanese))
- Rhodiola rosea (Golden root, rose root, arctic root)
- Salvia rosmarinus (Rosemary)
- Schisandra chinensis (Bei-Wuweizi, Schisandra, Chinese magnolia vine, Wu Wei Zi)
- Vinca minor (Periwinkle, lesser or common periwinkle)

Menopausal symptoms

- Angelica polymorpha (Dong quai, dang gui, Chinese angelica)
- Asparagus racemosus (Shatavari (Sanskrit), satavari (Hindi), satmuli (Bengali))
- Astragalus membranaceus (Astragalus, milk vetch, huang qi (Chinese), ogi (Japanese))
- Calendula officinalis (Calendula, marigold)
- Chamaelirium luteum (False unicorn root, helonias)
- Dioscorea spp. (Wild yam)
- Epimedium sagittatum (Horny goat weed, barrenwort, yin yang huo, Inyokaku)
- Glycine max (Soy, soy germ, soy isoflavones (genistein), phyto-oestrogens, tofu (bean curd))
- Humulus lupulus (Hops)
- Hypericum perforatum (St John's wort)
- Lavandula angustifolia (Lavender)
- Ligustrum lucidum (Glossy privet, nu zhen zi, joteishi)
- Paeonia lactiflora (Peony, white peony, Bai Shao)
- Panax ginseng (Ginseng, Ren Shen)
- Panax quinquefolium (American ginseng)
- Piper methysticum (Kava)
- Salvia officinalis (Sage)
- Tribulus terrestris (Tribulus, calthrops, puncture vine, Bai Ji Li)
- Trifolium pratense (Red clover, trifoil)
- Trigonella foenum-graecum (Fenugreek)
- Vitex agnus-castus (Chaste tree, chasteberry, Man Jing Zi)

Menopause

- Actaea racemosa (Black cohosh, squawroot, snakeroot)
- Alchemilla vulgaris (Lady's mantle)
- Capsella bursa-pastoris (Shepherd's purse)
- Hypericum perforatum (St John's wort)
- Scutellaria lateriflora (Blue skulcap)
- Trillium erectum (Beth root, birth root)
- Vitex agnus-castus (Chaste tree, chasteberry, Man Jing Zi)
- Withania somnifera (Ashwaghanda, winter cherry)

Menopause; Menorrhagia

- Viburnum opulus (Cramp bark)
- Vitex agnus-castus (Chaste tree, chasteberry)

Menopause; depression

- Lavandula angustifolia (Lavender)
- Piper methysticum (Kava)

Menopause; symptoms

- Actaea racemosa (Black cohosh, squawroot, snakeroot)
- Alchemilla vulgaris (Lady's mantle)

Menorrhagia

- Achillea millefolium (Yarrow)
- Alchemilla vulgaris (Lady's mantle)
- Capsella bursa-pastoris (Shepherd's purse)
- Dipsacus asper (Teasel root)
- Geranium maculatum (Cranesbill)
- Rubus idaeus (Raspberry leaf)
- Trillium erectum (Beth root, birth root)

Menstrual irregularity

- Achillea millefolium (Yarrow)
- Alchemilla vulgaris (Lady's mantle)
- Aletris farinosa (True unicorn root, white colic root)
- Angelica polymorpha (Dong quai, dang gui, Chinese angelica)
- Bupleurum falcatum (Bupleurum, sickle-leaved hare's ear)
- Calendula officinalis (Calendula, marigold)
- Caulophyllum thalictroides (Blue cohosh)
- Chamaelirium luteum (False unicorn root, helonias)
- Crocus sativus (Saffron)
- Epimedium sagittatum (Horny goat weed, barrenwort, yin yang huo, Inyokaku)
- Lamium album (White dead nettle)
- Mentha pulegium (Pennyroyal)
- Mentha x piperita (Peppermint, Bo He)
- Mitchella repens (Partridgeberry)
- Paeonia lactiflora (Peony, white peony, Bai Shao)
- Petroselinum crispum (Parsley root)
- Rehmannia glutinosa (Rehmannia, sheng di huang (uncured), shu di huang (cured), Chinese foxglove)
- Vitex agnus-castus (Chaste tree, chasteberry, Man Jing Zi)

Mental exhaustion

- Bacopa monnieri (Bacopa, brahmi)
- Ginkgo biloba (Maidenhair)
- Panax ginseng (Ginseng, Ren Shen)
- Panax quinquefolium (American ginseng)
- Schisandra chinensis (Bei-Wuweizi, Schisandra, Chinese magnolia vine, Wu Wei Zi)

Metabolic syndrome

- Coptis chinensis (Huanglian (China), makino (Japan))
- Fucus vesiculosus (Bladderwrack)
- Gymnema sylvestre (Gumar, meshashringi)

- Gynostemma pentaphyllum (Jiaogulan, xiancao)
- Humulus lupulus (Hops)
- Ligustrum lucidum (Glossy privet, nu zhen zi, joteishi)
- Magnolia officinalis (Magnolia, Hou po)
- Nigella sativa (Black cumin)
- Silybum marianum (St Mary's thistle, milk thistle, silymarin)
- Terminalia arjuna (Arjuna)

Metrorrhagia

- Angelica polymorpha (Dong quai, dang gui, Chinese angelica)
- Capsella bursa-pastoris (Shepherd's purse)
- Paeonia lactiflora (Peony, white peony, Bai Shao)
- Rehmannia glutinosa (Rehmannia, sheng di huang (uncured), shu di huang (cured), Chinese foxglove)
- Trillium erectum (Beth root, birth root)

Migraine

- Cola spp. (Kola nut, cola nut)
- Commiphora myrrha (Myrrh)
- Glycine max (Soy, soy germ, soy isoflavones (genistein), phyto-oestrogens, tofu (bean curd))
- Handroanthus impetiginosus (Pau d'arco, lapacho)
- Harpagophytum procumbens (Devil's claw)
- Macropiper excelsum (Kawakawa, New Zealand peppertree)
- Melissa officinalis (Lemon balm, Melissa)
- Paeonia lactiflora (Peony, white peony, Bai Shao)
- Piscidia piscipula (Jamaican dogwood)
- Stachys officinalis (Wood betony)
- Tanacetum parthenium (Feverfew)
- Tilia cordata (Lime tree, linden)
- Valeriana officinalis (Valerian, heliotrope, Mexican valerian (V. edulis))
- Verbena officinalis (Vervain)
- Vitex agnus-castus (Chaste tree, chasteberry, Man Jing Zi)

Miscarriage; repeated

- Chamaelirium luteum (False unicorn root, helonias)
- Vitex agnus-castus (Chaste tree, chasteberry)

Miscarriage; threatened

- Chamaelirium luteum (False unicorn root, helonias)
- Dioscorea spp. (Wild yam)
- Paeonia lactiflora (Peony, white peony, Bai Shao)
- Viburnum opulus (Cramp bark)
- Viburnum prunifolium (Black haw, Sweet viburnum)
- Vitex agnus-castus (Chaste tree, chasteberry)

Morning sickness

- Ballota nigra (Black horehound)
- Chamaelirium luteum (False unicorn root, helonias)

- Cinnamomum verum (Cinnamon, cassia bark, rou gui)
- Citrus reticulata (Chen pi, mandarin, tangerine)
- Dioscorea spp. (Wild yam)
- Mentha x piperita (Peppermint, Bo He)
- Zingiber officinale (Ginger, Sheng Jiang (fresh), Gan Jiang (dried))

Mucositis

- Plantago major (Plantain, broad-leaved plantain, Che Qian Zi)
- Rhodiola rosea (Golden root, rose root, arctic root)

Mumps

- Calendula officinalis (Calendula, marigold)
- Galium aparine (Clivers, cleavers)
- Isatis tinctoria (Isatis, ban lan gen, woad, Chinese indigo)
- Phytolacca americana (Poke root, pokeweed)

Muscular tension

- Achillea millefolium (Yarrow)
- Crocus sativus (Saffron)
- Dioscorea spp. (Wild yam)
- Piper methysticum (Kava)

Myalgia

- Bryonia dioica (Bryony)
- Capsicum spp. (Chilli, capsicum, pepper, paprika, cayenne)
- Paeonia lactiflora (Peony, white peony, Bai Shao)
- Rhodiola rosea (Golden root, rose root, arctic root)
- Salvia rosmarinus (Rosemary)
- Symphytum officinale (Comfrey)
- Viburnum opulus (Cramp bark)

Myocardial ischaemia

- Corydalis ambigua (Corydalis)
- Harpagophytum procumbens (Devil's claw)
- Inula racemosa (Inula)
- Panax notoginseng (Tienchi ginseng (san qi, tian qi – Mandarin) Yunnan bayou)
- Plectranthus barbatus (Coleus, makandi)
- Salvia miltiorrhiza (Dan shen, red root sage)
- Terminalia arjuna (Arjuna)
- Tilia cordata (Lime tree, linden)

Nausea

- Alpinia galanga (Greater galangal, Thai ginger)
- Ballota nigra (Black horehound)
- Cinnamomum verum (Cinnamon, cassia bark, rou gui)
- Citrus reticulata (Chen pi, mandarin, tangerine)
- Gentiana lutea (Gentian)
- Magnolia officinalis (Magnolia, Hou po)
- Matricaria chamomilla (Chamomile, German chamomile)

- Mentha x piperita (Peppermint, Bo He)
- Poria cocos (Hoelen, China root, sclerotium of tuckahoe, fu ling (Mandarin) and bukuryo (Japanese))
- Scutellaria baicalensis (Baikal skullcap, baical skullcap, Chinese skullcap, Huang qin (Mandarin), ogon (Japanese))
- Zingiber officinale (Ginger, Sheng Jiang (fresh), Gan Jiang (dried))

Nephritis

- Astragalus membranaceus (Astragalus, milk vetch, huang qi (Chinese), ogi (Japanese))
- Epimedium sagittatum (Horny goat weed, barrenwort, yin yang huo, Inyokaku)
- Poria cocos (Hoelen, China root, sclerotium of tuckahoe, fu ling (Mandarin) and bukuryo (Japanese))
- Salvia miltiorrhiza (Dan shen (Mandarin), red root sage)

Nerve damage

- Bacopa monnieri (Bacopa, brahmi)
- Hypericum perforatum (St John's wort)
- Salvia miltiorrhiza (Dan shen (Mandarin), red root sage)

Nervous exhaustion

- Angelica archangelica (European angelica, angelica)
- Avena sativa (green) (Oats, green oats, oat straw)
- Avena sativa (seed) (Oats, groats, oatmeal)
- Bacopa monnieri (Bacopa, brahmi)
- Crocus sativus (Saffron)
- Eschscholzia californica (Californian poppy)
- Hypericum perforatum (St John's wort)
- Poria cocos (Hoelen, China root, sclerotium of tuckahoe, fu ling (Mandarin) and bukuryo (Japanese))
- Rhodiola rosea (Golden root, rose root, arctic root)
- Withania somnifera (Ashwaghanda, winter cherry)
- Ziziphus jujuba var. spinosa (Zizyphus, sour Chinese date, jujube, Da Zao, Suan Zao Ren)

Nervous tachycardia

- Leonurus cardiaca (Motherwort)
- Lycopus spp. (Bugleweed, gypsy wort)
- Passiflora incarnata (Passion flower)
- Viscum album (Mistletoe)

Nervous tension

- Avena sativa (green) (Oats, green oats, oat straw)
- Avena sativa (seed) (Oats, groats, oatmeal)
- Crocus sativus (Saffron)
- Eschscholzia californica (Californian poppy)
- Hypericum perforatum (St John's wort)
- Piper methysticum (Kava)

- Piscidia piscipula (Jamaican dogwood)
- Poria cocos (Hoelen, sclerotium of tuckahoe, fu ling (Mandarin) and bukuryo (Japanese))
- Schisandra chinensis (Bei-Wuweizi, Schisandra, Chinese magnolia vine, Wu Wei Zi)
- Scutellaria lateriflora (Blue skulcap)
- Tilia cordata (Lime tree, linden)
- Turnera diffusa (Damiana)
- Valeriana officinalis (Valerian, heliotrope, Mexican valerian (V. edulis))
- Viscum album (Mistletoe)
- Ziziphus jujuba var. spinosa (Zizyphus, sour Chinese date, jujube, Da Zao, Suan Zao Ren)

Neuralgia

- Actaea racemosa (Black cohosh, squawroot, snakeroot)
- Avena sativa (seed) (Oats, groats, oatmeal)
- Capsicum spp. (Chilli, capsicum, paprika, cayenne)
- Harpagophytum procumbens (Devil's claw)
- Humulus lupulus (Hops)
- Hypericum perforatum (St John's wort)
- Melissa officinalis (Lemon balm, Melissa)
- Passiflora incarnata (Passion flower)
- Piscidia piscipula (Jamaican dogwood)
- Salvia rosmarinus (Rosemary)
- Stachys officinalis (Wood betony)

Neuralgia (topically)

- Angelica archangelica (European angelica, angelica)
- Capsicum spp. (Chilli, capsicum, pepper, paprika, cayenne)
- Salvia rosmarinus (Rosemary)

Neurasthenia

- Avena sativa (green) (Oats, green oats, oat straw)
- Bacopa monnieri (Bacopa, brahmi)
- Eschscholzia californica (Californian poppy)
- Leonurus cardiaca (Motherwort)
- Melissa officinalis (Lemon balm, Melissa)
- Reynoutria multiflora (He Shou Wu, Fo-Ti)
- Scutellaria lateriflora (Blue skulcap)
- Ziziphus jujuba var. spinosa (Zizyphus, sour Chinese date, jujube, Da Zao, Suan Zao Ren)

Neuritis

- Reynoutria multiflora (He Shou Wu, Fo-Ti)

Night blindness

- Atractylodes macrocephala (Atractylodes, bai zhu)
- Vaccinium myrtillus (Bilberry, blueberry)

Night cramps

- Centella asiatica (Gotu kola, brahmi, Indian pennywort)
- Piper methysticum (Kava)

Night sweats

- Astragalus membranaceus (Astragalus, milk vetch, huang qi (Chinese), ogi (Japanese))
- Salvia officinalis (Sage)
- Ziziphus jujuba var. spinosa (Zizyphus, sour Chinese date, jujube, Da Zao, Suan Zao Ren)

Non-alcoholic fatty liver disease (NAFLD)

- Centaurium erythraea (Centaury)
- Coptis chinensis (Huanglian (China), makino (Japan))
- Gynostemma pentaphyllum (Jiaogulan, xiancao)
- Picrorhiza kurroa (Kutki)

Nose bleeds

- Achillea millefolium (Yarrow)
- Capsella bursa-pastoris (Shepherd's purse)
- Vaccinium myrtillus (Bilberry, blueberry)

Obesity

- Coptis chinensis (Huanglian (China), makino (Japan))
- Glycine max (Soy, soy germ, soy isoflavones (genistein), phyto-oestrogens, tofu (bean curd))
- Gymnema sylvestre (Gumar, meshashringi)
- Gynostemma pentaphyllum (Jiaogulan, xiancao)
- Magnolia officinalis (Magnolia, Hou po)
- Nigella sativa (Black cumin)
- Silybum marianum (St Mary's thistle, milk thistle, silymarin)
- Trigonella foenum-graecum (Fenugreek)

Oedema; localised

- Aesculus hippocastanum (Horse chestnut)

Oligomenorrhoea

- Vitex agnus-castus (Chaste tree, chasteberry, Man Jing Zi)

Oliguria

- Taraxacum officinale folia (Dandelion leaf, Pu Gong Ying)

Organ prolapse

- Bupleurum falcatum (Bupleurum, sickle-leaved hare's ear)

Osteoarthritis

- Actaea racemosa (Black cohosh, squawroot, snakeroot)
- Artemisia annua (Sweet Annie, Chinese wormwood, qing hao)
- Dipsacus asper (Teasel root)
- Epimedium sagittatum (Horny goat weed, barrenwort, yin yang huo, Inyokaku)
- Galium aparine (Clivers, cleavers)
- Glycine max (Soy, soy germ, soy isoflavones (genistein), phyto-oestrogens, tofu (bean curd))
- Harpagophytum procumbens (Devil's claw)
- Rosa canina (Rosehip, dog rose)
- Salix spp. (Willow bark, white willow)
- Thuja occidentalis (Thuja, white cedar, arbor-vitae (American))
- Zingiber officinale (Ginger, Sheng Jiang (fresh), Gan Jiang (dried))

Osteoporosis/Osteopenia

- Berberis aristata (Daruharidra, Daruhaldi, Darvi, Chitra, Indian barberry)
- Dipsacus asper (Teasel root)
- Epimedium sagittatum (Horny goat weed, barrenwort, yin yang huo, Inyokaku)
- Glycine max (Soy, soy germ, soy isoflavones (genistein), phyto-oestrogens, tofu (bean curd))
- Ligustrum lucidum (Glossy privet, nu zhen zi, joteishi)
- Pueraria lobata (Kudzu)

Otitis media

- Verbascum thapsus (Mullein, candlewick plant, flannel-leaf, bunny's ears)

Ovarian and uterine pains

- Anemone pulsatilla (Pulsatilla)
- Dioscorea spp. (Wild yam)
- Viburnum opulus (Cramp bark)
- Viburnum prunifolium (Black haw, Sweet viburnum)

Ovarian cyst

- Glycyrrhiza spp. (Licorice, Liquorice, Gan Cao)
- Paeonia lactiflora (Peony, white peony, Bai Shao)
- Thuja occidentalis (Thuja, white cedar, arbor-vitae (American))
- Vitex agnus-castus (Chaste tree, chasteberry, Man Jing Zi)

Ovulation; eratic

- Angelica polymorpha (Dong quai, dang gui, Chinese angelica)
- Chamaelirium luteum (False unicorn root, helonias)
- Paeonia lactiflora (Peony, white peony, Bai Shao)
- Tribulus terrestris (Tribulus, calthrops, puncture vine, Bai Ji Li)
- Vitex agnus-castus (Chaste tree, chasteberry, Man Jing Zi)

Ovulation; painful

- Anemone pulsatilla (Pulsatilla)
- Chamaelirium luteum (False unicorn root, helonias)
- Vitex agnus-castus (Chaste tree, chasteberry, Man Jing Zi)

Palpitations

- Angelica polymorpha (Dong quai, dang gui, Chinese angelica)
- Astragalus membranaceus (Astragalus, milk vetch, huang qi (Chinese), ogi (Japanese))

- Salvia miltiorrhiza (Dan shen (Mandarin), red root sage)
- Ziziphus jujuba var. spinosa (Zizyphus, sour Chinese date, jujube, Da Zao, Suan Zao Ren)

Parasites
- Artemisia annua (Sweet Annie, Chinese wormwood, qing hao)
- Commiphora myrrha (Myrrh)
- Cryptolepis sanguinolenta (Yellow dye root, delboi)
- Juglans nigra (Black walnut)
- Punica granatum (Pomegranate)
- Syzygium aromaticum (Cloves)

Pelvic floor weakness
- Aletris farinosa (True unicorn root, white colic root)

Pelvic heaviness; congestion
- Aletris farinosa (True unicorn root, white colic root)

Periodontitis
- Commiphora myrrha (Myrrh)
- Lomatium dissectum (Fern-leaf biscuit root, tohza, desert parsley)
- Perilla frutescens (Perilla, su zi, shisu)
- Punica granatum (Pomegranate)
- Syzygium aromaticum (Cloves)

Peripheral vascular disease
- Angelica archangelica (European angelica, angelica)

Pertussis
- Actaea racemosa (Black cohosh, squawroot, snakeroot)
- Althaea officinalis (Marshmallow, white mallow)
- Asclepias tuberosa (Pleurisy root, butterfly weed)
- Drosera spp. (Sundew)
- Echinacea spp. (Echinacea)
- Euphorbia hirta (Euphorbia)
- Grindelia camporum (Gum weed)
- Inula helenium (Elecampane)
- Marrubium vulgare (White horehound)
- Pimpinella anisum (Aniseed)
- Prunus serotina (Wild cherry, black cherry)
- Thymus vulgaris (Thyme)
- Viola tricolor (Heartsease, wild pansy, viola)

Pharyngitis
- Baptisia tinctoria (Wild indigo)
- Bistorta officinalis (Bistort, common bistort, European bistort or meadow bistort)
- Commiphora myrrha (Myrrh)
- Echinacea spp. (Echinacea)
- Foeniculum vulgare (Fennel)
- Isatis tinctoria (Isatis, ban lan gen, woad, Chinese indigo)
- Pelargonium sidoides (African geranium, umckaloabo (severe cough in Zulu))
- Quercus robur (Oak bark)

Pleurisy
- Asclepias tuberosa (Pleurisy root, butterfly weed)
- Bryonia dioica (Bryony)
- Inula helenium (Elecampane)

Polycystic ovarian syndrome
- Actaea racemosa (Black cohosh, squawroot, snakeroot)
- Chamaelirium luteum (False unicorn root, helonias)
- Glycyrrhiza spp. (Licorice, Liquorice, Gan Cao)
- Humulus lupulus (Hops)
- Nigella sativa (Black cumin)
- Paeonia lactiflora (Peony, white peony, Bai Shao)
- Trigonella foenum-graecum (Fenugreek)

Post-viral syndromes
- Andrographis paniculata (Andrographis, kalmegh)
- Astragalus membranaceus (Astragalus, milk vetch, huang qi (Chinese), ogi (Japanese))
- Echinacea spp. (Echinacea)
- Eleutherococcus senticosus (Eleuthero, eleutherokokk, Siberian ginseng)
- Hypericum perforatum (St John's wort)
- Rhodiola rosea (Golden root, rose root, arctic root)

Pregnancy; to prepare uterus for labour
- Chamaelirium luteum (False unicorn root, helonias)
- Mitchella repens (Partridgeberry)
- Rubus idaeus (Raspberry leaf)

Premature ovarian failure
- Epimedium sagittatum (Horny goat weed, barrenwort, yin yang huo, Inyokaku)
- Vitex agnus-castus (Chaste tree, chasteberry, Man Jing Zi)

Premenstrual syndrome
- Angelica polymorpha (Dong quai, dang gui, Chinese angelica)
- Chamaelirium luteum (False unicorn root, helonias)
- Crocus sativus (Saffron)
- Dioscorea spp. (Wild yam)
- Hypericum perforatum (St John's wort)
- Passiflora incarnata (Passion flower)
- Piper methysticum (Kava)
- Scutellaria lateriflora (Blue skulcap)
- Valeriana officinalis (Valerian, heliotrope, Mexican valerian (V. edulis))
- Vitex agnus-castus (Chaste tree, chasteberry, Man Jing Zi)
- Withania somnifera (Ashwaghanda, winter cherry)

Prostatitis
- Agathosma betulina (Buchu)
- Arctostaphylos uva-ursi (Bearberry)

- Elymus repens (Couch grass)
- Equisetum arvense (Horsetail)
- Eutrochium purpureum (Gravel root, Joe Pye weed)
- Hydrangea arborescens (Hydrangea)
- Serenoa repens (Saw palmetto, cabbage palm, dwarf palmetto)
- Urtica dioica radix (Nettle root)
- Zea mays (Corn silk, maize)

Pruritus
- Calendula officinalis (Calendula, marigold)
- Hydrastis canadensis (Goldenseal)
- Scrophularia nodosa (Figwort)
- Stellaria media (Chickweed, starweed)

Pruritus ani (topically)
- Calendula officinalis (Calendula, marigold)
- Hydrastis canadensis (Goldenseal)
- Matricaria chamomilla (Chamomile, German chamomile)

Pruritus vulvae (douche)
- Alchemilla vulgaris (Lady's mantle)

Psoriasis
- Arctium lappa (Burdock)
- Berberis aquifolium (Oregon grape, mountain grape)
- Berberis vulgaris (Barberry)
- Calendula officinalis (Calendula, marigold)
- Coptis chinensis (Huanglian (China), makino (Japan))
- Curcuma longa (Turmeric)
- Echinacea spp. (Echinacea)
- Eutrochium purpureum (Gravel root, Joe Pye weed)
- Galium aparine (Clivers, cleavers)
- Ginkgo biloba (Maidenhair)
- Glycyrrhiza spp. (Licorice, Liquorice, Gan Cao)
- Iris versicolor (Blue flag)
- Isatis tinctoria (Isatis, ban lan gen, woad, Chinese indigo)
- Plectranthus barbatus (Coleus, makandi)
- Quercus robur (Oak bark)
- Rumex crispus (Yellow dock, curled dock)
- Scrophularia nodosa (Figwort)
- Smilax ornata (Sarsaparilla)
- Thuja occidentalis (Thuja, white cedar, arbor-vitae (American))
- Trifolium pratense (Red clover, trifoil)

Pulmonary fibrosis
- Salvia miltiorrhiza (Dan shen (Mandarin), red root sage)

Pyelitis
- Arctostaphylos uva-ursi (Bearberry)

Radiation; side effects of
- Aloe ferox (Aloe vera (gel), bitter aloes (resin))
- Calendula officinalis (Calendula, marigold)
- Centella asiatica (Gotu kola, brahmi, Indian pennywort)
- Panax ginseng (Ginseng, Ren Shen)
- Vitis vinifera (Grape vine, grapeseed extract)

Raynaud's syndrome
- Ginkgo biloba (Maidenhair)
- Pseudowintera colorata (Horopito)
- Zanthoxylum clava-herculis (Prickly ash)

Renal insufficiency
- Cordyceps militaris (Cordyceps, orange catapillar fungus, dong chong xia cao (China), hyakurakusou (Japan))
- Gynostemma pentaphyllum (Jiaogulan, xiancao)
- Rheum palmatum (Da Huang, Chinese rhubarb)
- Solidago virgaurea (Goldenrod)

Reproductive dysfunction
- Asparagus racemosus (Shatavari (Sanskrit), satavari (Hindi), satmuli (Bengali))
- Cordyceps militaris (Cordyceps, orange catapillar fungus, dong chong xia cao (China), hyakurakusou (Japan))

Respiratory catarrh
- Althaea officinalis (Marshmallow, white mallow)
- Angelica archangelica (European angelica, angelica)
- Justicia adhatoda (Basak, vasaka, Malabar nut)
- Pimpinella anisum (Aniseed)

Restlessness
- Humulus lupulus (Hops)
- Matricaria chamomilla (Chamomile, German chamomile)
- Melissa officinalis (Lemon balm, Melissa)
- Passiflora incarnata (Passion flower)
- Valeriana officinalis (Valerian, heliotrope, Mexican valerian (V. edulis))
- Ziziphus jujuba var. spinosa (Zizyphus, sour Chinese date, jujube, Da Zao, Suan Zao Ren)

Retinal blood flow disorders
- Ginkgo biloba (Maidenhair)
- Vaccinium myrtillus (Bilberry, blueberry)
- Vinca minor (Periwinkle, lesser or common periwinkle)

Retinal damage
- Ginkgo biloba (Maidenhair)
- Vaccinium myrtillus (Bilberry, blueberry)
- Vitis vinifera (Grape vine, grapeseed extract)

Rheumatism

- Actaea racemosa (Black cohosh, squawroot, snakeroot)
- Agathosma betulina (Buchu)
- Angelica archangelica (European angelica, angelica)
- Annona muricata (Graviola, soursop, guanábana)
- Apium graveolens (Celery seed, karafs)
- Asparagus racemosus (Shatavari (Sanskrit), satavari (Hindi), satmuli (Bengali))
- Caulophyllum thalictroides (Blue cohosh)
- Crocus sativus (Saffron)
- Dioscorea spp. (Wild yam)
- Ephedra sinensis (Ma-huang)
- Elymus repens (Couch grass)
- Eutrochium purpureum (Gravel root, Joe Pye weed)
- Filipendula ulmaria (Meadowsweet)
- Fucus vesiculosus (Bladderwrack)
- Guaiacum officinale (Guaiacum)
- Gynostemma pentaphyllum (Jiaogulan, xiancao)
- Harpagophytum procumbens (Devil's claw)
- Hedera helix (Ivy leaf, English ivy)
- Juniperus communis (Juniper)
- Ligustrum lucidum (Glossy privet, nu zhen zi, joteishi)
- Lomatium dissectum (Fern-leaf biscuit root, tohza, desert parsley)
- Macropiper excelsum (Kawakawa, New Zealand peppertree)
- Magnolia officinalis (Magnolia, Hou po)
- Peumus boldus (Boldo)
- Phytolacca americana (Poke root, pokeweed)
- Piscidia piscipula (Jamaican dogwood)
- Ruta graveolens (Rue)
- Smilax ornata (Sarsaparilla)
- Symphytum officinale (Comfrey)
- Syzygium aromaticum (Cloves)
- Taraxacum officinale radix (Dandelion root)
- Thuja occidentalis (Thuja, white cedar, arbor-vitae (American))
- Urtica dioica radix (Nettle root)
- Viola tricolor (Heartsease, wild pansy, viola)
- Zanthoxylum clava-herculis (Prickly ash)

Rheumatoid arthritis

- Actaea racemosa (Black cohosh, squawroot, snakeroot)
- Artemisia annua (Sweet Annie, Chinese wormwood, qing hao)
- Boswellia serrata (Boswellia, olibanum, frankincense)
- Dipsacus asper (Teasel root)
- Fucus vesiculosus (Bladderwrack)
- Glycine max (Soy, soy germ, soy isoflavones (genistein), phyto-oestrogens, tofu (bean curd))
- Guaiacum officinale (Guaiacum)
- Harpagophytum procumbens (Devil's claw)
- Hemidesmus indicus (Anantamul, Indian sarsparilla)
- Isodon rubescens (Dong ling cao, Chinese sage bush, rabdosia)
- Picrorhiza kurroa (Kutki)
- Salix spp. (Willow bark, white willow)
- Smilax ornata (Sarsaparilla)
- Thuja occidentalis (Thuja, white cedar, arbor-vitae (American))

Rhinitis

- Albizia lebbeck (Albizia, sirisha)
- Bidens tripartita (Burr marigold, water agrimony, gui zhen cao, longbacao)
- Ephedra sinensis (Ma-huang)
- Hydrastis canadensis (Goldenseal)
- Ocimum tenuiflorum (Tulsi, Holy basil)
- Perilla frutescens (Perilla, su zi, shisu)
- Plantago lanceolata (Ribwort, narrow-leaved plantain)
- Scutellaria baicalensis (Baikal skullcap, baical skullcap, Chinese skullcap, Huang qin (Mandarin), ogon (Japanese))
- Solidago virgaurea (Goldenrod)
- Vitis vinifera (Grape vine, grapeseed extract)

Rosacea, papulepostular

- Commiphora myrrha (Myrrh)

Schistosomiasis

- Commiphora myrrha (Myrrh)

Scleroderma

- Centella asiatica (Gotu kola, brahmi, Indian pennywort)
- Salvia miltiorrhiza (Dan shen (Mandarin), red root sage)

Senile macular degeneration

- Ginkgo biloba (Maidenhair)
- Vaccinium myrtillus (Bilberry, blueberry)

Sexual weakness

- Asparagus racemosus (Shatavari (Sanskrit), satavari (Hindi), satmuli (Bengali))
- Dulacia inopiflora (Muira puama)
- Epimedium sagittatum (Horny goat weed, barrenwort, yin yang huo, Inyokaku)
- Tribulus terrestris (Tribulus, calthrops, puncture vine, Bai Ji Li)

Shingles

- Avena sativa (green) (Oats, green oats, oat straw)

- Echinacea spp. (Echinacea)
- Hypericum perforatum (St John's wort)
- Isatis tinctoria (Isatis, ban lan gen, woad, Chinese indigo)
- Lomatium dissectum (Fern-leaf biscuit root, tohza, desert parsley)

Sinusitis

- Albizia lebbeck (Albizia, sirisha)
- Andrographis paniculata (Andrographis, kalmegh)
- Armoracia rusticana (Horseradish)
- Berberis aristata (Daruharidra, Daruhaldi, Darvi, Chitra, Indian barberry)
- Echinacea spp. (Echinacea)
- Ephedra sinensis (Ma-huang)
- Euphrasia officinalis (Eyebright)
- Hedera helix (Ivy leaf, English ivy)
- Hemidesmus indicus (Anantamul, Indian sarsparilla)
- Hydrastis canadensis (Goldenseal)
- Ocimum tenuiflorum (Tulsi, Holy basil)
- Pelargonium sidoides (African geranium, umckaloabo (severe cough in Zulu))
- Plantago lanceolata (Ribwort, narrow-leaved plantain)
- Sambucus nigra (Elder, elderflower, elderberry, sambuco)
- Scutellaria baicalensis (Baikal skullcap, baical skullcap, Chinese skullcap, Huang qin (Mandarin), ogon (Japanese))
- Solidago virgaurea (Goldenrod)

Sore throat (gargle)

- Althaea officinalis (Marshmallow, white mallow)
- Bistorta officinalis (Bistort, common bistort, European bistort or meadow bistort)
- Calendula officinalis (Calendula, marigold)
- Glycyrrhiza spp. (Licorice, Liquorice, Gan Cao)
- Myrica cerifera (Bayberry, candleberry, wax myrtle)
- Punica granatum (Pomegranate)
- Quercus robur (Oak bark)
- Salvia officinalis (Sage)
- Thymus vulgaris (Thyme)

Sperm count; low

- Panax ginseng (Ginseng, Ren Shen)
- Tribulus terrestris (Tribulus, calthrops, puncture vine, Bai Ji Li)

Splenic enlargement

- Bupleurum falcatum (Bupleurum, sickle-leaved hare's ear)
- Chionanthus virginicus (Fringe tree, old man's beard)
- Phyllanthus spp. (Phyllanthus)

Sprains (topically)

- Arnica montana (Arnica)

Stomatitis

- Baptisia tinctoria (Wild indigo)
- Bistorta officinalis (Bistort, common bistort, European bistort or meadow bistort)
- Propolis (Propolis)

Stress

- Asparagus racemosus (Shatavari (Sanskrit), satavari (Hindi), satmuli (Bengali))
- Atractylodes macrocephala (Atractylodes, bai zhu)
- Avena sativa (green) (Oats, green oats, oat straw)
- Avena sativa (seed) (Oats, groats, oatmeal)
- Bryonia dioica (Bryony)
- Codonopsis pilosula (Dang shen, codonopsis)
- Dulacia inopiflora (Muira puama)
- Eleutherococcus senticosus (Eleuthero, eleutherokokk, Siberian ginseng)
- Ganoderma lucidum (Reishi, lingzhi)
- Glycyrrhiza spp. (Licorice, Liquorice, Gan Cao)
- Panax ginseng (Ginseng, Ren Shen)
- Piper methysticum (Kava)
- Piscidia piscipula (Jamaican dogwood)
- Rhodiola rosea (Golden root, rose root, arctic root)
- Schisandra chinensis (Bei-Wuweizi, Schisandra, Chinese magnolia vine, Wu Wei Zi)
- Turnera diffusa (Damiana)
- Withania somnifera (Ashwaghanda, winter cherry)
- Ziziphus jujuba var. spinosa (Zizyphus, sour Chinese date, jujube, Da Zao, Suan Zao Ren)

Stroke; recovery after

- Bacopa monnieri (Bacopa, brahmi)
- Ginkgo biloba (Maidenhair)
- Vinca minor (Periwinkle, lesser periwinkle)

Surgery; recovery

- Centella asiatica (Gotu kola, brahmi, Indian pennywort)

Sweating; excessive

- Astragalus membranaceus (Astragalus, milk vetch, huang qi (Chinese), ogi (Japanese))
- Salvia officinalis (Sage)
- Ziziphus jujuba var. spinosa (Zizyphus, sour Chinese date, jujube, Da Zao, Suan Zao Ren)

Sweet cravings

- Gymnema sylvestre (Gumar, meshashringi)

Tachycardia

- Crataegus monogyna (Hawthorn)
- Grindelia camporum (Gum weed)
- Leonurus cardiaca (Motherwort)
- Lycopus spp. (Bugleweed, gypsy wort)

Thyroid gland; impaired
- Fucus vesiculosus (Bladderwrack)
- Plectranthus barbatus (Coleus, makandi)

Thyrotoxicosis with dyspnoea
- Lycopus spp. (Bugleweed, gypsy wort)

Tinea (topically)
- Phytolacca americana (Poke root, pokeweed)

Tinnitus
- Actaea racemosa (Black cohosh, squawroot, snakeroot)
- Ginkgo biloba (Maidenhair)
- Reynoutria multiflora (He Shou Wu, Fo-Ti)
- Vinca minor (Periwinkle, lesser periwinkle)

Tonsillitis
- Baptisia tinctoria (Wild indigo)
- Commiphora myrrha (Myrrh)
- Echinacea spp. (Echinacea)
- Hedera helix (Ivy leaf, English ivy)
- Isatis tinctoria (Isatis, ban lan gen, woad, Chinese indigo)
- Isodon rubescens (Dong ling cao, Chinese sage bush, rabdosia)
- Pelargonium sidoides (African geranium, umckaloabo (severe cough in Zulu))
- Phytolacca americana (Poke root, pokeweed)
- Quercus robur (Oak bark)
- Salvia officinalis (Sage)
- Thymus vulgaris (Thyme)
- Verbascum thapsus (Mullein, candlewick plant, flannel-leaf, bunny's ears)

Tracheitis
- Baptisia tinctoria (Wild indigo)
- Echinacea spp. (Echinacea)
- Glycyrrhiza spp. (Licorice, Liquorice, Gan Cao)
- Hedera helix (Ivy leaf, English ivy)
- Isodon rubescens (Dong ling cao, Chinese sage bush, rabdosia)
- Phytolacca americana (Poke root, pokeweed)
- Pimpinella anisum (Aniseed)
- Salvia officinalis (Sage)
- Thymus vulgaris (Thyme)
- Verbascum thapsus (Mullein, candlewick plant, flannel-leaf, bunny's ears)

Trichomoniasis vaginalis
- Commiphora myrrha (Myrrh)

Ulcer (topically)
- Althaea officinalis (Marshmallow, white mallow)
- Bistorta officinalis (Bistort, common bistort, European bistort or meadow bistort)
- Echinacea spp. (Echinacea)
- Geranium maculatum (Cranesbill)
- Isatis tinctoria (Isatis, ban lan gen, woad, Chinese indigo)
- Plantago lanceolata (Ribwort, narrow-leaved plantain)
- Propolis (Propolis)
- Stellaria media (Chickweed, starweed)
- Symphytum officinale (Comfrey)

Ulcer; gastrointestinal
- Alchemilla vulgaris (Lady's mantle)
- Aloe ferox (Aloe vera (gel), bitter aloes (resin))
- Althaea officinalis (Marshmallow, white mallow)
- Angelica archangelica (European angelica)
- Asparagus racemosus (Shatavari (Sanskrit), satavari (Hindi), satmuli (Bengali))
- Astragalus membranaceus (Astragalus, milk vetch, huang qi (Chinese), ogi (Japanese))
- Bidens tripartita (Burr marigold, water agrimony, gui zhen cao, longbacao)
- Bupleurum falcatum (Bupleurum, sickle-leaved hare's ear)
- Calendula officinalis (Calendula, marigold)
- Carica papaya (Paw paw, papaya)
- Centaurium erythraea (Centaury)
- Commiphora myrrha (Myrrh)
- Echinacea spp. (Echinacea)
- Filipendula ulmaria (Meadowsweet)
- Geranium maculatum (Cranesbill)
- Glycyrrhiza spp. (Licorice, Liquorice, Gan Cao)
- Hydrastis canadensis (Goldenseal)
- Matricaria chamomilla (Chamomile, German chamomile)
- Momordica charantia (Bitter melon, bitter gourd, African or wild cucumber)
- Propolis (Propolis)
- Salvia rosmarinus (Rosemary)
- Stellaria media (Chickweed, starweed)
- Symphytum officinale (Comfrey)
- Terminalia arjuna (Arjuna)
- Ulmus fulva (Slippery elm, red elm)
- Uncaria tomentosa (Cat's claw)

Ulcer; mouth
- Baptisia tinctoria (Wild indigo)
- Bistorta officinalis (Bistort, common bistort, European bistort or meadow bistort)
- Calendula officinalis (Calendula, marigold)
- Commiphora myrrha (Myrrh)
- Echinacea spp. (Echinacea)
- Plantago lanceolata (Ribwort, narrow-leaved plantain)
- Plantago major (Plantain, broad-leaved plantain)
- Propolis (Propolis)

Ulcerative colitis

- Althaea officinalis (Marshmallow, white mallow)
- Boswellia serrata (Boswellia, olibanum, frankincense)
- Mentha x piperita (Peppermint, Bo He)
- Propolis (Propolis)
- Symphytum officinale (Comfrey)
- Ulmus fulva (Slippery elm, red elm)

Urethritis

- Agathosma betulina (Buchu)
- Althaea officinalis (Marshmallow, white mallow)
- Arctostaphylos uva-ursi (Bearberry)
- Crateva magna (Varuna)
- Echinacea spp. (Echinacea)
- Elymus repens (Couch grass)
- Equisetum arvense (Horsetail)
- Eutrochium purpureum (Gravel root, Joe Pye weed)
- Hydrangea arborescens (Hydrangea)
- Zea mays (Corn silk, maize)

Urinary gravel

- Petroselinum crispum (Parsley root)
- Urtica dioica folia (Nettle leaf, stinging nettle)
- Zea mays (Corn silk, maize)

Urticaria

- Albizia lebbeck (Albizia, sirisha)
- Arctium lappa (Burdock)
- Berberis aquifolium (Oregon grape, mountain grape)
- Berberis vulgaris (Barberry)
- Ephedra sinensis (Ma-huang)
- Galium aparine (Clivers, cleavers)
- Scutellaria baicalensis (Baikal skullcap, baical skullcap, Chinese skullcap, Huang qin (Mandarin), ogon (Japanese))
- Stellaria media (Chickweed, starweed)
- Viola tricolor (Heartsease, wild pansy, viola)

Uterine bleeding; dysfunctional

- Aletris farinosa (True unicorn root, white colic root)
- Capsella bursa-pastoris (Shepherd's purse)
- Chamaelirium luteum (False unicorn root, helonias)
- Dioscorea spp. (Wild yam)
- Lamium album (White dead nettle)
- Mitchella repens (Partridgeberry)
- Paeonia lactiflora (Peony, white peony, Bai Shao)
- Panax notoginseng (Tienchi ginseng (san qi, tian qi – Mandarin) Yunnan bayou)
- Trillium erectum (Beth root, birth root)
- Viburnum opulus (Cramp bark)
- Vitex agnus-castus (Chaste tree, chasteberry, Man Jing Zi)

Uterine contractions

- Justicia adhatoda (Basak, vasaka, Malabar nut)
- Mitchella repens (Partridgeberry)
- Viburnum opulus (Cramp bark)
- Viburnum prunifolium (Black haw, Sweet viburnum)

Varicose veins

- Aesculus hippocastanum (Horse chestnut)
- Centella asiatica (Gotu kola, brahmi, Indian pennywort)
- Ruscus aculeatus (Butcher's broom, box holly)
- Vaccinium myrtillus (Bilberry, blueberry)
- Vitis vinifera (Grape vine, grapeseed extract)

Varicose veins (topically)

- Aesculus hippocastanum (Horse chestnut)
- Arnica montana (Arnica)
- Calendula officinalis (Calendula, marigold)
- Centella asiatica (Gotu kola, brahmi)
- Vaccinium myrtillus (Bilberry, blueberry)

Venous insufficiency

- Aesculus hippocastanum (Horse chestnut)
- Arnica montana (Arnica)
- Centella asiatica (Gotu kola, brahmi, Indian pennywort)
- Ginkgo biloba (Maidenhair)
- Pinus pinaster (Maritime bark)
- Ruscus aculeatus (Butcher's broom, box holly)
- Vaccinium myrtillus (Bilberry, blueberry)
- Vitis vinifera (Grape vine, grapeseed extract)

Venous leg ulcers

- Aesculus hippocastanum (Horse chestnut)
- Pinus pinaster (Maritime bark)

Vertigo

- Ginkgo biloba (Maidenhair)
- Vinca minor (Periwinkle, lesser or common periwinkle)

Viral pneumonia

- Isatis tinctoria (Isatis, ban lan gen, woad, Chinese indigo)
- Lomatium dissectum (Fern-leaf biscuit root)

Visceral pain

- Corydalis ambigua (Corydalis)
- Macropiper excelsum (Kawakawa, New Zealand peppertree)
- Symphytum officinale (Comfrey)

Visual fatigue

- Reynoutria multiflora (He Shou Wu, Fo-Ti)
- Vaccinium myrtillus (Bilberry, blueberry)

Warts

- Andrographis paniculata (Andrographis, kalmegh)
- Echinacea spp. (Echinacea)
- Thuja occidentalis (Thuja, white cedar, arbor-vitae (American))

Warts (topically)

- Chelidonium majus (Greater celandine)
- Lomatium dissectum (Fern-leaf biscuit root, tohza, desert parsley)
- Thuja occidentalis (white cedar, arbor-vitae)

Weight loss; to assist

- Aletris farinosa (True unicorn root, white colic root)
- Atractylodes macrocephala (Atractylodes, bai zhu)
- Capsicum spp. (Chilli, capsicum, pepper, paprika, cayenne)
- Chamaelirium luteum (False unicorn root, helonias)
- Cynara scolymus (Globe artichoke)
- Fucus vesiculosus (Bladderwrack)
- Glycine max (Soy, soy germ, soy isoflavones (genistein), phyto-oestrogens, tofu (bean curd))
- Gymnema sylvestre (Gumar, meshashringi)
- Humulus lupulus (Hops)
- Iris versicolor (Blue flag)
- Panax notoginseng (Tienchi ginseng (san qi, tian qi – Mandarin) Yunnan bayou)
- Plectranthus barbatus (Coleus, makandi)
- Ruscus aculeatus (Butcher's broom, box holly)
- Taraxacum officinale folia (Dandelion leaf, Pu Gong Ying)
- Taraxacum officinale radix (Dandelion root)
- Vitex agnus-castus (Chaste tree, chasteberry)
- Vitis vinifera (Grape vine, grapeseed extract)

Wounds

- Alchemilla vulgaris (Lady's mantle)
- Astragalus membranaceus (Astragalus, milk vetch, huang qi (Chinese), ogi (Japanese))
- Berberis aristata (Daruharidra, Daruhaldi, Darvi, Chitra, Indian barberry)
- Echinacea spp. (Echinacea)
- Filipendula ulmaria (Meadowsweet)
- Hypericum perforatum (St John's wort)
- Isatis tinctoria (Isatis, ban lan gen, woad, Chinese indigo)
- Plantago lanceolata (Ribwort, narrow-leaved plantain)
- Symphytum officinale (Comfrey)
- Vitis vinifera (Grape vine, grapeseed extract)

Wounds (topically)

- Alchemilla vulgaris (Lady's mantle)
- Aloe ferox (Aloe vera (gel), bitter aloes (resin))
- Althaea officinalis (Marshmallow, white mallow)

- Calendula officinalis (Calendula, marigold)
- Commiphora myrrha (Myrrh)
- Echinacea spp. (Echinacea)
- Hydrastis canadensis (Goldenseal)
- Hypericum perforatum (St John's wort)
- Lamium album (White dead nettle)
- Leptospermum scoparium (Manuka, tea tree)
- Lomatium dissectum (Fern-leaf biscuit root, tohza, desert parsley)
- Matricaria chamomilla (Chamomile, German chamomile)
- Plantago major (Plantain, broad-leaved plantain, Che Qian Zi)

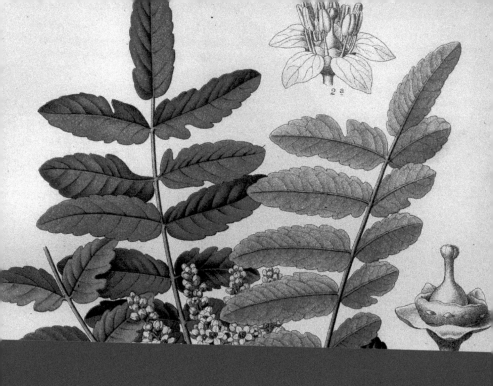

Glossary

Phytotherapy Desk Reference

Abortifacient

An agent that is used to terminate a pregnancy

Absorbent

Aids in the absorption of fluids

Acrid

Having a hot, biting taste

Action

The therapeutic activity of a remedy. Herbal medicines frequently exhibit more than one action

Active constituents

Chemical components of plants that have been shown to be responsible for or to contribute to the medicinal effect

Adaptogen

A nontoxic substance and especially a plant extract that is held to increase the body's ability to resist the damaging effects of stress and promote or restore normal physiological functioning

Adjuvant

An herb added to the mixture to aid the effect of the main one

Adrenal restorative

Aids in feeding and renewing the adrenal glands, promoting activity and reintegration in body function, particularly where there has been overexposure to stress leading to nervous exhaustion and debility

Aldose reductase inhibitor

Inhibits aldose reductase, an enzyme involved in the production of harmful sugar metabolites in diabetes

Alexipharmic

Herb warding off disease or the effect of poison

Alterative

See Depurative

Amebicide

Assists in treating bacterial infections

Amphoteric

Herb or entire plant extract which have opposite physiological actions, e.g., lowers and elevates blood pressure

AMPK-activator

AMP-activated protein kinase (AMPK) is an energy sensor and master regulator of cellular metabolism. Collectively, activation of AMPK in skeletal muscle, liver, and adipose tissue results in a favourable metabolic milieu for the prevention or treatment of T2D, i.e., decreased circulating glucose, reduced plasma lipid, and ectopic fat accumulation, as well as enhanced insulin sensitivity

Anaesthetising (mucous membranes)

Numbing effect on mucous membranes

Analgesic

An agent used to relieve pain when administered orally or topically. In herbal medicine, pain relief is largely a result of helping the body resolve the cause of pain

Anodyne

Pain reducing, usually used externally

Antacid

An agent used to neutralise acid in the stomach

Anthelmintic

Assists in killing or expelling intestinal worms or parasites

Antiallergic

Tempers the immune response, often by stabilising or inhibiting the degranulation of mast cells

Antiandrogenic

Agents used to block the production of male hormones

Antiangina

An agent intended to alleviate the symptoms of angina

Antiarrhythmic

An agent that normalises heart rhythm by counteracting irregular heart beat

Antiasthmatic

An agent that prevents or halts an asthmatic attack by alleviating the spasms of asthma

Antiatherosclerotic

A substance that reduces or inhibits the progression of atherosclerosis

Antibacterial

A substance that destroys or inhibits the growth of bacteria

Anticancer

A substance that counteracts the formation or growth of cancers

Anticarcinogenic

Having to do with preventing or delaying the development of cancer

Anticatarrhal

Reduces the formation of mucus

Anticholinergic

An agent that blocks the parasympathetic nerve impulse

Anticonvulsant

A type of drug used to prevent seizures, and commonly used in individuals with seizure disorders or epilepsy. Reducing or relieving convulsions or cramps

Antidepressant

An agent intended to alleviate the symptoms of depression

Antidiarrhoeal

Something that prevents or alleviate symptoms of diarrhoea

Antiemetic

Reduces the feelings of nausea, may relieve or prevent vomiting

Antifibrotic

Prevents the formation of fibrous tissue

Antifungal

A substance that destroys or stops the formation of fungi such as yeasts

Antigalactagogue

A substance that inhibits milk secretion

Antihaemorrhagic

A remedy that stems internal bleeding

Antihydrotic

A substance that reduces perspiration

Antihyperprostatic

Reduces enlargement of the prostate gland

Antihypertensive

Indicating a drug, supplement or mode of treatment that reduces the blood pressure of people with hypertension

Anti-inflammatory

A drug or supplement that fights inflammation, which is a response to injury, infection, or irritation that is characterised by redness, heat, swelling, and pain; an agent that counteracts inflammation; reducing inflammation by acting on body mechanisms, without directly acting on the cause of inflammation

Anti-implantation activity

Inhibits implantation of fertilised ovum

Antilithic

Reduces the formation of calculi in kidney, urinary system or joints

Antimicrobial

An agent that destroys or prevents the development of microorganisms; an agent that acts against bacteria, fungi, viruses, and parasites in the body

Antinociceptive

The action or process of blocking the detection of a painful or injurious stimulus by sensory neurons

Antiobesity

Reduces or prevents the accumulation of excessive fat in the body

Antioedematous

Reduces fluid retention and swelling by various mechanisms

Antionchotic

Reduces swelling

Antioxidant

Any substance that may prevent organ damage by scavenging free radicals and protecting against oxidation

Antiparasitic

Assists in killing or expelling parasites

Antiperiodic

Against fever

Antiphlogistic

A substance that prevents or counters inflammation

Antiplatelet

Reduces platelet aggregation

Antiproliferative

A substance that prevents or inhibits the growth and reproduction of similar cells

Antiprotozoal

A substance that kills or inhibits the growth of protozoa

Antipruritic

Reduces itching

Antipsoriatic

An agent that alleviates or prevents psoriasis, i.e., enhanced growth or dermal cells

Antipyretic

Reduces fever

Antirheumatic

Reduces the symptoms of rheumatism

Antisclerotic

Against atherosclerosis

Antiseptic

An agent used to prevent, resist and counteract infection

Antispasmodic

A substance that reduces muscular cramping, spasms and tension

Antithyroid

Relating to an agent that suppresses thyroid function

Antitumour

A substance that counteracts tumour formation or tumour growth (cancers)

Antitussive

Suppresses the cough reflex

Antiulcerogenic

Prevents and heals ulcers

Antiviral

An agent or procedure that prevents or inhibits viral infections

Anxiolytic

Reduces anxiety

Aperient

Mildly laxative

Aperitive

Improves appetite and digestion

Aphrodisiac

An agent used to stimulate sexual interest and desire

Apoptosis inducer

An agent that induces gene-directed cell death or programmed cell death that usually occurs when age, condition, or state of cell health dictates

Aromatic

Herbs with strong odour that stimulate digestive system

Astringent

Causes contraction of mucous membranes and exposed tissues

Balsam

A soothing and healing agent

Beta-blocker

An agent that decreases the rate and force of heart contractions and widens blood vessels, helping to reduce blood pressure

Bioflavonoid

A group of compounds; widely distributed in plants, that maintain the health of small blood vessel walls

Bitter tonic

A substance that promotes appetite, digestion and absorption by stimulating the secretion of digestive juices via reflexes from taste buds, gastrin and vagus

Bladder tonic

Maintains or restores health, vigour and function of the bladder

Blood sugar regulator

A substance that regulates the concentration of glucose in the blood

Blood tonic

Nourishes and restores health and function of the blood

Brain tonic

Maintains or restores health, vigour and function of the brain

Bronchodilator

An agent that increases the diameter of the pulmonary air passages

Calmative

Nourishes the entire body and nervous system

cAMP stimulant

An agent that stimulates the production and activation of cyclic adenosine monophosphate, a second messenger used for intracellular signal transduction and important in many biological processes including the regulation of glycogen, sugar and lipid metabolism

Cardioprotective

Decreases the risk of heart damage due to toxins or ischaemia

Cardiotonic

Increases the strength of the heart

Carminative

Relieves flatulence, usually by relaxing intestinal sphincter muscles

Cathartic

Strong laxative action

Chemoprotective

Protects against disease through the use of drugs or chemicals

Cholagogue

Increases the flow of bile

Choleretic

Increases the production and flow of bile

Circulatory stimulant

Improves peripheral circulation

Cognition enhancer

An agent that enhances mental activities associated with thinking, learning, and memory

Connective tissue regenerator

An agent that helps to regenerate tissue that performs the function of providing support, structure, and cellular cement to the body

Counter irritant

Produces a superficial inflammation of the skin. Often used to relieve a deeper inflammation by improving circulation. Used topically for inflammation and pain in muscles, ligaments and joints

Cytoprotective

Descriptive of a drug or agent protecting cells from damage expected to occur

Decoction

Water preparation where the bark, roots or other hardy or woody parts of a plant has simmered for some time, usually 15 to 30 minutes

Decongestant

Removes congestion of the mucous membranes

Demulcent

Soothes inflamed surfaces such as skin and mucous membranes.

Deobstruent

Loosing or removing obstructions in ducts. Could also refer to any obstruction, physical, mental or spiritual

Depurative

Improves detoxification of the body (by improving digestion, and the function of liver/gallbladder, kidney/bladder and/or the immune system); also known as alterative or 'blood purifiers'

Detersive

Cleaning of wounds or ulcers

Diaphoretic

Promotes sweating during a fever

Digestive stimulant

An agent that stimulates digestion

Discutient

Dispersing or absorbing of foreign or abnormal tissues

Diuretic

Increases urinary output and/or increases the excretion of metabolic waste products

Dopaminergic

An agent that enhances the action of dopamine or the neural or metabolic pathways in which it functions as a transmitter

Ecbolic

Aiding childbirth by increasing uterine contractions

Emetic

Causes vomiting

Emmenagogue

An herb that increases the strength and frequency of uterine contractions. Used in earlier times as a euphemism for abortifacient

Emollient

Reduces inflammation and irritation when applied to the skin

Epispastic

Prevents nosebleeds

Expectorant

Facilitates the removal of excess mucus by various means

Febrifuge

See antipyretic

Fibrinolytic

Prevents and reduces the development of insoluble fibrin clots

Fluid extract

A hydro-ethanolic extract of crude herbal material with a drug solvent ratio of 1:1 or 1:2 (1 part herb to 1 or 2 parts solvent)

Fresh plant tinctures (FPT)

An herbal extract made from fresh rather than dried plant material, using a mixture of water and alcohol as the menstruum.

Galactagogue

Promotes the production or flow of breast milk

Galenical

The crude botanic form of a drug

Glycetract

An herbal extract using glycerine and water as solvents

Glycetracta

Plant extracts in glycerine

Haemostatic

An agent that can arrest blood loss

Hepatic

A remedy that improves the function of the liver and normalises the flow of bile

Hepatoprotective

Protects the liver against damage from toxins

Hepatorestorative

Aids in nourishing and renewing the liver, promoting activity and reintegration in body function

Hepatotonic

Maintains or restores health, vigour and function of the liver

HPO regulator

Regulates the function of the hypothalamic-pituitary-ovarian axis

Hydragogue

Causing watery discharge

Hypnotic

An agent that induces deep and healing state of sleep

Hypocholesterolaemic

An agent that lowers blood cholesterol levels

Hypoglycaemic

An agent that lowers plasma glucose levels

Hypolipidaemic

An agent that lowers plasma lipid levels

Hypotensive

An agent that lowers blood pressure

Hypouricaemic

An agent that reduces the concentration of uric acid in the blood

Immunomodulator

An agent that assists in or is capable of modifying or regulating immune functions; an agent that causes an immunological adjustment, regulation or potentiation

Immunostimulant

Stimulates one or more aspects of the immune reaction, also called immunomodulating or immune-enhancing

Immunosuppressant

Reduces the immune response

Infused oil

An herbal extract using a fixed oil as the solvent

Infusion

Herbal tea prepared by pouring boiling water over flowers, leaves or other soft parts of a plant and leaving to steep for a short time usually in a covered vessel

Intract

Fresh plant extract

Laxative

Promotes the evacuation of the bowels

LH-RH antagonist

A substance that counteracts the action of luteinizing hormone-releasing hormone

Liniment

A soothing, oily, liquid preparation for rubbing on the skin

Lipogenesis-/Lipo-oxygenation inhibiting

Prevents or inhibits the production and deposition of fat, conversion of carbohydrate or protein to fatty acids, and oxygenation of lipids

Lithotryptic

Dissolving stones

Lymphatic

A remedy that improves the flow of lymphatic fluid or increases its detoxifying properties (lymphatic drainage)

Maceration

An extraction method where the cut herb is soaked in a solvent for some time before draining and pressing

Male tonic

Normalises reproductive function in males

Marc

The plant material left after an herbal extract has been made

Mel

Honey

Menstrual cycle regulator

An agent that acts to re-establish a periodic sequence whereby an egg cell is released from the ovary at four-weekly intervals

Menstruum

The solvent mixture used to make an herbal extract

Metabolic stimulant

A substance that acts to stimulate basal metabolic rate and general metabolism

Migraine prophylactic

An agent that acts to prevent migraine headaches

Mucilaginous

Contains mucins (complex carbohydrates) that are demulcent, emollient and soothing

Mucolytic

Breaks up or resolves mucus

Mucous membrane tonic

Normalises the function and secretions of mucous membranes

Natriuretic

Increases the excretion of sodium

Nerve stimulant

A substance that acts to stimulate the nervous system

Nervine/Tonic

Strengthens and nourishes the nervous system, usually with a relaxant effect

Nootropic

An agent that enhances mental activities associated with thinking, learning, and memory

Nutritive

Supplies biologically active optimum nourishment in the form of vitamins, minerals, trace elements, amino acids, carbohydrates and fats

Oestrogenic

Promotes the body's production of oestrogen and/or has the ability to stimulate oestrogen receptor sites

Oestrogen receptor modulating

An agent that modulates the activity and/or number of oestrogen receptors

Ovulation stimulant

A substance that acts to stimulate ovulation

Oxymel

Medicinal vinegar with added honey

Oxytocic

Stimulates uterine contractions

PAF inhibitor

A substance that inhibits the release or activity of platelet activating factor: PAF causes platelet aggregation and the release of blood-platelet substances (e.g., histamine), and is a mediator of inflammation (e.g., asthma) in that it reduces inflammation and contracts various involuntary muscles (e.g., airways)

Parturient

Induces or assists labour, facilitates proper delivery of the placenta

Partus praeparator

A herb prescribed in the last trimester of pregnancy to prepare and tone the uterus for labour

Percolation

An extraction method whereby the solvent is allowed to filter through powdered herb material packed in a cylindrical tube (percolator)

Phosphodiesterase-5 inhibitor

A phosphodiesterase type 5 inhibitor (PDE5 inhibitor) is a drug used to block the degradative action of cGMP-specific phosphodiesterase type 5 (PDE5) on cyclic GMP in the smooth muscle cells lining the blood vessels supplying various tissues

Photosensitising

Photosensitisers are photoactive molecules that absorb light energy and catalyse the formation of radical oxygen species (ROS) for phtodynamic therapy (PDT) in the treatment of infectious or proliferative skin disorders.

Phytotherapy

Plant therapy, modern term for scientifically validated herbal medicine

Postpartum tonic

Restores health, tone, vigour and function to the mother's body and assists in returning it to pre-pregnancy conditions in the period beginning immediately after the birth of a child

Preservative

A substance added to products or organic solutions to prevent chemical change or bacterial action

Prolactin inhibitor

Inhibits the action of prolactin, a hormone that stimulates a process called lactogenesis, which fills the breast with milk

Protective

Lessens damage from environmental pollution

Purgative

Promotes a stronger evacuation of the bowels than a laxative

Qi, chi

Vital energy, life force, also know as prana (India)

Refrigerant

Lowers body temperature without inducing sweating

Relaxant

Eases tension and pain in body and organs; non-sedative

Renal protective

Protects the kidneys against damage from toxins

Renal tonic

Maintains or restores health, vigour and function of the kidneys

Restorative

Restores normal function of the body, organ or system

Rhizome

Underground, fleshy stem that grows horizontally, as a food-storing organ. Rhizomes have nodes, buds and tiny leaves

Rubefacient

See Counter-irritant

Sedative

An agent that induces sleep

Sialagogue

A remedy that increases salivation

Soporific

A remedy that promotes sleep

Spasmolytic

See Antispasmodic

Spleen tonic

Maintains or restores health, vigour and function of the spleen

Stimulant

Term used in traditional herbal medicine to mean circulatory stimulant

Stomachic

A substance that promotes appetite and digestion

Styptic

Stems external bleeding

Succus

Plant juice

Sudorific

Producing profuse perspiration

Synergistic

When the combined action of two or more substances is greater than the action of the substances in isolation

Taste improver

A substance that acts to make an herbal preparation more palatable

Thymoleptic

Improves mood, antidepressant activity

Thyroid stimulant

A substance that acts to stimulate the thyroid gland

Tincture

A hydro-ethanolic extraction of crude herbal material, usually in the ratio of 1:5 (1 part herb extracted in 5 parts solvent)

Tonic

A substance that maintains or restores health, tone, vigour and function of a particular organ, usually over a period of time

Trophorestorative

Herb that restores function and morphology of the organ

Uterine tonic

Regulates the function of the uterus and the endometrium

Vasodilator

An agent that causes dilation of blood vessels

Vasoprotective

A substance given to promote venous drainage (e.g., in pregnancy)

Venotonic

Maintains the structure and integrity of veins and improves venous return

Vermifuge

Substance expelling worms

Visicant

Blister producing

Vital force

A life giving energy that permeates all living things, the energy that heals and repairs damaged tissue

Vulnerary

Promotes the healing of wounds

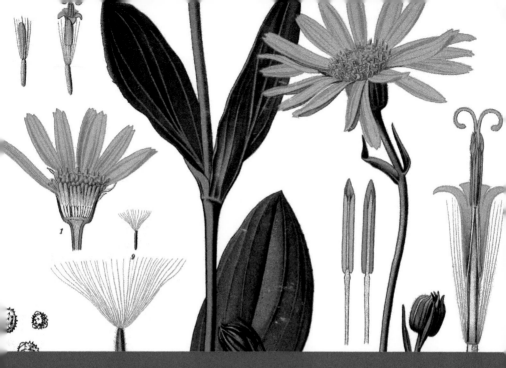

Bibliography

Phytotherapy Desk Reference

American Botanical Council, Expanded Commission E monographs, Eds. Blumenthal, M, Goldberg A, Brinckmann J. Amercial Botanical Council, Integrative Medicine Communicatins, 2000

Basch, E.M. Ulbricht, C.E. Natural Standard Herb and Supplement Handbook - The Clinical Bottom Line St Louis:Elsevier Mosby, 2005

Bensky, D. and Gamble, A. Chinese Herbal Medicine Materia Medica. Seattle: Eastland Press, 1986.

Blomenthal, M. The Complete German Commission E Monographs – Therapeutic.

Guides to Herbal Medicines. American Botanical Council. 1998.

Bone, K. M. Clinical Application of Ayurvedic and Chinese Herbs. Monographs for the Western Herbal Practitioner. Brisbane: Phytotherapy Press, 1996.

British Herbal Medicine Association. British Herbal Pharmacopoeia. Cowling: BHMA, 1983.

British Herbal Medicine Association. British Herbal Compendium, A handbook of scientific information on widely used plant drugs, Vol 1. Dorset: BHMA. 1992.

Braun, L. and Cohen, M. Herbs and Natural Supplements – An evidence-based guide 2nd Ed. Australia. Churchill Livingstone. Elsevier, 2008.

Culpeper, N. Culpeper's Complete Herbal. W. Fouscham and Co, New York.

Dwivedi, S. Terminalia arjuna Wight and Arn. - a useful drug for cardiovascular disorders. J Ethnopharmacol. 2007; 114(2):114-129.

European Medicines Agency, Community Herbal Monographs, Available online.

Fisher, C. and Painter, G. Materia Medica of Western Herbs for the Southern Hemisphere. 1996. ISBN: 0-473-03982-6.

Holmes, P. The Energetics of Western Herbs. Boulder, Colorado: Artemis Press, 1989.

Leung, A. Y. and Forster, S. Encyclopedia of Common Natural Ingredients used in Food, Drugs and Cosmetics, 2nd Ed. New York-Chichester: John Wiley, 1996.

Mills, S. Y. The Essential Book of Herbal Medicine. Harmondsworth, Middlesex: Penguin Arkana, 1993. (First published under the title Out of the Earth by Viking Arkana, 1991)

Mills, S.Y. The Dictionary of Modern Herbalism. A comprehensive guide to practical herbal therapy. Rochester, Vermont: Healing Arts Press. 1988.

Pole, S. Ayurvedic Medicine. The principles of traditional practice. Churchill Livingstone. Elsevier Ltd. 2006.

Trickey, R. Women, Hormones and the Menstrual Cycle. Melbourne: Trickey Enterprises, 2011.

Van Wyk, B.-E. and Wink, M. Medicinal Plants of the World. Briza Publications. South Africa. 2004.

Wichtl, M. (Ed). Herbal Drugs and Phytopharmaceuticals. A handbook for practice on a scientific basis. 3rd Ed. Stuttgart: Medpharm Scientific Publishers. Boca, Raton, London, New York, Washington DC: CRC Press. 2004.

World Health Organisation, WHO Monographs on Selected Medicinal Plants, Volumes 1-3, WHO Press 1999 to 2007